Appetite and Food Intake

Behavioral and Physiological Considerations

Appetite and Food Intake

Behavioral and Physiological Considerations

Edited by

Ruth B.S. Harris

Richard D. Mattes

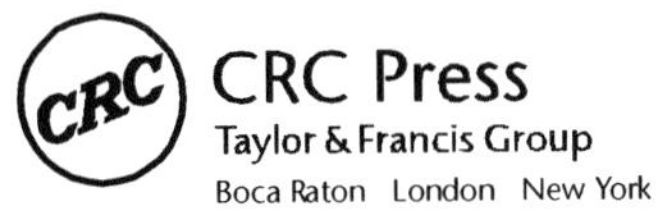

CRC Press is an imprint of the
Taylor & Francis Group, an **informa** business

CRC Press
Taylor & Francis Group
6000 Broken Sound Parkway NW, Suite 300
Boca Raton, FL 33487-2742

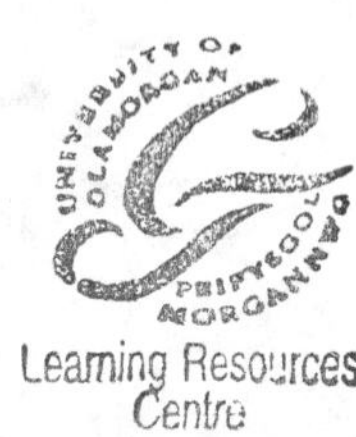

Printed in the United States of America on acid-free paper
10 9 8 7 6 5 4 3 2 1

International Standard Book Number-13: 978-1-4200-4783-7 (Hardcover)

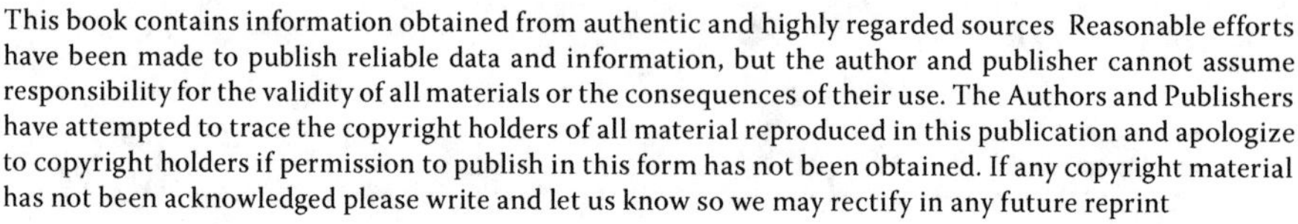

Library of Congress Cataloging-in-Publication Data

Appetite and food intake : behavioral and physiological considerations / [edited by]
Ruth B.S. Harris and Richard Mattes.
p. ; cm.
Includes bibliographical references and index.
ISBN 978-1-4200-4783-7 (hardcover : alk. paper)
1. Ingestion--Regulation. 2. Appetite--Physiological aspects. 3. Appetite disorders. 4. Food habits--Psychological aspects. I. Harris, Ruth B. S. II. Mattes, Richard.
[DNLM: 1. Appetite--physiology. 2. Eating--physiology. 3. Eating--psychology. 4. Food Habits--physiology. 5. Food Habits--psychology. 6. Nutrition Disorders. WI 102 A64553 2008]

QP147.A66 2008
612.3'1--dc22 2007045100

Visit the Taylor & Francis Web site at
http://www.taylorandfrancis.com

and the CRC Press Web site at
http://www.crcpress.com

Contents

Preface

Globally, there are more than 1 billion obese people and another 800 million are chronically undernourished. Nearly 30,000 (half of them children) die everyday from malnutrition. In more affluent nations, these problems are exacerbated by eating disorders and food insecurity. In the United States, as many as 10 million females and 1 million males have an eating disorder such as anorexia or bulimia. Approximately 25 million more have binge eating disorder. An estimated 35.1 million people live in households deemed food insecure and 10.8 million are considered food insecure with hunger. These problems stem from the interplay of political, economic, agricultural, nutritional, psychological, physiological, and social forces. Of course, each of these areas is also multifaceted, but all intersect on one key point: all influence ingestive behavior (when, where, what, and how much we choose to eat). As a result, expertise in each of these areas must be brought to bear on the problem of malnutrition (i.e., under- and overnutrition). This book focuses on the psychological and biological determinants of feeding, the governing influences when food availability is not limiting.

When asked to edit a book on food intake, the editors believed it was an opportunity not only to develop a volume that summarizes current knowledge of the factors that guide food selection and consumption, but to do so in a way that highlights the synergies and gaps between approaches using animal models or human trials. As you read the book, you will come across pairs of chapters that address the same topic, but are surprisingly diverse in their interpretation of scientific knowledge. These different perspectives are often complimentary to one another but also provide the reader with an appreciation of advantages and limitations that are provided by clinical/applied versus basic research. We hope that this will leave researchers working at different levels along this continuum with a greater appreciation of the challenges that each face and where future efforts, hopefully collaborations, may be most productive and challenging.

The organization of the book is such that we start with whether, or not, there are mechanisms that control food intake and the role played by appetitive cues. Next, preingestive motivational, cognitive, and orosensory processes that influence food acquisition, as well as the processing of ingesta, are considered. This is followed by chapters addressing intestinal, and postabsorptive signaling systems and metabolism. The final contributions focus on the micro- and macronutrient composition of foods linked to ingestive behavior and the physiologic consequences of consumption. The chapters are contributed by scientists who are driving current research and thinking on each of these topics. The range of topics discussed in this book highlights the diverse nature of food intake research, ranging from cellular neurobiology to measures of human behavior. This is an ever-evolving area of study that continues to incorporate more disciplines as the complexity of the reward and appetitive systems continues to unravel. As you progress through the book, it will also become apparent that there is some overlap in the topics that are discussed by each author, reflecting how complex the interactions are between different processes that influence food choice and consumption.

We anticipate that this book will be a useful reference tool for individuals who range from experts in the field to those who are simply interested in how an individual decides what foods to eat and how much to eat. In addition, this should be a useful overview for graduate students entering the field as a specialization and to others in professions, such as nursing or dietetics, where the greater emphasis is on translating the science into practice. Making appropriate food choices and maintaining an adequate intake is a perennial challenge to the survival of all organisms. More recently, the problems of inappropriate food choices and overconsumption have become major global health issues. Therefore, understanding how food intake is determined has important practical and economic implications at the individual and population levels. The information in this book summarizes current understanding of how the environment, food composition, and individual physiological status influence our food choices.

Editors

Ruth B.S. Harris, Ph.D., is professor of foods and nutrition at the University of Georgia. She has a long-standing interest in the role of circulating factors in the regulation of energy balance. This was initiated during her graduate studies working under the guidance of professor G.R. Hervey, University of Leeds, England, and continues today with studies on the effects of leptin on peripheral metabolism and adipocyte development. A more recent interest has been in the effect of acute stress on long-term regulation of body weight. She has published more than 100 research papers in peer-reviewed journals and holds membership in the American Physiology Society, Society for Neuroscience, American Nutrition Society, Society for the Study of Ingestive Behavior, and Society for Experimental Biology and Medicine. Dr. Harris has served on the National Institutes of Health (NIH) Integrative Physiology and Obesity Related Disorders (IPOD) Study Section, as an associate editor for *Experimental Biology and Medicine* and on the editorial board of the *Journal of Nutrition*, the *American Journal of Physiology, Regulatory, Comparative and Integrative Physiology*, and *Adipocyte*.

Richard Mattes, Ph.D., is professor of foods and nutrition at Purdue University, adjunct associate professor of medicine at the Indiana University School of Medicine, and affiliated scientist at the Monell Chemical Senses Center. His research focuses on the areas of hunger and satiety, regulation of food intake in humans, food preferences, human cephalic phase responses, and taste and smell. At Purdue University, Dr. Mattes is associate director of the Ingestive Behavior Research Center; he directs the Analytical Core Laboratory for the Botanical Center for Age Related Diseases and chairs the Human Subjects Review Committee. He also holds numerous external responsibilities including coexecutive editor of *Appetite*, editorial board of *Ear, Nose and Throat Journal*, past chair of the Research Dietetic Practice Group of the American Dietetic Association, member of the Scientific Advisory Committee to the International Life Science Institute, North America, and secretary of the Rose Marie Pangborn Sensory Science Scholarship Fund. Dr. Mattes has authored more than 135 publications. He earned an undergraduate degree in biology and a masters degree in public health from the University of Michigan as well as a doctorate degree in human nutrition from Cornell University. He conducted postdoctoral studies at the Memorial Sloan-Kettering Cancer Center and the Monell Chemical Senses Center.

Contributors

John Beard
Department of Nutritional Sciences
The Pennsylvania State University
University Park, Pennsylvania

Emma J. Bertenshaw
Department of Psychology
University of Sussex
Brighton, United Kingdom

Miriam E. Bocarsly
Department of Psychology
Drexel University
Philadelphia, Pennsylvania

Didier Chapelot
Physiologie du Comportement Alimentaire
Université Paris 13
Bobigny, France

Mihai Covasa
Department of Nutritional Sciences
The Pennsylvania State University
University Park, Pennsylvania

Angelo Del Parigi
Pfizer Global Research and Development
Ann Arbor, Michigan

Dianne Figlewicz Latteman
VA Puget Sound Health Care System and Department of Psychiatry and Behavioral Science
University of Washington
Seattle, Washington

Mark I. Friedman
Monell Chemical Senses Center
Philadelphia, Pennsylvania

Nori Geary
Center for Integrative Human Physiology
University of Zurich
Zurich, Switzerland

Carolyn Gunther
Department of Human Nutrition
Ohio State University
Columbus, Ohio

Chirag Kapadia
Childrens Hospital of Philadelphia
Philadelphia, Pennsylvania

Allen S. Levine
Minnesota Obesity Center
VA Medical Center
Minneapolis, Minnesota

David A. Levitsky
Division of Nutritional Sciences and Department of Psychology
Cornell University
Ithaca, New York

Jeanine Louis-Sylvestre
UFR Santé Médecine et Biologie Humaine Léonard de Vinci
Bobigny, France

Michael R. Lowe
Department of Psychology
Drexel University
Philadelphia, Pennsylvania

Thomas A. Lutz
Institute of Veterinary Physiology
University of Zurich
Zurich, Switzerland

Nik Mazlan Mamat
Kulliyyah of Allied Health Sciences
International Islamic University Malaysia
Bandar Indera Mahkota, Malaysia

Claire M. Mathes
Department of Psychology
University of Florida
Gainesville, Florida

David J. Mela
Unilever Food and Health Research Institute
Vlaardingen, The Netherlands

Pawel K. Olszewski
Minnesota Obesity Center
VA Medical Center
Minneapolis, Minnesota

Nicola Pannacciulli
Amylin Pharmaceuticals, Inc.
San Diego, California

Harry P.F. Peters
Unilever Food and Health Research Institute
Vlaardingen, The Netherlands

Neil E. Rowland
Department of Psychology
University of Florida
Gainesville, Florida

Gary J. Schwartz
Albert Einstein School of Medicine
New York, New York

Thomas R. Scott
San Diego State University
San Diego, California

James Stubbs
Slimming World
Alfreton, England

P. Antonio Tataranni
Sanofi-Aventis
Bridgewater, New Jersey

Dorothy Teegarden
Department of Foods and Nutrition
Purdue University
West Lafayette, Indiana

Karen L. Teff
Monell Chemical Senses Center
Philadelphia, Pennsylvania

Stephen Whybrow
The Rowett Research Institute
Aberdeen, Scotland

Martin R. Yeomans
Department of Psychology
University of Sussex
Brighton, United Kingdom

1 Food Intake: Control, Regulation, and the Illusion of Dysregulation

Mark I. Friedman

CONTENTS

The cause of every need of a living being is also the cause of the satisfaction of the need.

Eduard F.W. Pflüger, 1877

1.1 INTRODUCTION

Research to understand the determinants of food intake has its roots in the field of regulatory physiology, which originated from the work of Claude Bernard and Walter Cannon. Bernard, the great mid-nineteenth-century French physiologist, was struck by the constancy of the body's internal environment, leading him to conclude that "The fixity of the internal environment is the requirement for a free life." About 50 years later, Cannon coined the term "homeostasis" to refer to this state of stability and to the physiological processes that maintain it.[1] Soon after, Curt Richter extended Cannon's concept to include a behavioral component that also serves to maintain the constancy of the internal milieu.[2] Thus, for example, the loss of sodium not only triggers secretion of hormones that cause sodium retention by the kidneys, but also elicits an appetite for this electrolyte. Other homeostatic systems with a behavioral component include those for blood pressure (hypovolemic thirst), blood osmolality (osmotic thirst), and body temperature (thermotaxis).

Food intake has been viewed traditionally within the framework of energy homeostasis and as the behavioral contributor to maintenance of body fat content and energy balance. There has been a long debate over the extent to which food intake is influenced by such regulatory factors as opposed to nonregulatory determinants associated with the food environment, like food palatability and cognitive influences. This issue has become particularly acute in recent years with the increase in research on human food intake, which often generates results that do not appear to fit with a regulatory role for eating behavior.[3] It is within this context that I was asked to address in this chapter the question of "whether there is regulation of food intake."

Regulation and control are inherent in the concept of homeostasis. In common parlance the terms "control" and "regulation" are used interchangeably with no consequence. In discussions of physiological systems, however, indiscriminate use of these words can distort our understanding of those systems. I begin this chapter by clarifying the meaning of "control" and "regulation" in physiological systems and then present a model describing the role of food intake in energy homeostasis, which focuses on energy production as the regulated variable instead of body weight or energy balance. From this perspective, I discuss how this "energostatic" model helps explain the mistaken impression that food intake is dysregulated or poorly controlled, and I examine the utility of the distinction between regulatory and nonregulatory control of food intake.

1.2 REGULATION AND CONTROL

Although "regulation" and "control" are used synonymously in the vernacular, the contrast between the common meanings of the terms can be quite pointed. Consider, for example, the difference between "government regulation" versus "government control" of scientific research. Within the field of biology, definitions of these terms vary depending on the discipline, subject matter, and level of analysis (molecular, population). In physiology, "regulation" and "control" have particular meanings.

"Regulation" refers to the capacity to maintain the constancy of a physiological parameter in the face of variations in the internal and external environments.[4] In this sense, regulation refers to the performance of a variable, not to the existence of specific mechanisms.[5] Besides constancy, Brobeck[6] added another important feature to the meaning of physiological regulation — the existence of a sensor that directs responses that serve to preserve the regulated parameter. To use his definition, regulation "... denotes the preservation of a relatively constant value by means of physiological mechanisms which include a specialized detector for the value or some function of it."

There are several aspects of Brobeck's definition that are noteworthy. For one, he recognizes the impossibility of maintaining a truly constant physiological state by referring to a "relative constancy." In this regard, it is interesting that the concept of homeostasis, or its application to certain physiological variables such as body weight, has been criticized for its emphasis on constancy despite recognition early on that such stability is not perfect. In fact, Cannon[1] made the point that he allowed for such variability when he coined the term "homeostasis" by using the prefix *homeo* (from *homoio*), meaning "like" or "similar," rather than *homo*, meaning "same." Brobeck's definition also captures the dynamic nature of regulation by inclusion of a feedback mechanism. This seems self-evident, because it is difficult to imagine physiological regulation without a means for feedback and even more difficult to think of a feedback mechanism without a sensor. Finally, in keeping with Pflüger's quote at the beginning of this chapter, Brobeck acknowledges that it is the regulated variable that activates the sensor. In other words, that which is regulated is that which is sensed.

"Control" refers to the exercise of influence or direction over a process or response. In contrast to regulation, which refers to the performance of a system, control, as Brobeck[6] puts it, "describes management." In the context of homeostasis, such management is exerted in the service of a regulated variable; for example, respiration is controlled in the service of acid-base balance, and heart rate is controlled to maintain blood pressure. Unlike regulation, control does not imply stability. Rather, a controlled process or response can vary widely in order to help maintain the relative constancy of the regulated variable. In other words, physiological (homeostatic) regulation is achieved through the operation of controlled processes and responses, and if Pflüger and Brobeck are correct, the regulated variable or something closely tied to it is exercising this control.

1.2.1 Is There Regulation of Food Intake?

In their invitation to contribute a chapter for this book, the editors asked me to address the question of "whether there is regulation of food intake." It should be clear from the preceding discussion that, from a physiological point of view, the answer to this question is "no." Food intake is not maintained at a constant level in spite of changes in the internal and external environment. It varies widely in response to all kinds of environmental perturbations, such as those in ambient temperature, the nutritional value of the food, and reproductive and metabolic status. The idea that food intake would remain relatively constant in the face of environmental challenges seems nonsensical. At worst, such constancy could be fatal if, for example, food intake failed to increase in the cold.

The fact that food intake is not held steady in the face of changes in the internal and external environments, but rather varies considerably, in itself indicates that food consumption is managed and not regulated. Thus, the more complete answer to the question of whether food intake is regulated is, "No, it is controlled." Presumably, it is controlled as a means to regulate some physiological variable; food intake regulates, but is not regulated. Knowing what variable food intake regulates is likely to tell us what controls it.

1.3 CONTROL OF ENERGY INTAKE BY ENERGY METABOLISM

Food intake is affected by a wide range of naturally occurring and experimentally induced changes in the internal and external environments, but by far the largest and most persistent changes in food intake are associated with alterations in energy homeostasis. For example, a sustained, near doubling of food intake is seen in response to decreased ambient temperature, caloric dilution of the diet, lactation, and experimental diabetes mellitus. Even the dramatic hyperphagia following lesions to the ventromedial hypothalamus can be attributed to the peripheral metabolic effects of such brain damage.[7] Since manipulations of brain neurochemistry also produce changes in peripheral metabolism it is possible that even these treatments stimulate feeding by altering energy homeostasis.

Food contains nutrients which are necessary for survival besides those that provide energy. With an otherwise adequate diet, however, a lack of these essential nutrients is not felt, and certainly would not be fatal, for some period of time. Without food, you would die from a lack of calories long before you would from a lack of essential vitamins or fatty acids. Modifying the content of vitamins, minerals, and essential fatty acids in food produces little or no change in food intake, although it might affect the selection of diet if an appropriate choice is available. In contrast, variation in the energy content of food can result in pronounced, inverse changes in food intake that serve to maintain energy intake over a wide range of dietary energy content.[8] It was this robust compensatory response to changes in dietary energy density that led Adolph to conclude that "animals eat for calories."[8]

It is unlikely that animals eat for food calories *per se;* that is, for the potential energy in food that can be measured using a bomb calorimeter. Instead, they eat for the energy that is extracted from food. This is clearly illustrated by the finding that rats with experimental diabetes mellitus, which cannot readily oxidize carbohydrate, but do easily burn fat for energy, increase food intake when their high-fat diet is "diluted" with glucose much like normal rats do when their food is diluted with non-nutritive cellulose.[9] Adolph's conclusion is therefore only partially correct. It is more accurate to say that "animals eat for calories they can use."

The energy derived from food is realized by the breakdown of carbohydrates, fats, and some amino acids through intracellular metabolic pathways, which ultimately lead to the generation of adenosine triphosphate (ATP), the primary biochemical form of energy. The constancy of ATP production is not only a requirement for the free life, it is necessary for any life at all. A highly complex system of physiological, endocrine, and biochemical mechanisms assures an adequate supply of energy-yielding substrates to tissues and precisely controls the intracellular processing of those fuels to yield ATP in sufficient amounts to meet demands. Production of ATP is tightly coupled with demand, resulting in relatively stable ATP levels. Because energy-yielding substrates are continually utilized for ATP production, the supply of metabolic fuels ultimately needs to be replenished from the external sources. Food intake serves this purpose.

Given the crucial importance of maintaining energy production, it is possible that some aspect of ATP metabolism is the regulated variable that food intake serves to help keep steady and that also provides the feedback stimulus that controls energy intake. The most well-known theories for the metabolic control of food intake are based on signals generated by substrates, namely glucose and fat or fatty acids. However, all fuels are eventually broken down to intermediates that enter the final common metabolic pathways of energy production. Although less well known, the idea that processes beyond the level of individual fuel metabolism generate a signal controlling food intake is not new. Ugolev and Kassil[10] suggested almost 50 years ago that an intermediate in the tricarboxylic acid (Krebs) cycle may be such a signal. Since then, others have discussed an "energostatic" control of food intake,[11] and along similar lines, Nicolaidis[12] posited an "ischymetric" (from *ischys* = power) control of food intake that involves sensing basal metabolic rate. Others still have focused on oxidative metabolism as a source of the controlling signal.[7,13]

Although an energostatic control of food intake is appealing for a number of reasons, not the least of which is its explanatory power,[7,14] the idea did not gain much currency for a number of years because its mechanism was ill-defined. Hence, references to an "unidentified" or "hypothetical" energostat.[15] More recently, however, direct evidence that changes in ATP production can affect food intake has been forthcoming. In addition to putting the focus on ATP metabolism as a source for a stimulus controlling food intake, studies have also indicated that this stimulus is detected in the liver.

The liver sits at the crossroads of metabolism, processing fuels consumed in food in the postabsorptive state and mobilized from storage during fasting. Unlike other cells, hepatocytes do not express creatine kinase[16] and therefore do not synthesize phosphocreatine, which buffers decreases in ATP. This apparently makes hepatocyte ATP concentrations more labile and more vulnerable to reduction. Thus, in contrast to other cells, hepatocyte ATP falls during a relatively short fast[17] and is depleted very rapidly during ischemia and hypoxia.[16]

Considerable evidence suggests that these changes in hepatic liver energy status generate or constitute a stimulus that controls food intake in rats. For example, a variety of metabolic inhibitors that reduce liver ATP stimulate feeding behavior,[18–20] and preventing the decrease also prevents the eating response.[21] The decrease in liver energy status precedes the eating response, and the eating response wanes as liver energy status is restored.[22] Fasting reduces liver ATP levels, and the restoration of liver energy status during refeeding tracks the compensatory hyperphagia after fasting.[17]

1.4 AN ENERGOSTATIC MODEL FOR THE CONTROL OF FOOD INTAKE

Because generation of cellular energy depends on the supply of metabolic fuels, the function of any sensor of energy production must be viewed within a larger context of bodily fuel fluxes. Figure 1.1 illustrates the relationships between pathways of fuel partitioning and a sensor of energy production that controls energy intake. According to this model, metabolic fuels have three fates: they can be (1) shunted into storage from which they also can be mobilized, (2) expended, for example, as heat or muscular activity, or (3) metabolized in the energy sensor. The supply of fuels to the energy sensor can therefore be increased or decreased depending on the degree to which fuels are shunted into storage, mobilized from storage, and oxidized to supply energy to cells other than those monitoring energy production (to brown fat cells, myocytes, etc.).

In addition to partitioning fuels among tissues (e.g., adipose tissue, muscle), fuels can also be partitioned among metabolic pathways. This could be especially

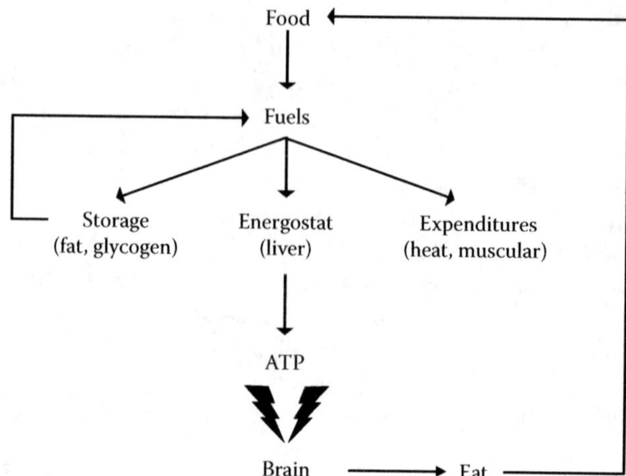

FIGURE 1.1 Fuel partitioning and the signal to eat under baseline or steady-state conditions. Under these conditions, there is a balance or equilibrium between the flux of fuels into storage, to meet the demand for expenditures, and through the energostat.

important if hepatocytes are energy sensors, given that these cells are in the business of synthesizing fat and glycogen and processing fuels mobilized from storage. Presumably, shifts in hepatocellular fuel partitioning could affect fuel flux through oxidative, energy-yielding pathways, resulting in a changing signal to eat.

As portrayed in Figure 1.1, changes in hepatocyte energy production generate a signal that is communicated to the brain to control food intake. Considerable evidence indicates that this is a neural signal carried by vagal afferent neurons.[23] The signal could be bloodborne as well, although there are no data ruling this possibility in or out. How changes in hepatocyte energy metabolism are transformed into a neural (or humoral) signal is unknown. Langhans and Scharrer[13] suggested that perturbations in ATP could alter hepatocyte membrane potential by modifying the activity of the sodium pump. Consistent with their hypothesis, we have shown that the fructose analogue, 2,5-anhydro-d-mannitol (2,5-AM), which stimulates feeding by reducing liver energy status, increases intracellular sodium in hepatocytes in vitro.[24] In addition, we have found that 2,5-AM increases hepatocellular calcium concentration,[25] which could alter hepatocyte potential or cause the secretion of a paracrine or endocrine signal.

It has probably not escaped the reader's attention that the energostatic model described here does not include the usual endocrine and peptide suspects that play a crucial role in many models for control of food intake. There are several reasons for this omission. First, the energostatic model presented here does not require inclusion of endocrine or peptide signaling to explain changes in food intake under a variety of conditions.[7,14] Second, hormones (for example, insulin, leptin, ghrelin) thought to control food intake by acting as signals have metabolic actions by their direct effects on peripheral tissues, but also via their effect in the brain,[26–28] which we have known since the days of Claude Bernard controls peripheral metabolism. It is therefore unclear whether these hormones affect food intake by acting as signals or as metabolic modifiers. Third, while it is clear that manipulation of various brain peptides (neuropeptideY, proopiomelanocortin, etc.) can affect food intake, this does not necessarily mean they do so by being a part of a "feeding circuit." Like peripherally secreted hormones, these peptides may be part of the machinery that controls peripheral metabolism. Indeed, manipulations of at least some of these brain peptides, as well as centrally acting metabolic hormones, can have direct effects on hepatic metabolism,[29–32] which, in keeping with the model presented here, could generate a signal causing changes in food intake.

Although many questions remain about how an energy sensor functions, the overall fuel partitioning model presented here offers a single framework for understanding changes in food intake across a range of naturally occurring and experimental conditions. It is not the purpose of this chapter to discuss this model's explanatory power, which can be found elsewhere.[7,14] Rather, in keeping with the charge to address the question of whether food intake is regulated, I will use this model to explain why food intake can sometimes mistakenly appear to be poorly controlled or, as sometimes described, "dysregulated."

1.5 THE ILLUSION OF DYSREGULATION

The results of animal experiments performed over the years have led us to expect that food intake changes predictably under various experimental and natural conditions. Food intake typically decreases after a period of overfeeding and increases after a fast. Intake changes in an inverse manner with variation in the caloric density of the diet or ambient temperature, and in a direct fashion with increased exercise. Often these changes in food consumption compensate precisely for the energetic perturbation and result in restoration of body weight or, more specifically, body fat content. When food intake changes or fails to change as expected, it is considered "dysregulated" or poorly controlled. Similarly, it is also seen as dysregulated when it changes in response to "nonregulatory" factors such as the palatability of the diet, the amount of food provided, or social circumstances.

It is premature to conclude that food intake is poorly controlled when we do not yet fully understand what controls it or what in fact food intake regulates. It might be more accurate to say that it is not doing what we expect or is not following the rules. However, being faced with unmet expectations does not necessarily lead to the conclusion that there is an actual breakdown of control; it may be the expectations or rules that are faulty, not the control of food intake. I believe this is the case. In particular, I think that the misperception — the illusion — of dysregulation is rooted largely in erroneous assumptions about the relationship between body weight (fat) and food intake and the role of food intake in energy balance. The energostatic model outlined provides a framework to understand the apparent discrepancies and reconcile them with a properly functioning regulatory control of food intake.

1.5.1 Regulatory "Failures"

The traditional, "lipostatic" model for control of food intake postulates a direct link between food consumption and body fat content; body fat content is a regulated

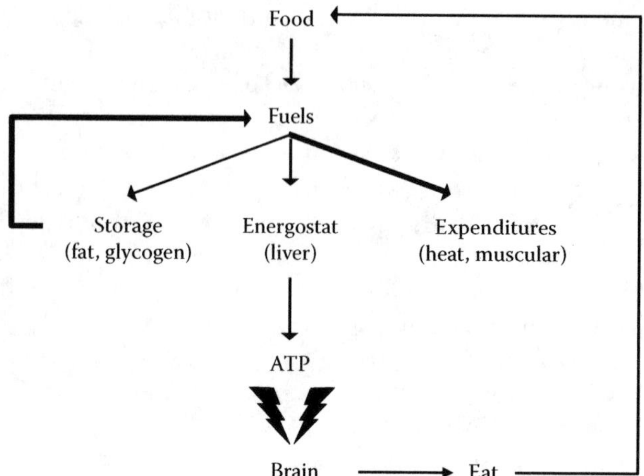

FIGURE 1.2 Partitioning of fuels under conditions in which the supply of fuels to meet the demands of increased expenditures is met through mobilization of stored fuels at the expense of a reduction in stored fuels mainly in the form of fat. In this scenario, the supply of fuels to the energostat is unaffected, and food intake does not change.

variable, and food intake is controlled by body fat to regulate it. Consequently, when food intake does not change sufficiently to maintain or restore body weight to a normal or expected level, it can be seen as poorly controlled. The energostatic model presented here differs markedly from this lipostatic perspective. In contrast to a direct control of food intake by body fat stores, the energostatic model assumes that fuel storage affects food intake *indirectly* by altering the supply of fuels to or the provisioning of fuels within the energy sensor.

Such uncoupling of body fat content from control of food intake means that food intake does not necessarily have to change in an inverse manner when body weight is gained or lost. Thus, rats with experimental diabetes mellitus can lose most of their body fat yet eat normal amounts of food if their diet contains sufficient amounts of fat, a fuel these animals can ready oxidize.[9] Weight loss associated with increased thermogenesis does not have to be fully compensated by increased food intake if the demand for fat fuels from brown fat is satisfied by mobilization of fat stores instead of increased consumption of food (see Figure 1.2). Similarly, high energy intakes can be maintained when muscular activity is reduced from a sustained high level if the fuels otherwise oxidized in muscle are stored in adipose tissue rather than supplied to the energostat (see Figure 1.2) at the expense of weight gain.

The consumption and storage of metabolic fuels are two solutions to the same physiological problem of maintaining cellular energy production. Food consumption supplies energy-yielding substrates from the external environment, whereas fuel stores in the form of glycogen and, to a much greater extent, fat provide energy when fuels from the outside are unavailable. If there are different solutions to the same problem, it stands to reason that when a problem is solved by any one solution there is less need to solve it in other ways. This kind of trade-off is seen when food intake decreases under conditions of rapid weight loss either from obese levels after

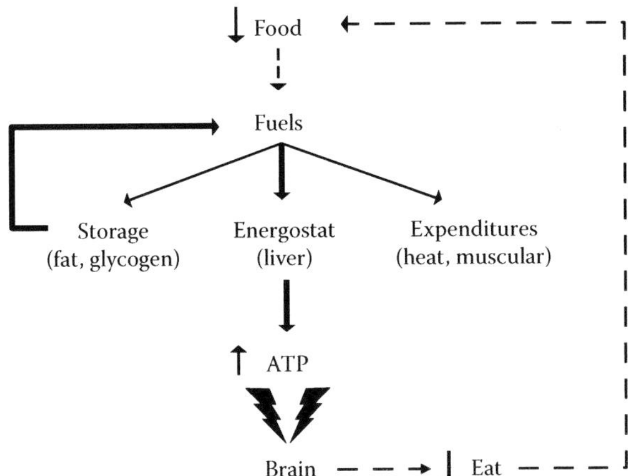

FIGURE 1.3 Partitioning of fuels during excessive mobilization of body fat. In this scenario, the increased supply of fuels from adipose tissue increases the flux of fuels through the energostat, thereby reducing the signal to eat.

overfeeding or from normal levels when insulin levels are reduced (see Figure 1.3). In both cases, oxidation of fat fuels mobilized from storage is sufficient to maintain energy production in the energostat, which dampens the stimulus for feeding. To put it simply, there is less need to eat food if you are eating yourself.

The overeating that accompanies the development and maintenance of obesity is another case in which food intake is seen as dysregulated or poorly controlled. This hyperphagia is typically thought to result from a lack of, or insensitivity to, a negative feedback signal associated with body fat content (the role of environmental factors such as access to a variety of palatable foods is discussed in a later section). The uncoupling between body fat content and food intake raises doubts that overeating is due to a failure in a direct control of food intake by body fat. Studies showing that body fat content is restored to normal after lipectomy or adipose tissue transplant reinforce this conclusion because this restoration is achieved without changes in food intake.[33,34]

The model presented here offers an alternative explanation for the overeating associated with obesity that does not depend on a breakdown in the mechanism(s) controlling food intake. In practically every animal model of obesity in which overeating is present there is a shift in fuel partitioning toward storage that is independent of the hyperphagia. Such a shift in metabolism has been observed prior to overeating during development in genetic models[35] and after lesions of the ventromedial hypothalamus (VMH).[36] In addition, in Zucker rats,[37] a genetic model of obesity, and in rats with VMH lesions,[38] body fat accumulates even when overeating is prevented. As shown in Figure 1.4, this shift toward fat deposition would be expected to increase food intake by diverting metabolic fuels away from oxidation in the energy sensor. In this way, the hyperphagia of obesity is no different than that which can occur in cold ambient temperatures or with intense exercise, except that instead of fuels being lost as heat or in muscular work they are lost to adipose tissue.

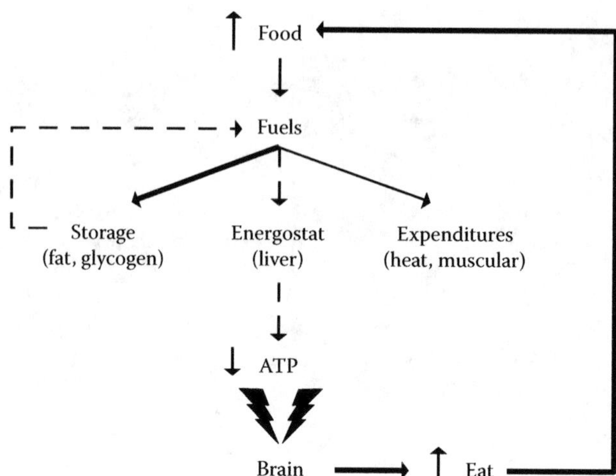

FIGURE 1.4 Partitioning of fuels during the development of obesity. In this scenario, a primary shift in the flux of fuels into storage compromises the supply of fuels to the energostat and increases the signal to eat.

Obesity induced by eating a high-fat diet — diet-induced obesity — is difficult to explain from a lipostatic perspective because it is not clear why a change in diet would affect the presumed negative feedback control of food intake exerted by the amount of body fat or why there is such extreme individual variability in the susceptibility to diet-induced overeating and obesity. In rats, consumption of high-fat diets results in overeating and obesity when the diet is also high in carbohydrate content; a high-fat, low-carbohydrate diet does not cause diet-induced hyperphagia and excess weight gain.[39] These observations are consistent with the energostatic model, given that carbohydrates stimulate the secretion of insulin, which fosters fat storage and inhibits fat oxidation. More recent studies indicate that individual differences in the propensity to overeat and become obese on such high-fat diets are related to a preexisting capacity to oxidize fatty acids.[40,41] The more limited the ability to burn fat, the greater the overeating and weight gain during high-fat feeding. This suggests that, in addition to increased fuel storage, diet-induced hyperphagia and obesity may result from a preexisting deficit in the oxidation of fatty acids, an important fuel for the liver.

The energostatic model turns the lipostatic explanation of overeating in obesity on its head. According to the lipostatic hypothesis, overeating is an attempt to increase body fat to a higher than normal level and thereby increase the negative feedback signal for food intake; in other words, you overeat in order to become obese. In contrast, from the perspective of the energostatic model, you overeat because you are becoming obese; that is, overeating is a response to the loss of fuels into fat stores. Thus, the hyperphagia associated with obesity is not due to a malfunctioning control of food intake, but rather to a disordered metabolism that shunts an excess of fuels into storage. The control of food intake is not broken, but in fact works too well, because it is responding appropriately to a loss of oxidizable fuel and energy production. Unfortunately, the fuels are "lost" to adipose tissue where it can be seen and where it may result in health problems.

One could claim that overeating is poorly controlled eating because there is a gain in body weight that can be detrimental to health and well being, but it seems hardly fair to blame food intake when a disordered metabolism is at fault. That would be analogous to blaming the hammer rather than the carpenter for missing a nail. Seeing food intake as dysregulated because it is not restrained in the face of weight gain also presupposes that a gain in body fat is necessarily a bad thing. From an evolutionary perspective, there may be little downside to gaining weight, especially if you are not, like humans, a prey species when it might slow you down running from predators[42] or if weight gain occurs well into or beyond reproductive age before the detrimental health effects of obesity are manifest. In short, depending on the timing and degree, we can probably afford to gain weight and body fat without much downside. From an evolutionary perspective, weight gain may be neither good nor bad, but simply just a matter of fact.

1.5.2 Is Body Energy Balance a Useful Concept?

Food intake is often viewed in terms of its role in the regulation of body energy balance, but is it controlled by energy balance, and for that matter, is energy balance regulated?

Energy balance is described by the formula,

$$\Delta E_b = E_i - E_e$$

wherein ΔE_b is a change in body energy content, E_i is energy intake, and E_e is energy expenditure. This formula is a restatement of the First Law of Thermodynamics, which pertains to the conservation of energy (the amount of energy in a system is equal to the energy added to the system minus the energy lost from it). The concept of energy balance is, in essence, descriptive rather than explanatory — the energy in the body *must* add up to the difference between what energy comes in and what goes out.

Even though obesity is often cast in terms of a disturbance in energy balance, strictly speaking it makes little sense to talk of being out of energy balance because, by definition, living organisms, like physical systems, must always be in energy balance or they would violate the Laws of Thermodynamics. If animals are always in energy balance, it is difficult to think of energy balance as a regulated variable which is maintained by changes in food intake because there would be nothing to regulate. It is equally challenging to imagine what the feedback signal would be or how it would be monitored other than from outside the organism because it is a theoretical construct and not a physiological event.

What is probably meant in most cases by being "out of energy balance" is that food intake has exceeded or fallen short of expenditure, resulting in, respectively, a gain or loss of body weight (fat). Again this is simply a statement of fact and does little to offer an explanation or mechanism. From the perspective of physiological regulation, the static nature of the energy balance equation masks dynamic relationships between body fat, food intake, and expenditure that involve complex biochemical, endocrine, and physiological feedback mechanisms. When invoked in the context of body fat maintenance, the energy balance formula communicates a less than dynamic situation and implies that the content of body fat is a passive result of variations in energy intake and expenditure. Body energy (fat) is the dependent variable, and intake and expenditure are the independent variables.

We know, of course, that adipose tissue is not just a static depository for fat, but is a very active tissue, which both stores and mobilizes fat fuels and secretes hormones with metabolic actions throughout the body. Keeping these "independent" capabilities of adipose tissue in mind, it is possible to portray the energostatic model in terms of the energy balance formula. In this case, we solve for energy intake rather than a change in body energy or fat content as in

$$E_i = \Delta E_b - E_e$$

and allow body energy to vary freely, independently of food intake. In the case of obesity, body energy increases as more fuels are routed to fat stores, and if energy expenditure remain constant, food intake increases as a result.

1.5.3 "Nonregulatory" Food Intake

A distinction is often made between "regulatory" and "nonregulatory" controls of food intake. Regulatory, or sometimes "homeostatic," controls are associated with the internal environment, with physiological regulations and signals. Nonregulatory (nonhomeostatic) controls are associated with external influences (e.g., the palatability, variety, composition, and availability of food) and cognitive or cultural factors (e.g., learning, craving, meal timing). Observation of an apparently poor control of food intake in response to energetic manipulations has lead to the conclusion that nonhomeostatic controls may override or take precedence over regulatory controls, especially in humans, and are largely responsible for determining how much food is consumed on a day-to-day basis. Nonregulatory factors, particularly those associated with food palatability, variety, portion size, and accessibility, are also thought responsible for overeating and obesity in humans.

Undoubtedly, there are a number of external factors that affect feeding behavior, but what impact do they have on intake over a long-term, nutritionally significant interval? And are they truly nonregulatory? To date, there remains very little scientific evidence that an abundance and variety of palatable food drives overeating over the long-term. The idea that food palatability can cause obesity stems from "cafeteria" studies in which rats became obese when fed cookies, peanut butter, and other appealing (at least to the experimenter) foods in addition to their regular rat chow.[43] A problem with these kinds of experiments, as well as those in which rats are given sucrose solutions along with chow, is that food palatability is confounded with a change in diet composition. In the case of cafeteria diets, the change was from a low-fat, high-carbohydrate chow to a high-fat, high-carbohydrate diet, which, as discussed earlier, can cause overeating and obesity. This change in diet composition appears critical, because no overeating and obesity is observed when rats are fed a variety of palatable foods while holding diet composition constant.[44] In addition, rats still overeat and become obese when fed a food, which by virtue of its composition causes overeating and weight gain, even if it is made extremely unpalatable.[45]

To conclude that the sensory and hedonic properties of food are truly nonregulatory controls of intake, it would be necessary for the taste, flavor, and palatability of food to have no physiological or metabolic consequences. But we know they do. These food stimuli trigger endocrine and metabolic responses that affect metabolism, in some cases for hours,[46] and also can increase food intake in the short term.[47] Such cephalic-phase reflexes appear to prepare the body for an influx of nutrients. Cephalic-phase insulin secretion, for example, promotes a shift in metabolism from a catabolic to anabolic state, including the inhibition of fatty acid oxidation and the synthesis and storage of fat. Under these conditions, the energostatic model would predict an increase in the "metabolic" signal to eat. Thus, the effects of food flavor and palatability on food intake may be due to their regulatory effects, which could elicit eating or permit continued intake as oxidizable fuels are shunted into storage. Perhaps the palatable taste of dessert "makes room" in the fuel supply to sustain or pique our appetite despite a full stomach.

Nonregulatory cognitive controls of food intake include learned habits and food cues. For example, people often claim they eat not because they are hungry, but because it is mealtime. If we eat only because it is time for breakfast, lunch, or dinner, then our metabolic state should be unaffected by the timing of meals. This is not the case; there is a vast literature showing that the timing of meals greatly affects metabolic feeding and fasting cycles.[48] It seems plausible that, with regular meal timing, both the readiness and metabolic signals to eat appear according to schedule. In addition, the absence of perceived hunger does not mean there is not metabolic hunger. The areas of the brain stem that receive sensory input from the liver in the control of food intake, for example, are the same as those that receive signals monitoring other homeostatic parameters of which we are unaware, such as blood pressure. Indeed, such a disconnect between unconscious metabolic hunger and perceived hunger may help account for the poor relationship between reported hunger and food intake.

Food itself can cause food intake, and an overabundance of food and food cues in the environment are thought to contribute to overeating and obesity. Whether such a food-rich environment in fact causes overeating and obesity remains to be determined through experimentation. Animal studies are not encouraging in this regard. Rats can be trained to eat in response to an external stimulus and will do so repeatedly throughout the day whenever that stimulus is presented.[49] However, these animals do not increase energy intake on a daily basis, because they reduce their intake of maintenance diet to compensate.[49] And again, it is not clear that the eating that occurs in response to food or food-related stimuli is truly nonregulatory, because food and learned food cues[50] elicit cephalic-phase responses.

1.6 IMPLICATIONS FOR RESEARCH ON HUMANS

There is substantial evidence for a metabolic control of food intake in humans, perhaps involving signaling of liver energy status. Injection of insulin or the glucose analogue, 2-deoxy-d-glucose, triggers hunger and stimulates eating in human subjects.[51,52] Cognitive functions related to food stimuli are enhanced during insulin-induced hypoglycemia in humans,[53] a finding which is consistent with the contention that metabolic factors can underlie or modulate cognitive controls of food intake. Healthy human subjects reduce energy intake in a compensatory fashion during intravenous feeding.[54] This finding provides strong evidence for a metabolic control of food intake independent of the sensory features of food. In humans, the level of liver ATP or the degree of restoration of liver ATP after an experimentally induced reduction is inversely correlated with body mass index (BMI).[55,56] Whether this intriguing relationship is a cause or effect of obesity, and whether it is related to differences in food intake, remains to be seen.

More detailed studies of the metabolic control of feeding in humans are sorely needed, especially as our understanding of this control in animals has progressed beyond the notions of "glucostatic" and "lipostatic" mechanisms. A recent study using human subjects, for example, revealed relationships between blood leptin levels and hunger and food intake that were independent of circulating glucose and insulin concentrations.[57] Experiments on the metabolic control of food intake in humans are difficult in many respects, not the least of which is the need for invasive procedures involved in manipulating and measuring metabolic variables. Clearly, more noninvasive, or minimally invasive, techniques need to be developed and used. The use of magnetic resonance spectrometry to measure liver ATP in conscious humans[55,56] is an example that is relevant to the energostatic model discussed here. The use of noninvasive techniques would improve subject compliance and also might permit more ecologically valid "field" studies of the metabolic control of food intake in humans.

One methodological issue regarding experiments on the metabolic control of food intake in humans that could be dealt with now pertains to the nearly invariable use of fasted subjects, although there are exceptions.[58] Human subjects in metabolic studies, including those involving measures of food intake or appetite, are typically fasted overnight in order to minimize variability of metabolic parameters; however, with the exception of breakfast, people usually eat before such prolonged food deprivation. Because the amount of food consumed may be determined by the metabolism of that food, it is possible that metabolic measurements taken during fasting would miss critical relationships between metabolism and food intake. Studies of metabolism under normal eating conditions might provide a more ecologically and physiologically valid picture of the metabolic control of food intake.

Whereas some studies fail to demonstrate complete compensation of energy intake in response to changes in dietary energy content,[59] others find good compensation.[60,61] The basis for this discrepancy is unclear, although it seems that studies finding good compensation tend to be those in which subjects are living in the laboratory under tightly controlled conditions. This environment is similar to that of laboratory rats, which appear to control food intake more precisely in response to variation in dietary energy density than do free living humans. As discussed earlier in this chapter, this may simply reflect a difference in how these two species respond to energetic challenges; rats may be more inclined to deal with such challenges by modifying food intake, whereas humans may do so by changing energy storage and expenditure as well as intake. It is also possible that experience with food may affect how accurately rats and humans control food intake.

Adult humans living in developed countries, who constitute practically all of the subjects used in experiments on control of food intake in humans, have a long history of associating a wide variety of foods or classes of foods with their metabolic effects. This stands in stark contrast to adult laboratory rodents, which have an extremely limited food experience, most often restricted to only one food with a relatively constant composition and energy density. Typically, dietary manipulations in human studies are covert in order to minimize potentially confounding changes in the sensory properties of the food. Therefore, expecting adult humans to vary intake in response to changes in dietary energy density (or other dietary manipulations) is asking them to unlearn food–metabolism relationships formed over many years of a rich and varied food experience. It may be the lack of such experience that accounts for the finding that children very accurately alter food intake in response to changes in dietary energy content.[62] It would be interesting to see if adult humans eating a single, nutritionally complete diet — a people "chow" — over a long period of time compensated more accurately for changes in its energy density than those with a varied food history given familiar foods with unfamiliar caloric densities. Conversely, would rats with a long history of eating a variety of foods with different energy densities compensate less well?

I have heard more than a few presentations describing results from experiments on nonregulatory controls of food intake that conclude by raising the possibility that the abundance of a varied and palatable food supply contributes to the high rates of obesity seen in many developed countries. When the speakers are asked on what basis they would even entertain this conclusion, the typical response is something like, "Because I look out in the world and see all this food and all these obese people." Unfortunately, that is pretty much the extent of the scientific evidence that overeating in humans is caused by food availability and palatability. I am aware of only one study[63] that has examined the effects of palatability on food intake in human subjects over more than a few hours and observed an increase in energy intake. Even in this case, the effect was found in a subset of subjects (lean, but not obese), and the exposure to palatable food lasted only one week, and, in the longer term, the role of diet palatability in humans seems to be overridden by postingestive consequences of eating.[64] If an excess of a variety of palatable food is an important cause of overeating and obesity, it should be demonstrable in an experimental context. Again, such long-term studies in humans are difficult to do with respect to methodology, logistics, and compliance, but they need to be done for experimental evidence to take the place of hand waving.

1.7 CONCLUSIONS

The issues discussed in this chapter — including the basic one of whether there is regulation of food intake — revolve around perceptions. How we think about regulation and control can shape our understanding of food intake; for example, if food intake is thought to be regulated, it can also be seen as dysregulated. If food intake is viewed as regulating body fat content, then the mechanisms for control of intake are thought to be broken or out of control when changes in body weight and food intake are uncoupled. Overeating in obesity, for example, is considered the result of a faulty feedback control from body fat or a disordered mechanism for feeding behavior. In contrast, seeing body fat storage and food intake as two solutions to the problem of maintaining energy production leads to different conclusions. From this energostatic perspective, dissociation between body fat and food intake does not mean that the control of intake is broken; indeed, overeating that is associated with the development of obesity results because the mechanism for control of intake works too well.

Expectations affect perceptions. If food intake fails to change in response to an energetic challenge as expected, we see it is as poorly controlled or dysregulated. But as with the uncoupling of food intake and body weight, this dysregulation can be illusory if the source of control is misplaced (i.e., body fat versus energy production) or if the variable regulated by food intake can also be regulated by other means (e.g., mobilization or storage of fat). Distinctions between regulatory and nonregulatory controls of food intake are warranted if based on the initial source of the controlling stimulus (e.g., intero- versus exteroceptive, cognitive versus physiological). It is unquestionable that nonregulatory controls are involved in determining food intake in the short-term, but it is at best premature to conclude that nonregulatory controls supplant or override regulatory controls over the long-term. Given that metabolic changes can affect food-related cognitive processes and cephalic stimuli affect metabolism, the extent to which nonregulatory controls are truly nonregulatory remains to be resolved.

Although, as Claude Bernard wrote, the constancy of the internal environment is a requirement for the free life, constancy is not a sufficient condition. After all, sessile animals must maintain homeostasis to survive, but one could hardly consider them free. The ability to modify behavior is also necessary for a truly free life. For those who study the control of food intake, it is the variability in food consumption that we seek to explain. If, as Pflüger tells us, we can identify the regulated variable that is kept constant by variations in food intake, we should know what controls food intake. In this chapter, I have offered an alternative to commonly held views by suggesting that food intake serves to regulate energy production, not body fat content or energy balance. This framework explains findings that are anomalous for more traditional theories and in doing so erases misperceptions and avoids premature abandonment of regulatory explanations for the control of food intake.

ACKNOWLEDGMENTS

The author thanks Charles Horn, Marcia Pelchat, Danielle Reed, and Michael Tordoff for their helpful comments and stimulating discussions during the preparation of this chapter.

REFERENCES

1. Canon, W.B., Organization for physiological homeostasis, *Physiol. Rev.*, 9, 399, 1929.
2. Moran, T.H. and Schulkin, J., Curt Richter and regulatory physiology, *Am. J. Physiol. Regul. Integr. Comp. Physiol.*, 279, R357, 2000.
3. Levitsky, D.L., The non-regulation of food intake in humans: Hope for reversing the epidemic of obesity, *Physiol. Behav.*, 86, 623, 2005.
4. Hue, L., From control to regulation: A new prospect for metabolic control analysis, in *Technological and Medical Implications of Metabolic Control Analysis,* Cornish-Bowden, A. and Cárdenas, M.L., Eds., Kluwer Academic Publishers, Dordrecht, 2000, p. 329.

5. Hofmeyr, J.-H.S. and Cornish-Bowden, A., Quantitative assessment of regulation in metabolic systems, *Eur. J. Biochem.,* 200, 223, 1991.
6. Brobeck, J.R., Exchange, control, and regulation, in *Physiological Controls and Regulations,* Yamamoto, W.S. and Brobeck, J.R., Eds., W.B Saunders, Philadelphia, 1965, p. 1.
7. Friedman, M.I. and Stricker, E.M., The physiological psychology of hunger: a physiological perspective, *Psychol. Rev.,* 83, 409, 1976.
8. Adolph, E.F., Urges to eat and drink in rats, *Am. J. Physiol.,* 151, 110, 1947.
9. Friedman, M.I., Hyperphagia in rats with experimental diabetes mellitus: A response to a decreased supply of utilizable fuels. *J. Comp. Physiol. Psychol.,* 92, 109, 1978.
10. Ugolev, A.M. and Kassil, V.G., Fiziologiia appetite, *Usp. Soy. Biol.,* 51, 352, 1961.
11. Booth, D.A., Postabsorptively induced suppression of appetite and the energostatic control of feeding, *Physiol. Behav.,* 9, 199, 1972.
12. Nicolaidis, S. and Even, P.C., The ischemytric control of feeding, *Int. J. Obes.,* 14 (Suppl. 3), 35, 1990.
13. Langhans, W. and Scharrer, E., Metabolic control of eating, *World Rev. Nutr. Diet.,* 70, 1, 1992.
14. Friedman, M.I., Metabolic control of calorie intake, in *Chemical Senses, Volume 4: Appetite and Nutrition,* Friedman, M.I., Tordoff, M.G., and Kare, M.R., Eds., Marcel Dekker, New York, 1991, p. 19.
15. Van Itallie, T.B. and Kissileff, H.R., Physiology of energy intake: An inventory control model, *Am. J. Clin. Nutr.,* 42, 914, 1985.
16. Miller, K., Halow, J., and Koretsky, A.P., Phosphocreatine protects transgenic mouse liver expressing creatine kinase from hypoxia and ischemia, *Am. J. Physiol. Cell Physiol.,* 265, C1544, 1993.
17. Ji, H. and Friedman, M.I., Compensatory hyperphagia after fasting tracks recovery of liver energy status, *Physiol. Behav.,* 68, 181, 1999.
18. Rawson, N.E. et al., Hepatic phosphate trapping, decreased ATP and increased feeding after 2,5-anhydro-d-mannitol, *Am. J. Physiol. Regul. Integr. Comp. Physiol.,* 266, R112, 1994.
19. Rawson, N.E., Ulrich, P.M., and Friedman, M.I., l-Ethionine, an amino acid analogue, stimulates eating in rats, *Am. J. Physiol. Regul. Integr. Comp. Physiol.,* 267, R612, 1994.
20. Friedman, M.I. et al., Fatty acid oxidation affects food intake by altering hepatic energy status, *Am. J. Physiol. Regul. Integr. Comp. Physiol.,* 276, R1046, 1999.
21. Rawson, N.E. and Friedman, M.I., Phosphate-loading prevents the decrease in ATP and increase in food intake produced by 2,5-anhydro-d-mannitol, *Am. J. Physiol. Regul. Integr. Comp. Physiol.,* 266, R1792, 1994.
22. Koch, J.E., et al., Temporal relationships between eating behavior and liver adenine nucleotides in rats treated with 2,5-anhydro-d-mannitol, *Am. J. Physiol. Regul. Integr. Comp. Physiol.,* 274, R610, 1998.
23. Horn, C.C., Tordoff, M.G., and Friedman, M.I., Role of vagal afferent innervation in feeding and brain Fos expression produced by metabolic inhibitors, *Brain Res.,* 919, 198, 2001.
24. Friedman, M.I. et al., 2,5-Anhydro-d-mannitol increases hepatocyte sodium: transduction of a hepatic hunger stimulus?, *Biochim. Biophys. Acta,* 1642, 53, 2003.
25. Rawson, N.E., Ji, H., and Friedman, M.I., 2,5-Anhydro-d-mannitol increases hepatocyte calcium: implications for a hepatic hunger stimulus, *Biochim. Biophys. Acta,* 1642, 59, 2003.
26. Plum, L., Belgardt, B.F., and Bruning, J.C., Central insulin action in energy and glucose homeostasis, *J. Clin. Invest.,* 116, 1761, 2006.

27. Otukonyong, E.E. et al., Central leptin differentially modulates ultradian secretory patterns of insulin, leptin and ghrelin independent of effects on food intake and body weight, *Peptides,* 26, 2559, 2005.
28. Theander-Carrillo, C. et al., Ghrelin action in the brain controls adipocyte metabolism, *J. Clin. Invest.,* 116, 1983, 2006.
29. Zarjevski, N. et al., Chronic intracerebroventricular neuropeptide-Y administration to normal rats mimics hormonal and metabolic changes of obesity, *Endocrinology,* 133, 1753, 1993.
30. Adage, T. et al., Hypothalamic, metabolic, and behavioral responses to pharmacological inhibition of CNS melanocortin signaling in rats, *J. Neurosci.,* 21, 3639, 2001.
31. Pocai, A. et al., Central leptin acutely reverses diet-induced hepatic insulin resistance, *Diabetes,* 54, 3182, 2005.
32. Inoue, H. et al., Role of hepatic STAT3 in brain-insulin action on hepatic glucose production, *Cell Metab.,* 3, 267, 2006.
33. Mauer, M.M., Harris, R.B., and Bartness, T.J., The regulation of total body fat: lessons learned from lipectomy studies, *Neurosci. Biobehav. Rev.,* 25, 15, 2001.
34. Rooks, C., Compensation for an increase in body fat caused by donor transplants into mice, *Am. J. Physiol. Regul. Integr. Comp. Physiol.,* 286, R1149, 2004.
35. Markewicz, B., Kuhmichel, G., and Schmidt, I., Onset of excess fat deposition in Zucker rats with and without decreased thermogenesis, *Am. J. Physiol. Endo. Met.,* 265, E478, 1993.
36. Hustvedt, B.-E. and Løvø, A., Rapid effect of ventromedial hypothalamic lesions on lipogenesis in rats, *Acta Physiol. Scand.,* 87, 28A, 1973.
37. Zucker, L.M., Efficiency of energy utilization by the Zucker hereditarily obese rat "fatty," *Proc. Soc. Exp. Biol. Med.,* 148, 498, 1975.
38. Han, P.W., Hypothalamic obesity in rats without hyperphagia, *Trans. N.Y. Acad. Sci.,* 30, 229, 1967.
39. Ramirez, I. and Friedman, M.I., Dietary hyperphagia in rats: role of fat, carbohydrate and energy content, *Physiol. Behav.,* 47, 1157, 1990.
40. Ji, H. and Friedman, M.I., Fasting plasma triglyceride levels and fat oxidation predict dietary obesity in rats, *Physiol. Behav.,* 78, 767, 2003.
41. Ji, H. and Friedman, M.I., Reduced capacity for fatty acid oxidation in rats with inherited susceptibility to diet-induced obesity, *Metabolism,* 56, 1124, 2007.
42. Speakman, J.R., Obesity: the integrated roles of environment and genetics, *J. Nutr.,* 134 (Suppl), 2090S, 2004.
43. Sclafani, A. and Springer, D., Dietary obesity in adult rats: similarities to hypothalamic and human obesity syndromes, *Physiol. Behav.,* 17, 461, 1976.
44. Naim, M. and Kare, M.R., Sensory and postingestional components of palatability in dietary obesity: an overview, in *Chemical Senses, Volume 4: Appetite and Nutrition,* Friedman, M.I., Tordoff, M.G., and Kare, M.R., Eds., Marcel Dekker, New York, 1991, p. 109.
45. Ramirez, I., Overeating, overweight and obesity induced by an unpreferred diet, *Physiol. Behav.,* 43, 501, 1988.
46. Teff, K.L. and Engelman, K., Oral sensory stimulation improves glucose tolerance in humans: effects on insulin, C-peptide, and glucagons, *Am. J. Physiol. Regul. Integr. Comp. Physiol.,* 270, R1371, 1996.
47. Tordoff, M.G. and Friedman, M.I., Drinking saccharin increases food intake and preference: IV. Cephalic phase and metabolic factors, *Appetite,* 12, 37, 1989.
48. Fuller, R.W. and Diller, E.R., Diurnal variation in liver glycogen and plasma free fatty acids in rats fed *ad libitum* or single daily meal, *Metabolism,* 19, 226, 1970.
49. Weingarten, H.P., Meal initiation controlled by learned cues: basic behavioral properties, *Appetite,* 5, 147, 1984.

50. Strubbe, J.H., Parasympathetic involvement in rapid meal-associated conditioned insulin secretion in the rat, *Am. J. Physiol. Regul. Integr. Comp. Physiol.*, 263, R615, 1992.
51. Thompson, D.A. and Campbell, R.G., Hunger in humans induced by 2-deoxy-d-glucose: glucoprivic control of taste preference and food intake, *Science*, 198, 1065, 1977.
52. Dewan, S. et al., Effects of insulin-induced hypoglycaemia on energy intake and food choice at a subsequent test meal, *Diabetes Metab. Res. Rev.*, 20, 405, 2004.
53. Schultes, B. et al., Processing of food stimuli is selectively enhanced during insulin-induced hypoglycemia in healthy men, *Psychoneuroendocrinology*, 30, 496, 2005.
54. Gil, K.M. et al., Parenteral nutrition and oral intake: effect of branched-chain amino acids, *Nutrition*, 6, 291, 1990.
55. Cortez-Pinto, H. et al., Alterations in liver ATP homeostasis in human nonalcoholic steatohepatitis, *JAMA*, 282, 1659, 1999.
56. Nair, S. et al., Hepatic ATP reserve and efficiency of replenishing: comparison between obese and nonobese normal individuals, *Am. J. Gastroenterol.*, 98, 466, 2003.
57. Teff, K.L. et al., 48-h Glucose infusion in humans: effect on hormonal responses, hunger and food intake, *Physiol. Behav.*, 90, 733, 2007.
58. Teff, K.L. et al., Dietary fructose reduces circulating insulin and leptin, attenuates postprandial suppression of ghrelin, and increases triglycerides in women, *J. Clin. Endocrinol. Metab.*, 89, 2963, 2004.
59. Bell, E.A., Energy density of foods affects energy intake in normal-weight women, *Am. J. Clin. Nutr.*, 67, 412, 1998.
60. Foltin, R.W. et al., Compensation for caloric dilution in humans given unrestricted access to food in a residential laboratory, *Appetite*, 10, 13, 1988.
61. Goldberg, G.R. et al., Dietary compensation in response to covert imposition of negative energy balance by removal of fat or carbohydrate, *British J. Nutr.*, 80, 141, 1998.
62. Birch, L.L. and Deysher, M., Caloric compensation and sensory specific satiety: Evidence for self regulation of food intake by young children, *Appetite*, 7, 323, 1986.
63. Stubbs, R.J. et al., Effect of altering the variety of sensorially distinct foods, of the same macronutrient content, on food intake and body weight in men, *Eur. J. Clin. Nutr.*, 55, 19, 2001.
64. Stubbs, R.J. and Whybrow, S., Energy density, diet composition and palatability: Influences on overall food energy intake in humans, *Physiol. Behav.*, 81, 755, 2004.

2 The Control of Food Intake and the Regulation of Body Weight in Humans

David A. Levitsky

CONTENTS

2.1 INTRODUCTION

A common belief among the vast majority of researchers and practitioners involved in the control of food intake of humans is that body weight is regulated through the control of food intake. Implicit in this belief are two assumptions: (1) body weight is physiologically regulated, and (2) it is regulated specifically through the control of energy intake. These assumptions originate deep in the history of animal physiology and psychology and have been seldom questioned. Yet the veracity of these assumptions will determine the success of our efforts to stem the surge of overweight and obesity so evident throughout the world.

There are three arguments that are used to support the notion that body weight of humans is regulated through the control of food intake. These three arguments stem from the fundamental properties of body weight, which are typical of physical regulatory systems: (1) body weight remains constant for long periods of time, despite variations in energy intake and expenditure, (2) after periods of excessive energy intake and weight gain, voluntary energy intake is reduced and body weight returns to pre-overfeeding levels, and (3) after periods of food restriction and subsequent weight loss, voluntary energy intake is increased and body weight recovers to its predeprivation values.

2.1.1 Classic Argument for the Regulation of Body Weight through the Control of Food Intake

2.1.1.1 Constancy of Body Weight

There are several variations of this argument. One popular version is that if we eat an extra chocolate cookie everyday (250 kcal), we will gain about 25 pounds in 1 year and that, because such a large weight gain rarely happens, this is evidence that control of intake must prevent us from gaining so much weight. A variation of this argument is illustrated in Figure 2.1. The average American eats approximately 2200 kcal/day. Over a period of a year, this intake amounts to approximately 800,000 kcal. If energy regulation were perfect, then at the end of a year, body weight will match energy expenditure exactly, and no gain or loss in body weight should occur. Unfortunately that is not what happens in reality. The upper right insert in Figure 2.1

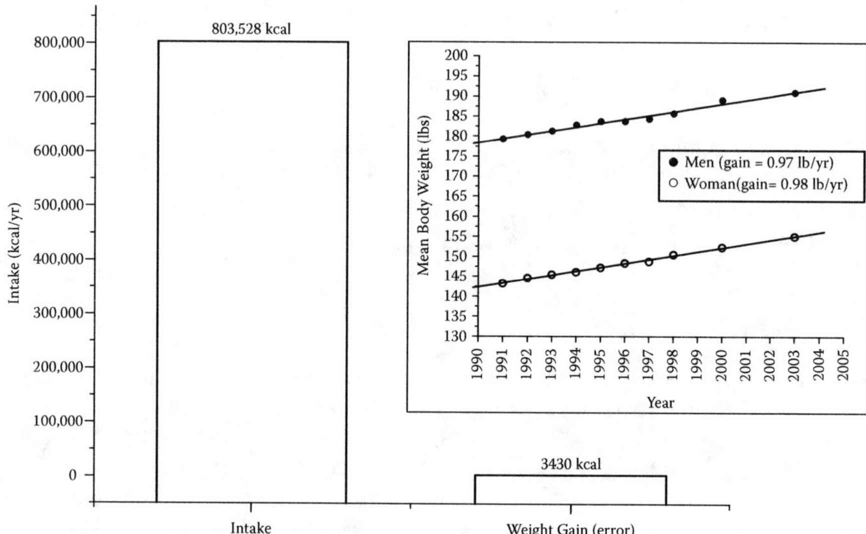

FIGURE 2.1 Inset: Mean body weight for males and females corrected for age estimated from HANES surveys. (Adapted from Zhang, Q. and Wang, Y., *Obes. Res.*, 12, 1622–1632, 2004. With permission.) Main figure: Theoretical difference in energy balance at the end of a year for a person who consumed 2200 kcal each day and gained 0.98 lbs (average yearly weight gain of Americans[81,86]).

shows estimates of mean body weight for American males and females taken over the past 15 years.[143] As is evident from this figure, both males and females are getting bigger. However, the increase in body weight is slightly less than a pound per year (0.98 lb/yr).[81,86] The gain in body weight can be converted to the amount of energy required to gain this amount of weight by multiplying it by the well accepted value of 3500 kcal/lb to yield a value of 3430 kcal. Expressing this "error" in terms of the large amount of energy consumed per year (3430 kcal/802,528 kcal) results in an error of less than 0.5%. Clearly, the argument goes, such precision could not occur without some physiological, regulatory mechanism operating to prevent changes in body weight.

This argument is valid only to the extent that an alternative mechanism to weight regulation cannot account for the data. Such an alternative explanation has been proposed. Levitsky[70] constructed a computer simulation of changes in body weight across time based upon three assumptions: (1) daily energy intake is a random process having a normal distribution and a mean of 2200 kcal/day, (2) the amount of daily energy expenditure is also a random process having a normal distribution with a mean of 2200 kcal per day, (3) daily energy expenditure increases as a function of body mass. This third assumption can be validated on the basis of two arguments. First, as body mass increases, the energy needed to move the larger body mass the same distance must also increase. Second, as an adult increases body weight, nearly half of the weight gain is lean body mass, which has a relatively high energy requirement. The computer model sampled daily from a normal distribution for intake and expenditure and, based on the differences, either increased or decreased body mass. The model repeatedly produced an energetic error at the end of 1 year of less than 0.5%. Because a model of the constancy of body weight can be constructed assuming random distribution of both energy intake and energy expenditure, and without the proposed properties of physiological regulation, the argument that stability of human body weight proves the existence of physiological regulation cannot be made.

2.1.1.2 Response to Food Deprivation

The deprivation of food has long served as a model procedure for stimulating eating behavior and the motivation to eat. Indeed, the inability to refrain from eating while "dieting" is widely believed to be the major reason why dieting is so ineffective a means of controlling body weight.[46,94,128,140] Despite these common observations and the fact that being deprived of food almost always leads to an increase in hunger sensations,[134] there is very little evidence that being deprived of food causes overeating in humans. In one study, spontaneous food consumption measured after skipping lunch (6-hour food deprivation) resulted in greater intake than intake after eating 1 hour prior.[127] But it is not clear whether the food deprivation stimulated intake or whether the consumption of the meal 1 hour prior to testing suppressed eating. In a subsequent study,[1] 14-hour food deprivation increased intake relative to a 2-hour deprivation. However, imposing a "negative" mood on the subjects completely eliminated the deprivation effect on food intake.

In a study of eating-disordered patients, very little effect of imposing a 19-hour food deprivation was found on subsequent food intake, except for one of the

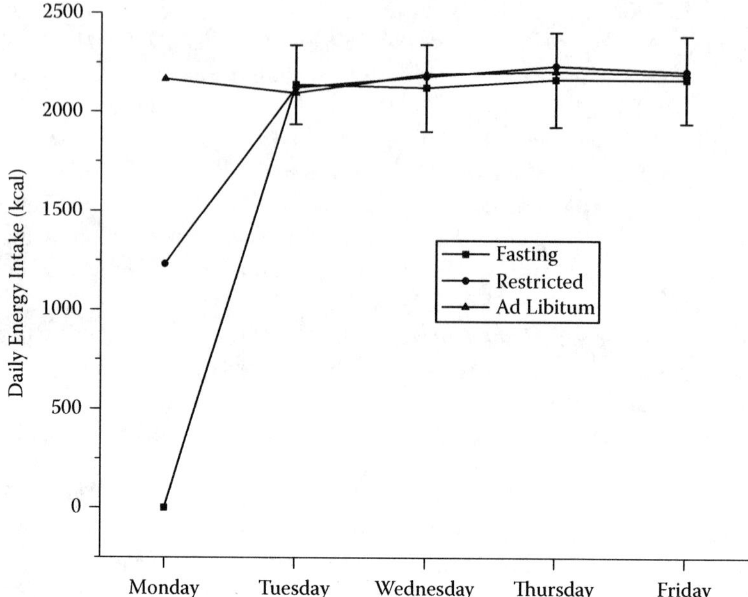

FIGURE 2.2 Mean and standard error of daily energy intake from Monday to Friday following either (a) ad lib. consumption, (b) 1200 kcal consumption, or (c) total fasting on Monday. (Adapted from Levitsky, D.A., *Physiol. Behav.,* 86, 623–632, 2005. With permission.)

three groups of patients.[52] Following a 36-hour fast, participants found food intake increased only about 20% when compared to testing after no fasting.[61]

Figure 2.2 displays the results of a study conducted in our lab in which *ad libitum* food intake was measured from Monday to Friday for 3 weeks. On Monday of each week, the subjects either (a) consumed food *ad libitum,* (b) consumed only 1200 kcal, or (c) were totally fasted. *Ad libitum* intake was measured from Tuesday to Friday. As is clearly evident in this figure, energy intake following the dietary manipulation did not differ between any of the deprivation conditions. Interestingly, body weight totally recovered following the restricted and total fasting condition.

Consequently, there is little evidence from the literature supporting the view that food intake in humans is increased proportionally to the degree of food deprivation.

2.1.1.3 Response to Overfeeding

Overfeeding presents an ideal mode for demonstrating the critical role that the control of food intake is proposed to play in the regulation of body weight. Inducing weight gain by overfeeding rats is followed by a significant reduction in subsequent food intake and a loss of body weight.[56] Despite the existence of this relatively direct test of the role of the control of food intake in the regulation of body weight, very few studies have used overfeeding to examine the regulation of food intake in humans. In one study, men of different ages were subjected to 21 days of overfeeding.[105] Following the period of overfeeding, the intake of young men decreased, whereas the intake of the older men remained constant. For the young men, different foods were

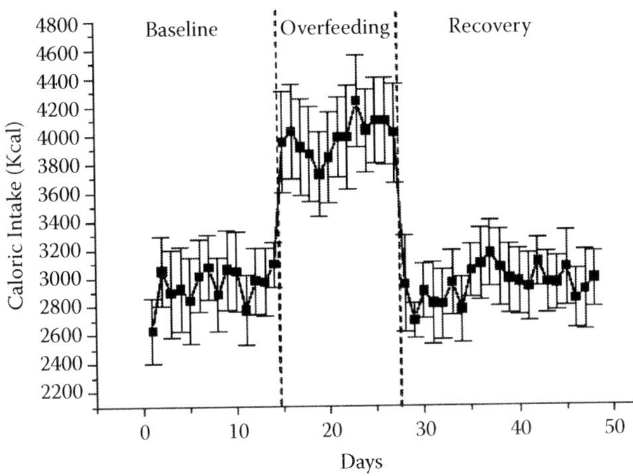

FIGURE 2.3 Mean and standard error of daily energy intake during (a) 2 weeks of baseline, (b) 2 weeks of overeating by 33%, and (c) during the 3-week period of recovery. (Adapted from Levitsky, D.A., Obarzanek, E., Mrdjenovic, G., and Strupp, B.J., *Physiol. Behav.*, 84, 669–675, 2005. With permission.)

served during the baseline period and following overfeeding, making it difficult to draw conclusions as to whether, or not, the decreased intake was due to the overfeeding or to the difference in the foods offered.

In another study, we performed a direct comparison of the effects of overfeeding on *ad libitum* food intake in humans in our lab.[74] Subjects were overfed each day by about 33% for 13 days, and then allowed to eat *ad libitum* for the next 3 weeks. Figure 2.3 shows the results. Despite producing a significant increase in body weight and complaints from the subjects that they couldn't eat any more, on the very next day, following the termination of overfeeding, the subjects returned to their normal level of food intake. Interestingly, the subjects all lost weight during the recovery period. What is important to recognize, however, is that the return to normal body weight was not accomplished through the control of food intake, since after overfeeding, subjects did not eat less than their normal intakes.

2.1.2 Response to Energy Density of the Diet

If physiological regulation of body weight operates to control human food intake, then eating behavior should be sensitive to changes in energy density of the food. Otherwise, consumption of energy-dense diets should cause obesity, and consumption of energy-sparse diets should cause starvation. The effect of changes in the energy density of diet on spontaneous food consumption is very clear: humans do not respond to changes in energy density by making appropriate adjustments in food intake. (For a more complete review see References [4,69].) Despite many claims to the contrary, when people eat foods having a decreased energy density, they do not increase their subsequent energy intake sufficiently to maintain body weight. Figure 2.4 shows the results of a within-subject, weighed-food-intake study of the effects of feeding the same foods that differed only in the amount of dietary fat for

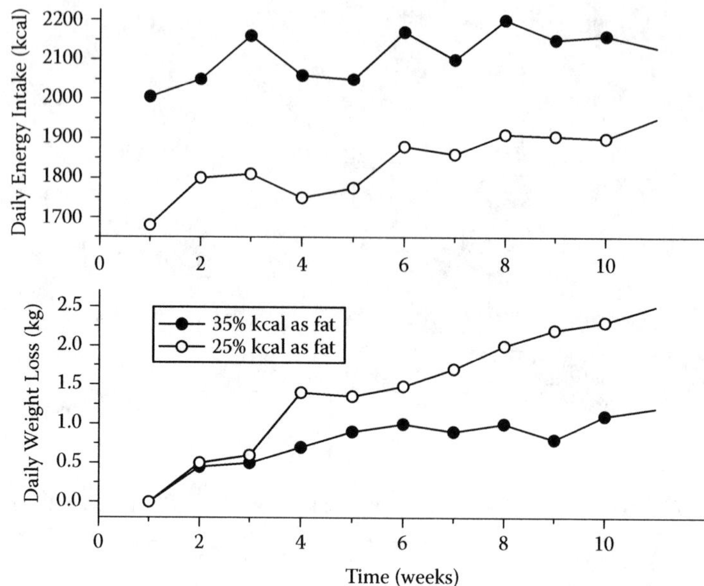

FIGURE 2.4 Mean and stardard error of daily energy intake and body weight loss measured across 11 weeks after eating the same foods differing only in fat content. (Adapted from Kendall, A., Levitsky, D.A., Strupp, B.J., and Lissner, L., Weight loss on a low-fat diet: consequence of the imprecision of the control of food intake in humans, *Am. J. Clin. Nutr.*, 53, 1124–1129, 1991. With permission.)

11 weeks.[62] Not only is there no indication that subjects receiving the low-fat food increased intake over time, but the incomplete compensation resulted in a significant difference in weight loss between groups.

Although change in dietary fat is one of the most effective ways to change energy density of the diet,[85] the lack of compensation for change in energy density is not limited to fat, but has been demonstated also when energy density is changed by varying water and fiber content.[7,107] Indeed, this lack of an adjustment of food intake to changes in energy density has been observed in epidemiological data[68] as well as in experimental studies.

There is very little evidence that humans display precise physiological regulation of energy intake. When deprived of food, they do not increase intake proportionally to the deficit. When overfed, they do not decrease intake. When the energy density of the diet is altered, they do not make adjustments to food intake to maintain a constant energy intake.

2.2 OPPORTUNITY NOT REGULATION

How can this be? Is it not true that humans regulate their energy balance? An enormous amount of data has been published in recent years documenting exquisite physiological pathways through the gastrointestinal track, from adipose tissue, and through many layers of brain-linking detectors of food and body stores to powerful stimulators and inhibitors of food intake. Have we biologically evolved so quickly that we do not use these fundamental, biological processes that determine our eating behavior? Perhaps we have been viewing the question from the wrong perspective.

Inherent in the concept of intake regulation is an energy depletion/repletion model of eating behavior. Regulation describes systems that attempt to maintain some entity constant. While no one would deny the necessity of eating to maintain a sufficient store of energy in the body to sustain and propagate life, it does not necessarily follow that the behavior of eating is controlled only by that system. George Collier was one of the first to suggest that, although the depletion/repletion model may have allowed us to identify and track the biology of eating related to energy depletion, it may have obscured the effects of many powerful, yet subtle, environmental stimuli that affect the eating behavior of animals.[17,18] Whereas Collier's formulations were directed more toward a general understanding of animal behavior in its own environment, Harvey Weingarten developed a similar idea, but related it more directly to eating behavior. He suggested that eating behavior was controlled by two motivational systems.[135] One system was controlled by the internal signals and generated biological signals from the classical depletion/repletion regulatory model of feeding system. The other, like Collier's, was driven by external, environmental stimuli associated with food and eating. Weingarten hypothesized that these two systems were controlled by different neural substrates and presented several very clever experiments to support this view. More recently, Berridge and Robinson[12] proposed a similar, yet broader theory of eating, but placed it into the context of reward. They suggested that the neurochemical systems underlying reward (food) in the mammalian brain may be divided into three parts: (1) a learning system that involves knowledge about the reward, (2) a homeostatic "need" that is driven by a physiological regulatory system involved in energy balance, and (3) a hedonic "want" or "desire" system that is independent of physiological regulation, but that might drive the behavior toward the consumption of food just as strongly as the homeostatic one. A similar but elaborate version of this theory that has recently been proposed by Lowe and Levine[79] expands the theory to encompass the human "dieting" literature as well. Although all three of these models suggest a nonregulatory aspect of eating behavior, none actually explains how the two systems that are suggested to control eating interact with each other.

Two models of eating behavior have been proposed that do attempt to show how classical depletion/repletion regulation and nonregulation eating integrate into a single conceptual framework. These models are depicted in Figure 2.5. Herman and Polivy[49] suggest that a boundary exists within the entire range of an individual's intake. Either a very low food intake (food deprivation) may elicit a biological signal that will cause eating to occur, or a very high food intake (gorging) will cause the biological signal of the depletion/repletion regulatory system to promote the cessation of eating. Levitsky[72] suggests that a range of body weight exists (Settling-Zone) for each individual. Biology plays two roles in this model. First, genetics determines where on the scale of body weights an individual's Settling-Zone lies. Second, biological regulatory mechanisms are activated whenever actual body weight either exceeds or drops below the Settling-Zone. What is common to both models, however, is that with either the "boundary" or the "Settling-Zone" human food intake is controlled primarily by external stimuli.

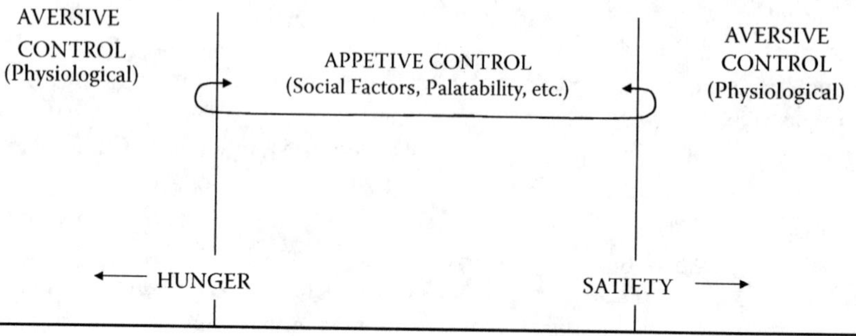

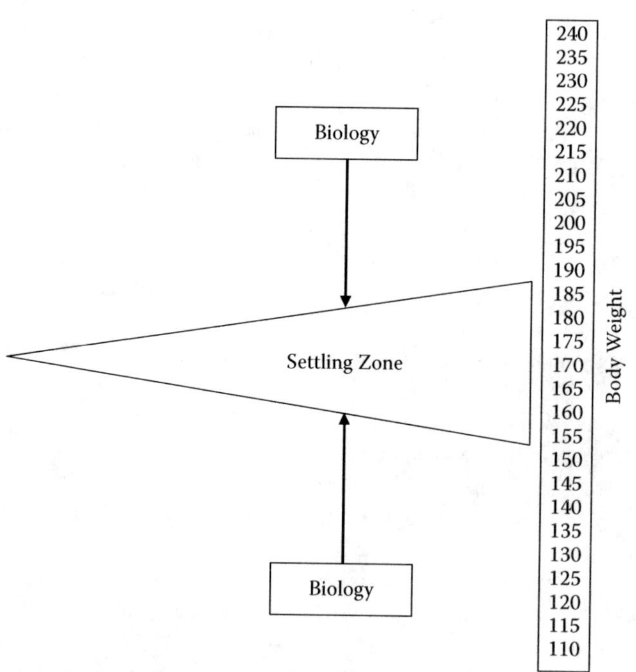

FIGURE 2.5 Boundary model of Herman and Polivy. (Adapted from Herman, C. and Polivy, J., in *Eating and Its Disorders.*, Stunkard, A.J. and Stellar, E., Eds., Raven Press, New York, 1984, pp. 141–156. With permission.) Settling zone model of Levitsky. (Adapted from Levitsky, D.A., Putting behavior back into feeding behavior: a tribute to George Collier, *Appetite,* 38, 143–148, 2002. With permission.)

2.3 EVIDENCE OF THE NONREGULATION OF HUMAN FEEDING BEHAVIOR

2.3.1 Portion Size Effect

Perhaps one of the most powerful demonstrations of an external stimulus affecting human food intake is the portion size effect. The effect is quite simple: the more food you put on a person's plate, the more the person eats. The effect was first noted by Siegel,[119] but has received little attention until fairly recently. Booth[14] reported that serving a larger lunch resulted in greater food consumption. Edelman published a study with army recruits[38] showing that the more food that was put on their plate, the more they ingested.

In the last 10 years, a considerable amount of laboratory data has substantiated the robustness of the portion size effect. It is evident in children,[88,108] when all the foods of a meal are altered[75] or when a single component of the meal is altered.[66,109] The phenomenon occurs whether or not the foods are discrete, such as sandwiches,[111] or amorphous such as snacks,[44,111,132] or a liquid, such as soup[75,133] or drinks.[42] The phenomenon occurs not just in the laboratory but has been observed under more "free-living" restaurant environments.[34]

The portion size effect is neither trivial nor transitory. Increasing the size of the portion served at a single meal can increase energy intake by as much as 50%, or about 1000 kcal.[75] A recent study by Rolls[110] demonstrated the effect of changing portion size lasts at least 2 days, and a recently completed study in our lab showed the effect of decreasing portion size for lunch remained for 2 weeks.

The inability of humans to adjust energy intake when served an altered portion size probably can account for the remarkable success of meal replacements as an aid to weight reduction.[53] Meal replacements usually are packaged, liquid foods of fixed size, containing less energy than is normally consumed at a meal. They are typically used to "replace" one or two meals during the day. The third meal consists of normal foods, and the size is usually determined by the subject, though usually restricted in energy density and or volume. Meal replacements are at least as effective,[43,57,90,100,131] and in most cases, superior[3,35,76] to conventional methods of dietary restriction in producing weight loss. Meal replacements were also found to be just as effective as treatment with Orlistat for producing weight loss.[58]

Most importantly, the use of meal replacements appears to be quite effective in maintaining weight loss.[36,116,41] Figure 2.6 is adapted from the Flechtner-Mors study. The meal replacement group used liquid meals to replace two meals and a snack during the first 3 months of initial weight loss, and then replaced just one meal and one snack for the 4 years of the study. Both the meal replacement group and the control group received conventional dietary advice. Although there was some recovery of body weight in the group receiving the meal replacements during the maintenance period, their body weight remained about 8 kg less than baseline body weight. Also embedded in this figure are the results of a recent meta-analysis of weight loss techniques.[37] The investigators estimated that conventional nutritional and lifestyle changes result in a loss of 5 kg or less at the end of 2 to 4 years, and that pharmacological therapy produces a weight loss of between 5 and 10 kg at the end of 2 years.

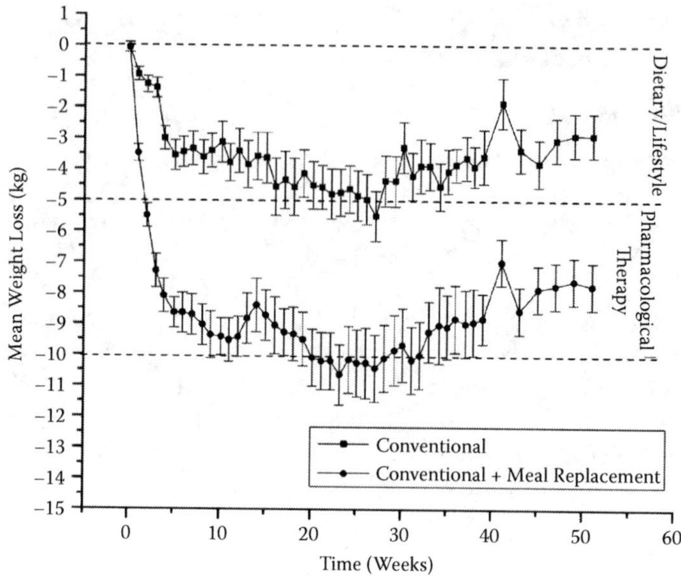

FIGURE 2.6 Mean weight loss in groups placed on a conventional low calorie diet and those placed on on the same low calorie diet but also given access to meal replacements. (Adapted from Flechtner-Mors, M., Ditschuneit, H.H., Johnson, T.D., Suchard, M.A., and Adler, G., *Obes. Res.*, 8, 399–402, 2000. With permission.)

The degree of maintained weight loss in the meal replacement groups was equivalent to that in groups undergoing pharmacological treatment.

These studies of meal replacements have important implications for the concept of body weight regulation and the control of food intake in humans. First, the meal replacement effect is not limited to liquid diets. Substituting ready-to-eat cereals for a meal has been shown to produce a significant loss in body weight.[63,80] What is particularly interesting about these two studies is that the subjects were not trying to lose weight. The weight loss resulted from a failure of humans to adjust to the reduced number of calories served at the meal. Providing people with portion-controlled meals consisting of ordinary foods has also been found to be effective in producing a greater weight loss than conventional therapy alone.[59,82,137,138]

What appears to be the critical factor for the meal replacement effect is that the meal is served as a visual package and is consumed as a structured visual unit comprised of the package and the portion. Humans seem to determine the size of their meal in terms of visual food units rather than through the use of any physical property of food that may be a surrogate for energy.[31,44] Vision, not energy regulation, appears to determine human food intake. It is particularly interesting that removing vision from sighted people reduces their food intake by about 23%.[5,78]

2.3.2 Variety Effect

Another very powerful controller of human food intake that does not appear to conform to biological regulation is the food variety effect. Food variety can be divided

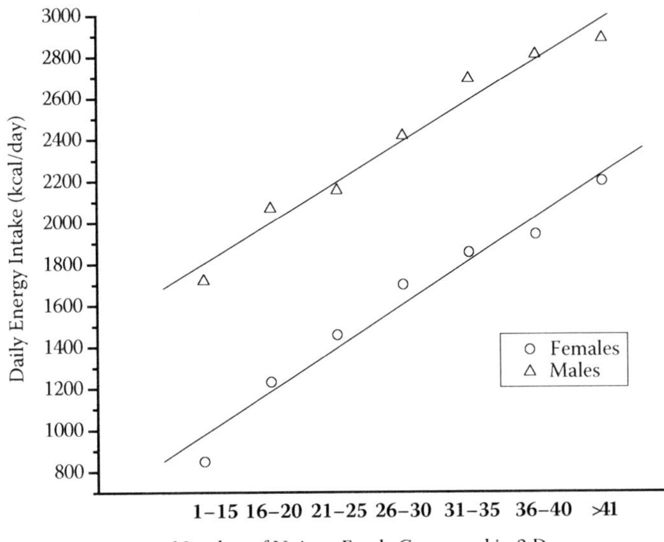

FIGURE 2.7 Mean daily energy intake of males and females who consumed different number of foods within a 3-day interval. (Adapted from Smiciklas-Wright, H., Krebs-Smith, S., and Krebs-Smith, J., in *What Is America Eating?: Proceedings of a Symposium*, National Research Council Food and Nutrition Board, National Academy Press, Washington, DC, 1986, pp. 126–140. With permission.)

into at least two different phenomena: the "food monotony effect" and "sensory-specific satiety." The older of these phenomena, the "monotony effect," was first reported in a series of military studies by Pilgrim.[117,120] They demonstrated that, when military recruits are offered the same or similar meals daily, a significant reduction in daily energy intake occurs compared to having access to varied meals every day. The effect has been replicated many times.[15,39,45,55,67,84,93,142] The effect is not trivial and may be responsible, in part, for the weight-reducing effects of commercial liquid diets. Although some of the effect is probably caused by reduced portion size, as discussed above, there are several studies that demonstrate that the amount consumed actually decreases with continued use when the liquid diet is the only food available.[15,48]

Whereas the "monotony effect" refers to a decline in energy intake with repetitive meals, "sensory-specific satiety" refers to a reduction in energy intake within a meal.* When different foods are presented either sequentially, like meal courses, or simultaneously,[6,91,124] energy intake is greater than when the same food is offered repeatedly within a meal.[60,98,112–114]

Like the portion size effect, the variety effect is not trivial. Figure 2.7 is adapted from an analysis of U.S. Department of Agriculture's (USDA) 1977–1978 Nationwide

* Although a considerable amount of work on stimulus-specific satiety has focused on the perceived changes in satiety and taste, this discussion is limited to those studies that measured directly food consumed.

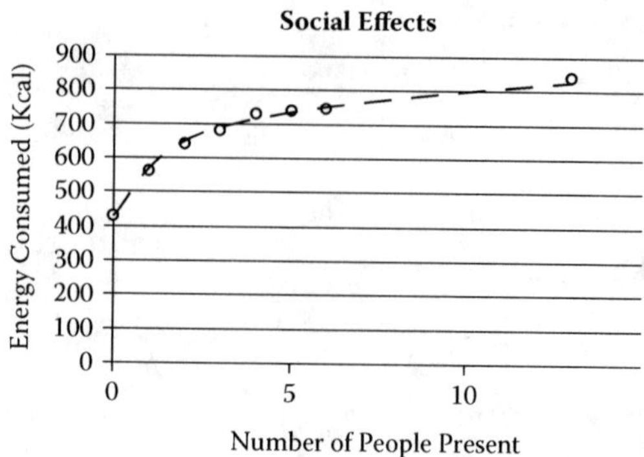

FIGURE 2.8 Mean amount of food a person consumes at a meal as a function of the number of people with whom they eat. (Adapted from de Castro, J.M., *Appetite,* 24, 260, 1995. With permission.)

Food Consumption Survey[128] and shows the relationship between the number of different foods consumed in 3 days and the average daily energy intake. It is quite evident from this figure that daily energy intake increases markedly with the number of different foods that are consumed. Even more striking is that the increase in the variety of foods consumed, both within a meal and between meals, and the total amount eaten is sustained across days[126] and may ultimately result in an increase in fat composition.[83,106,141]

Whether or not variety increases body weight (fatness) depends on the kinds of foods to which the variety is linked. McCrory and her colleagues[83] point out that, whereas an increase in variety increases the consumption of all kinds of foods, increases in the variety of energy-dense foods such as sweets, snacks, and entrées are associated with increased body weight. In addition, an increase in the variety of foods with low energy density, such as vegetables, was found to be related to body fat, a finding further supported by more recent studies.[118,141]

The variety effect appears sufficiently robust that it has been used successfully as an adjunct to weight reduction programs. Reducing the variety of energy-dense foods was effective in causing a greater reduction in food intake and a greater rate of weight loss than a standard weight reduction program[103] and may have improved the ability of people to sustain weight loss following treatment.[102]

2.3.3 Social Effect*

One of the most powerful modulators of human eating behavior is the social environment. As indicated in Figure 2.8, the more people humans eat with, the greater their food intake. As this figure shows, the social facilitation effect is not trivial, but can actually produce a change of intake on the order of about 50%. Although the bulk of this work was carried out by John de Castro and his associates using food diaries,[9,21,22,24,25,27–30,104] the social facilitation effect has been observed by others using different methods.[16,38,54,65]

* See Herman et al.[51] for an excellent review.

The amount of food intake of others in the environment can also influence the amount of an individual's food intake.[19,50,89,97] The social effect on eating is not always positive. When people have reason to believe that overeating may be viewed negatively, the presence of others actually depresses intake.[99] People also tend to eat more in the presence of family than in the presence of strangers,[23] or when eating with people of the same, rather than opposite, gender.[87] The visual stimulus of the presence of another person is not essential to affect eating, but can be construed within a person's mind. Thus, simply telling people how much food others have eaten is sufficient to affect the amount that they eat.[19,96,115]

The latter effect of the presence of other people during an eating occasion may explain, in part, the social facilitation caused by eating with more people. The presence of more people eating together increases the length of time it takes to complete a meal, as assessed by correlation studies,[8,21,95,123] or in a situation where the number of people is experimentally manipulated.[16] Extending the time available for eating increases the opportunity to see others eating, and the chance of seeing a food that one has not eaten, and and distracts from feelings of being full. All of these variables have been found to increase human food intake.

2.4 STIMULUS-BOUND EATING: AN ALTERNATIVE TO REGULATION THEORY

As indicated by the previous discussion, there is abundant evidence that human feeding behavior is influenced to a large extent by external stimuli or by cognitive cues that have nothing to do with physiological regulation, but rather, human expectation. Human eating behavior, to a very large extent, appears to be elicited, rather than driven.

If this is true, then human eating may be elicited by more abstract stimuli, such as food advertisements. Indeed, many investigators have pointed out a strong correlation between television watching and obesity.[2,11,32,33,92,101,129] Although some of this relationship may be due to a reduction in activity, there is evidence that a significant correlation exists between watching television and energy intake.[13,125,136] Although some of the increase in food intake while watching television may be due to distraction from feelings of fullness,[10] Halford provided the most convincing evidence that watching food commercials actually causes an increase in food intake in children.[47] Figure 2.9 shows the results of their study. A group of school children watched video advertisements (taken from commercial TV), and then were given a plate of snacks to eat as much or as little as they liked. As can be seen in the figure, after watching food commercials, the children ate significantly more snacks than after viewing nonfood commercials.

About 40 years ago, Elliot Valenstein introduced the term stimulus-bound eating into the literature to explain the nonspecificity of hypothalamic stimulation to affect specific behaviors in the rat.[130] Stimulus-bound eating may not only explain the portion size effect, but may also be a cause of the obesity epidemic that is so evident throughout the world. Rather than focus on the nonspecificity of induced behaviors, the term can be used to describe the power of external or cognitive signals to elicit eating behavior in humans, much along the lines of Weingarten's notion of the stimulus control of eating.[20,135] It may also explain why attempts at restricting food intake

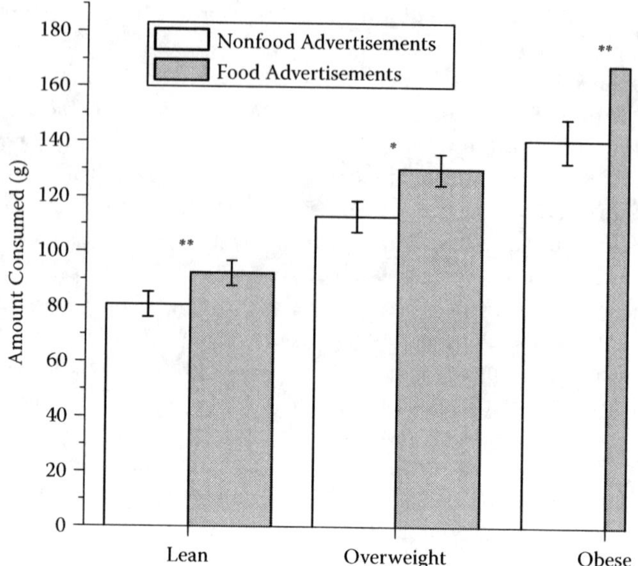

FIGURE 2.9 Mean and standard error of the amount of food consumed of children after they watched either a television advertisement about food or one without food. (Adapted from Halford, J.C., Gillespie, J., Brown, V., Pontin, E.E., and Dovey, T.M., *Appetite,* 42, 221–225, 2004. With permission.)

are so futile in this "obesigenic environment," where escaping visual food cues is almost impossible. The increasing omnipresence of food cues in the human environment may explain the increase of body weight seen everywhere in the world where food is abundant.

Stimulus-bound eating is subtle and weak, but the food-related stimuli are ubiquitous and unrelenting. Only a very small and infrequent capitulation to these food cues is sufficient to cause a significant increase in body weight. An estimate of how small the indulgences may be can be gleaned from Figure 2.1. The upper right figure indicates that we are gaining weight at a rate of 0.98 lbs per year. Converting to energy, this amounts to 3430 kcal per year. On a daily basis, this increase in weight can be caused by an increase in energy intake of less than 10 kcal a day.

2.5 A POSSIBLE SOLUTION: REGULATION THROUGH COGNITION

Without physiological regulation, what can be done to prevent the slow slide toward obesity? Daily monitoring of body weight may be the kind of tool that contemporary people need to help them in the battle of the bulge. While daily body weight is a crude indicator of the weight of body tissue (because of the variability imposed by fluctuations in body water, glycogen, and intestinal contents), when plotted over time, the trend in daily body weight is a very good estimator of energy balance. Using freshman weight gain as a model to study the slow insidious increase in body weight, we

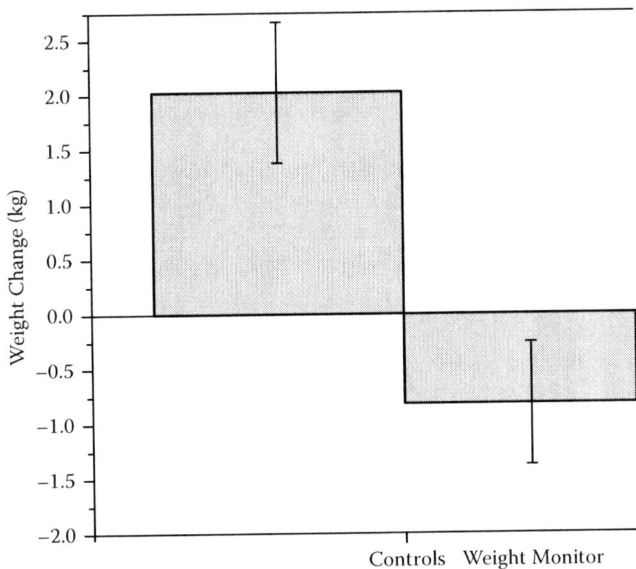

FIGURE 2.10 Mean and stardard error of the weight change of freshmen across the first 12 weeks of their first semester as function of whether or not they used daily weight monitoring. (Adapted from Levitsky, D.A., Garay, J., Nausbaum, M., Neighbors, L., and Dellavalle, D.M., *Int. J. Obes. (Lond.)*, 30, 1003–1010, 2006. With permission.)

provided one group with conventional bathroom scales and instructed them to weigh themselves every morning, and to email their weights to our staff.[73] Staff then plotted the weight and returned information about the weight trends during the past week. The change in subjects' weight during the first 12 weeks of the semester is plotted in Figure 2.10. The group that weighed themselves every day gained no weight, whereas the control group members, who were weighed at the beginning and end of the semester, gained approximately 2 kg. When interviewed at the end of the trial, the weight-monitoring group said that when they saw their weight increasing they decreased the amount of food they put on their plate, reduced the number of foods they put on their plate, skipped dessert, and even skipped a meal, depending upon how that change fit into their lifestyle. Other researchers, too, have found that daily weight monitoring is helpful for maintaining a loss in body weight.[64,77,139]

Monitoring of daily trends in body weight may provide the feedback required to help individuals approximate how much to eat on any given day in order to maintain their weight at a certain level. Acting in this way, daily weight monitoring may become part of an external regulatory system that controls our eating behavior and, ultimately, determines our body weight.

REFERENCES

1. Agras, W.S. and Telch, C.F., The effects of caloric deprivation and negative affect on binge eating in obese binge-eating disordered women, *Behav. Ther.*, 29, 491–503, 1998.

2. Andersen, R.E., Crespo, C.J., Bartlett, S.J., Cheskin, L.J., and Pratt, M., Relationship of physical activity and television watching with body weight and level of fatness among children: Results from the Third National Health and Nutrition Examination Survey, *JAMA*, 279, 938–942, 1998.
3. Ashley, J.M., St Jeor, S.T., Perumean-Chaney, S., Schrage, J., and Bovee, V., Meal replacements in weight intervention, *Obes. Res.*, 9, 312S–320S, 2001.
4. Astrup, A., Grunwald, G.K., Melanson, E.L., Saris, W.H., and Hill, J.O., The role of low-fat diets in body weight control: a meta-analysis of *ad libitum* dietary intervention studies, *Int. J. Obes. Relat. Metab. Disord.,* 24, 1545–1552, 2000.
5. Barkeling, B., Linne, Y., Melin, E., and Rooth, P., Vision and eating behavior in obese subjects, *Obes. Res.,* 11, 130–134, 2003.
6. Beatty, W.W., Dietary variety stimulates appetite in females but not in males, *Bull. Psychon. Soc.,* 19, 212–214, 1982.
7. Bell, E.A., Castellanos, V.H., Pelkman, C.L., Thorwart, M.L., and Rolls, B.J., Energy density of foods affects energy intake in normal-weight women, *Am. J. Clin. Nutr.,* 67, 412–420, 1998.
8. Bell, R. and Pliner, P.L., Time to eat: the relationship between the number of people eating and meal duration in three lunch settings, *Appetite,* 41, 215–218, 2003.
9. Bellisle, F., Dalix, A.M., and de Castro, J.M., Eating patterns in French subjects studied by the "weekly food diary" method, *Appetite,* 32, 46–52, 1999.
10. Bellisle, F., Dalix, A.M., and Slama, G., Non food-related environmental stimuli induce increased meal intake in healthy women: comparison of television viewing versus listening to a recorded story in laboratory settings, *Appetite,* 43, 175–180, 2004.
11. Berkey, C.S., Rockett, H.R., Field, A.E., Gillman, M.W., Frazier, A.L., Camargo, C.A., Jr., and Colditz, G.A., Activity, dietary intake, and weight changes in a longitudinal study of preadolescent and adolescent boys and girls, *Pediatrics,* 105, E56, 2000.
12. Berridge, K.C. and Robinson, T.E., Parsing reward, *Trends Neurosci.,* 26, 507–513, 2003.
13. Blass, E.M., Anderson, D.R., Kirkorian, H.L., Pempek, T.A., Price, I., and Koleini, M.F., On the road to obesity: television viewing increases intake of high-density foods, *Physiol. Behav.,* 88, 597–604, 2006.
14. Booth, D., Juller, J., and Lewis, V., Human control of body weight: Cognitive or physiological? Some energy-related perceptions and misperceptions, in *The Body Weight Regulatory System: Normal and Disturbed Mechanisms,* Cioffi, L.A., James, W.P.T., and Van Itallie, T.B., Eds. Raven Press, New York, 1981, pp. 305–314.
15. Cabanac, M. and Rabe, E.F., Influence of a monotonous food on body weight regulation in humans, *Physiol. Behav.,* 17, 675–8, 1976.
16. Clendenen, V.I., Herman, C.P., and Polivy, J., Social facilitation of eating among friends and strangers, *Appetite,* 23, 1–13, 1994.
17. Collier, G., Hirsch, E., and Hamlin, P.H., The ecological determinants of reinforcement in the rat, *Physiol. Behav.,* 9, 705–716, 1972.
18. Collier, G. and Johnson, D.F., Who is in charge? Animal versus experimenter control, *Appetite,* 29, 159–180, 1997.
19. Conger, J.C., Conger, A.J., Costanzo, P.R., Wright, K.L., and Matter, J.A., The effect of social cues on the eating behavior of obese and normal subjects, *J. Pers.,* 48, 258–271, 1980.
20. Cornell, C.E., Rodin, J., and Weingarten, H., Stimulus-induced eating when satiated, *Physiol. Behav.,* 45, 695–704, 1989.
21. de Castro, J.M., Social facilitation of duration and size but not rate of the spontaneous meal intake of humans, *Physiol. Behav.*, 47, 1129–1135, 1990.
22. de Castro, J., Brewer, E.M., Elmore, D.K., and Orozco, S., Social facilitation of the spontaneous meal size of humans occurs regardless of time, place, alcohol or snacks, *Appetite,* 15(2), 89–101, 1990.

23. de Castro, J.M., Family and friends produce greater social facilitation of food-intake than other companions, *Physiol. Behav.,* 56, 445–455, 1994.
24. de Castro, J.M., Family and friends produce greater social facilitation of food intake than other companions, *Physiol.Behav.,* 56, 445–455, 1994.
25. de Castro, J.M., Social facilitation of duration and size but not rate of the spontaneous meal intake of humans, *Physiol. Behav.,* 47, 1129–1135, 1990.
26. de Castro, J.M., Social facilitation of food intake in humans, *Appetite,* 24, 260, 1995.
27. de Castro, J.M., Social facilitation of the spontaneous meal size of humans occurs on both weekdays and weekends, *Physiol. Behav.,* 49, 1289–1291, 1991.
28. de Castro, J.M., Bellisle, F., Feunekes, G.I.J., Dalix, A.M., and DeGraaf, C., Culture and meal patterns: a comparison of the food intake of free-living American, Dutch, and French students, *Nutr. Res.,* 17, 807–829, 1997.
29. de Castro, J.M., Brewer, E.M., Elmore, D.K., and Orozco, S., Social facilitation of the spontaneous meal size of humans occurs regardless of time, place, alcohol or snacks, *Appetite,* 15, 89–101, 1990.
30. de Castro, J.M. and de Castro, E.S., Spontaneous meal patterns of humans — influence of the presence of other people, *Am. J. Clin. Nutr.,* 50, 237–247, 1989.
31. Devitt, A.A. and Mattes, R.D., Effects of food unit size and energy density on intake in humans, *Appetite,* 42, 213–220, 2004.
32. Dietz, W.H. and Gortmaker, S.L., TV or not TV: fat is the question, *Pediatrics,* 91, 499–501, 1993.
33. Dietz, W.H., Jr., and Gortmaker, S.L., Do we fatten our children at the television set? Obesity and television viewing in children and adolescents, *Pediatrics,* 75, 807–812, 1985.
34. Diliberti, N., Bordi, P.L., Conklin, M.T., Roe, L.S., and Rolls, B.J., Increased portion size leads to increased energy intake in a restaurant meal, *Obes. Res.,* 12, 562–568, 2004.
35. Ditschuneit, H.H., Do meal replacement drinks have a role in diabetes management? *Nestle Nutr. Workshop Ser. Clin. Perform. Programme,* 11, 171–179; discussion 179–181, 2006.
36. Ditschuneit, H.H. and Flechtner-Mors, M., Value of structured meals for weight management: risk factors and long-term weight maintenance, *Obes. Res.,* 9 (Suppl. 4), 284S–289S, 2001.
37. Douketis, J.D., Macie, C., Thabane, L., and Williamson, D.F., Systematic review of long-term weight loss studies in obese adults: clinical significance and applicability to clinical practice, *Int. J. Obes. (Lond.),* 29, 1153–1167, 2005.
38. Edelman, B., Engell, D., Bronstein, P., and Hirsch, E., Environmental effects on the intake of overweight and normal-weight men, *Appetite,* 7, 71–83, 1986.
39. Essed, N.H., van Staveren, W.A., Kok, F.J., Ormel, W., Zeinstra, G., and deGraaf, C., The effect of repeated exposure to fruit drinks on intake, pleasantness and boredom in young and elderly adults, *Physiol. Behav.,* 89, 335–341, 2006.
40. Flechtner-Mors, M., Ditschuneit, H.H., Johnson, T.D., Suchard, M.A., and Adler, G., Metabolic and weight loss effects of long-term dietary intervention in obese patients: four-year results, *Obes. Res.,* 8, 399–402, 2000.
41. Flechtner-Mors, M., Ditschuneit, H.H., Johnson, T.D., Suchard, M.A., and Adler, G., Metabolic and weight loss effects of long-term dietary intervention in obese patients: four-year results, *Obes. Res.,* 8, 399–402, 2000.
42. Flood, J.E., Roe, L.S., and Rolls, B.J., The effect of increased beverage portion size on energy intake at a meal, *J. Am. Diet. Assoc.,* 106, 1984–1990; discussion 1990–1991, 2006.
43. Fontaine, K.R., Yang, D., Gadbury, G.L., Heshka, S., Schwartz, L.G., Murugesan, R., Kraker, J.L., Heo, M., Heymsfield, S.B., and Allison, D.B., Results of soy-based meal replacement formula on weight, anthropometry, serum lipids & blood pressure during a 40-week clinical weight loss trial, *J. Nutr.,* 2, 14, 2003.

44. Geier, A.B., Rozin, P., and Doros, G., Unit Bias. A new heuristic that helps explain the effect of portion size on food intake, *Psychol. Sci.,* 17, 521–525, 2006.
45. Gerrish, C.J. and Mennella, J.A., Flavor variety enhances food acceptance in formula-fed infants, *Am. J. Clin. Nutr.,* 73, 1080–1085, 2001.
46. Gibson, L.J., Peto, J., Warren, J.M., and Dos Santos Silva, I., Lack of evidence on diets for obesity for children: a systematic review, *Int. J. Epidemiol.,* 35, 1544–1552, 2006.
47. Halford, J.C., Gillespie, J., Brown, V., Pontin, E.E., and Dovey, T.M., Effect of television advertisements for foods on food consumption in children, *Appetite,* 42, 221–225, 2004.
48. Hashim, S.A. and Van Itallie, T.B., Studies in normal and obese subjects with a monitored food dispensing device, *Ann. N. Y. Acad. Sci.,* 131, 654–661, 1965.
49. Herman, C. and Polivy, J., A boundry model for the retulation of eating, in *Eating and Its Disorders.,* Stunkard, A.J. and Stellar, E., Eds., Raven Press, New York, 1984, pp. 141–156.
50. Herman, C.P., Koenig-Nobert, S., Peterson, J.B., and Polivy, J., Matching effects on eating: do individual differences make a difference? *Appetite,* 45, 108–109, 2005.
51. Herman, C.P., Roth, D.A., and Polivy, J., Effects of the presence of others on food intake: a normative interpretation, *Psychol. Bull.,* 129, 873–886, 2003.
52. Hetherington, M.M., Stoner, S.A., Andersen, A.E., and Rolls, B.J., Effects of acute food deprivation on eating behavior in eating disorders, *Int. J. Eat. Disord.,* 28, 272–283, 2000.
53. Heymsfield, S.B., van Mierlo, C.A., van der Knaap, H.C., Heo, M., and Frier, H.I., Weight management using a meal replacement strategy: meta and pooling analysis from six studies, *Int. J. Obes. Relat. Metab. Disord.,* 27, 537–549, 2003.
54. Hirsch, E.S. and Kramer, F.M., Situational influences on food intake, in *Nutritional Needs in Hot Environments,* Marriott, B.M., Ed., A report of the Committee on Military Nutrition Research, Food and Nutrition Board, Institute of Medicine, National Academy Press, Washington, DC, 1993, pp. 215–243.
55. Hirsch, E.S., Matthew Kramer, F., and Meiselman, H.L., Effects of food attributes and feeding environment on acceptance, consumption and body weight: lessons learned in a twenty-year program of military ration research US Army Research (Part 2), *Appetite,* 44, 33–45, 2005.
56. Hoebel, B.G. and Teitelbaum, P., Weight regulation in normal and hypothalamic hyperphagic rats, *J. Comp. Physiol. Psychol.,* 61, 189–193, 1966.
57. Huerta, S., Li, Z., Li, H.C., Hu, M.S., Yu, C.A., and Heber, D., Feasibility of a partial meal replacement plan for weight loss in low-income patients, *Int. J. Obes. Relat. Metab. Disord.,* 28, 1575–1579, 2004.
58. Jebb, S.A. and Goldberg, G.R., Efficacy of very low-energy diets and meal replacements in the treatment of obesity, *J. Hum. Nutr. Diet.,* 11, 219–225, 1998.
59. Jeffery, R.W., Wing, R.R., Thorson, C., Burton, L.R., Raether, C., Harvey, J., and Mullen, M., Strengthening behavioral interventions for weight loss: a randomized trial of food provision and monetary incentives, *J. Consult. Clin. Psychol.,* 61, 1038–1045, 1993.
60. Johnson, J. and Vickers, Z.M., Effects of flavor and macronutrient composition of food servings on liking, hunger and subsequent intake, *Appetite,* 21, 25–39, 1993.
61. Johnstone, A.M., Faber, P., Gibney, E.R., Elia, M., Horgan, G., Golden, B.E., and Stubbs, R.J., Effect of an acute fast on energy compensation and feeding behaviour in lean men and women, *Int. J. Obes.,* 26, 1623–1628, 2002.
62. Kendall, A., Levitsky, D.A., Strupp, B.J., and Lissner, L., Weight loss on a low-fat diet: consequence of the imprecision of the control of food intake in humans, *Am. J. Clin. Nutr.,* 53, 1124–1129, 1991.
63. Kirk, T., Crombie, N., and Cursiter, M., Promotion of Dietary Carbohydrate as an approach to weight maintenance after initial weight loss: a pilot study, *J. Hum. Nutr. Diet.,* 13, 277–285, 2000.

64. Klem, M.L., Wing, R.R., McGuire, M.T., Seagle, H.M., and Hill, J.O., A descriptive study of individuals successful at long-term maintenance of substantial weight loss, *Am. J. Clin. Nutr.*, 66, 239–246, 1997.
65. Klesges, R.C., Bartsch, D., Norwood, J.D., Kautzman, D., and Haugrud, S., The effects of selected social and environmental variables on the eating behavior of adults in the natural-environment, *Int. J. Eat. Disord.*, 3, 35–41, 1984.
66. Kral, T.V., Roe, L.S., and Rolls, B.J., Combined effects of energy density and portion size on energy intake in women, *Am. J. Clin. Nutr.*, 79, 962–968, 2004.
67. Kramer, F.M., Lesher, L.L., and Meiselman, H.L., Monotony and choice: repeated serving of the same item to soldiers under field conditions, *Appetite*, 36, 239–240, 2001.
68. Ledikwe, J.H., Blanck, H.M., Kettel Khan, L., Serdula, M.K., Seymour, J.D., Tohill, B.C., and Rolls, B.J., Dietary energy density is associated with energy intake and weight status in US adults, *Am. J. Clin. Nutr.*, 83, 1362–1368, 2006.
69. Levitsky, D., Macronutrient intake and the control of body weight, in *Nutrition in the Prevention and Treatment of Disease*, Coulston, A.M. et al., Eds., Academic Press, San Diego, CA, 2001, pp. 499–516.
70. Levitsky, D.A., Constancy of body weight does not mean physiological regulation, paper presented at the Annual Meeting of the Society for the Study of Ingestive Behavior, Naples, FL, 2006.
71. Levitsky, D.A., The non-regulation of food intake in humans: hope for reversing the epidemic of obesity, *Physiol. Behav.*, 86, 623–632, 2005.
72. Levitsky, D.A., Putting behavior back into feeding behavior: a tribute to George Collier, *Appetite*, 38, 143–148, 2002.
73. Levitsky, D.A., Garay, J., Nausbaum, M., Neighbors, L., and Della Valle, D.M., Monitoring weight daily blocks the freshman weight gain: a model for combating the epidemic of obesity, *Int. J. Obes. (Lond.)*, 30, 1003–1010, 2006.
74. Levitsky, D.A., Obarzanek, E., Mrdjenovic, G., and Strupp, B.J., Imprecise control of energy intake: absence of a reduction in food intake following overfeeding in young adults, *Physiol. Behav.*, 84, 669–675, 2005.
75. Levitsky, D.A. and Youn, T., The more food young adults are served, the more they overeat, *J. Nutr.*, 134, 2546–2549, 2004.
76. Li, Z., Hong, K., Saltsman, P., DeShields, S., Bellman, M., Thames, G., Liu, Y., Wang, H.J., Elashoff, R., and Heber, D., Long-term efficacy of soy-based meal replacements vs an individualized diet plan in obese Type II DM patients: relative effects on weight loss, metabolic parameters, and C-reactive protein, *Eur. J. Clin. Nutr.*, 59, 411–418, 2005.
77. Linde, J.A., Jeffery, R.W., French, S.A., Pronk, N.P., and Boyle, R.G., Self-weighing in weight gain prevention and weight loss trials, *Ann. Behav. Med.*, 30, 210–216, 2005.
78. Linne, Y., Barkeling, B., Rossner, S., and Rooth, P., Vision and eating behavior, *Obes. Res.*, 10, 92–95, 2002.
79. Lowe, M.R. and Levine, A.S., Eating motives and the controversy over dieting: eating less than needed versus less than wanted, *Obes. Res.*, 13, 797–806, 2005.
80. Mattes, R.D., Ready-to-eat cereal used as a meal replacement promotes weight loss in humans, *J. Am. Coll. Nutr.*, 21, 570–577, 2002.
81. Maynard, L.M., Serdula, M.K., Galuska, D.A., Gillespie, C., and Mokdad, A.H., Secular trends in desired weight of adults, *Int. J. Obes.*, 30, 1375–1381, 2006.
82. McCarron, D.A., Oparil, S., Chait, A., Haynes, R.B., Kris-Etherton, P., Stern, J.S., Resnick, L.M., Clark, S., Morris, C.D., Hatton, D.C., Metz, J.A., McMahon, M., Holcomb, S., Snyder, G.W., and Pi-Sunyer, F.X., Nutritional management of cardiovascular risk factors. a randomized clinical trial, *Arch. Intern. Med.*, 157, 169–177, 1997.
83. McCrory, M.A., Fuss, P.J., McCallum, J.E., Yao, M., Vinken, A.G., Hays, N.P., and Roberts, S.B., Dietary variety within food groups: association with energy intake and body fatness in men and women, *Am. J. Clin. Nutr.*, 69, 440–447, 1999.

84. Meiselman, H.L., deGraaf, C., and Lesher, L.L., The effects of variety and monotony on food acceptance and intake at a midday meal, *Physiol. Behav.,* 70, 119–125, 2000.
85. Mela, D. and Rogers, P., *Food, Eating and Obesity: The Psychobiological Basis of Appetite and Weight Control,* Chapman & Hall, London. 1998.
86. Mokdad, A.H., Serdula, M.K., Dietz, W.H., Bowman, B.A., Marks, J.S., and Koplan, J.P., The spread of the obesity epidemic in the United States, 1991–1998, *JAMA,* 282, 1519–1522, 1999.
87. Mori, D., Chaiken, S., and Pliner, P., "Eating lightly" and the self-presentation of femininity, *J. Pers. Soc. Psychol.,* 53, 693–702, 1987.
88. Mrdjenovic, G. and Levitsky, D.A., Children eat what they are served: the imprecise regulation of energy intake, *Appetite,* 44, 273–282, 2005.
89. Nisbett, R. and Storms, M., Cognitive and social determinants of food intake, in *Thought and Feeling: Cognitive Alternation of Feeling States,* London, H. and Nishbett, R.E., Eds., Aldine, Chicago, 1974, pp. 190–208.
90. Noakes, M., Foster, P.R., Keogh, J.B., and Clifton, P.M., Meal replacements are as effective as structured weight-loss diets for treating obesity in adults with features of metabolic syndrome, *J. Nutr.,* 134, 1894–1899, 2004.
91. Norton, G.N.M., Anderson, A.S., and Hetherington, M.M., Volume and variety: relative effects on food intake, *Physiol. Behav.,* 87, 714–722, 2006.
92. Obarzanek, E., Schreiber, G.B., Crawford, P.B., Goldman, S.R., Barrier, P.M., Frederick, M.M., and Lakatos, E., Energy intake and physical activity in relation to indexes of body fat: the National Heart, Lung, and Blood Institute Growth and Health Study, *Am. J. Clin. Nutr.,* 60, 15–22, 1994.
93. Pelchat, M.L. and Schaefer, S., Dietary monotony and food cravings in young and elderly adults, *Physiol. Behav.,* 68, 353–359, 2000.
94. Pirozzo, S., Summerbell, C., Cameron, C., and Glasziou, P., Advice on low-fat diets for obesity, *Cochrane Database Syst. Rev.* CD003640, 2002.
95. Pliner, P., Bell, R., Hirsch, E.S., and Kinchla, M., Meal duration mediates the effect of "social facilitation" on eating in humans, *Appetite,* 46, 189–198, 2006.
96. Pliner, P. and Mann, N., Influence of social norms and palatability on amount consumed and food choice, *Appetite,* 42, 227–37, 2004.
97. Pliner, P. and Mann, N., Influence of social norms and palatability on amount consumed and food choice, *Appetite,* 42, 227–237, 2004.
98. Pliner, P., Polivy, J., Herman, C.P., and Zakalusny, I., Short-term intake of overweight individuals and normal weight dieters and non-dieters with and without choice among a variety of foods, *Appetite,* 1, 203–213, 1980.
99. Polivy, J., Herman, C.P., Hackett, R., and Kuleshnyk, I., The effects of self-attention and public attention on eating in restrained and unrestrained subjects, *J. Pers. Soc. Psychol.,* 50, 1253–1260, 1986.
100. Poston, W.S., Haddock, C.K., Pinkston, M.M., Pace, P., Karakoc, N.D., Reeves, R.S., and Foreyt, J.P., Weight loss with meal replacement and meal replacement plus snacks: a randomized trial, *Int. J. Obes. (Lond.),* 29, 1107–1114, 2005.
101. Proctor, M.H., Moore, L.L., Gao, D., Cupples, L.A., Bradlee, M.L., Hood, M.Y., and Ellison, R.C., Television viewing and change in body fat from preschool to early adolescence: the Framingham Children's Study, *Int. J. Obes. Relat. Metab. Disord.,* 27, 827–833, 2003.
102. Raynor, H.A., Jeffery, R.W., Phelan, S., Hill, J.O., and Wing, R.R., Amount of food group variety consumed in the diet and long-term weight loss maintenance, *Obes. Res.,* 13, 883–890, 2005.
103. Raynor, H.A., Jeffery, R.W., Tate, D.F., and Wing, R.R., Relationship between changes in food group variety, dietary intake, and weight during obesity treatment, *Int. J. Obes. Relat. Metab. Disord.,* 28, 813–820, 2004.

104. Redd, M. and de Castro, J.M., Social facilitation of eating — effects of social instruction on food-intake, *Physiol. Behav.,* 52, 749–754, 1992.
105. Roberts, S.B., Fuss, P., Dallal, G.E., Atkinson, A., Evans, W.J., Joseph, L., Fiatarone, M.A., Greenberg, A.S., and Young, V.R., Effects of age on energy expenditure and substrate oxidation during experimental overfeeding in healthy men, *J. Gerontol. A Biol. Sci. Med. Sci.,* 51, B148–B157, 1996.
106. Roberts, S.B., Hajduk, C.L., Howarth, N.C., Russell, R., and McCrory, M.A., Dietary variety predicts low body mass index and inadequate macronutrient and micronutrient intakes in community-dwelling older adults, *J. Gerontol. A Biol. Sci. Med. Sci.,* 60, 613–621, 2005.
107. Rolls, B.J., Bell, E.A., Castellanos, V.H., Chow, M., Pelkman, C.L., and Thorwart, M.L., Energy density but not fat content of foods affected energy intake in lean and obese women, *Am. J. Clin. Nutr.,* 69, 863–871, 1999.
108. Rolls, B.J., Engell, D., and Birch, L.L., Serving portion size influences 5-year-old but not 3-year-old children's food intakes, *J. Am. Diet. Assoc.,* 100, 232–234, 2000.
109. Rolls, B.J., Morris, E.L., and Roe, L.S., Portion size of food affects energy intake in normal-weight and overweight men and women, *Am. J. Clin. Nutr.,* 76, 1207–1213, 2002.
110. Rolls, B.J., Roe, L.S., and Meengs, J.S., Reductions in portion size and energy density of foods are addictive and lead to sustained decreases in energy intake, *Am. J. Clin. Nutr.,* 83, 11–17, 2006.
111. Rolls, B.J., Roe, L.S., Meengs, J.S., and Wall, D.E., Increasing the portion size of a sandwich increases energy intake, *J. Am. Diet. Assoc.,* 104, 367–372, 2004.
112. Rolls, B.J., Rowe, E.A., and Rolls, E.T., How sensory properties of foods affect human feeding-behavior, *Physiol. Behav.,* 29, 409–417, 1982.
113. Rolls, B.J., Rowe, E.A., Rolls, E.T., Kingston, B., Megson, A., and Gunary, R., Variety in a meal enhances food intake in man, *Physiol. Behav.,* 26, 215–221, 1981.
114. Rolls, B.J., Van Duijvenvoorde, P.M., and Rolls, E.T., Pleasantness changes and food intake in a varied four-course meal, *Appetite,* 5, 337–348, 1984.
115. Roth, D.A., Herman, C.P., Polivy, J., and Pliner, P., Self-presentational conflict in social eating situations: a normative perspective, *Appetite,* 36, 165–171, 2001.
116. Rothacker, D.Q., Five-year self-management of weight using meal replacements: comparison with matched controls in rural Wisconsin, *Nutrition,* 16, 344–348, 2000.
117. Schutz, H.G. and Pilgrim, F.J., A field-study of food monotony, *Psychol. Rep.,* 4, 559–565, 1958.
118. Sea, M.M.M., Woo, J., Tong, P.C.Y., Chow, C.C., and Chan, J.C.N., Associations between food variety and body fatness in Hong Kong Chinese adults, *J. Am. Coll. Nutr.,* 23, 404–413, 2004.
119. Siegel, P.S., The completion compulsion in human eating, *Psychol. Rep.,* 3, 15–16, 1957.
120. Siegel, P.S. and Pilgrim, F.J., The effect of monotony on the acceptance of food, *Am. J. Psychol.,* 71, 756–759, 1958.
121. Smiciklas-Wright, H., Krebs-Smith, S., and Krebs-Smith, J., Variety in foods, in *What Is America Eating?: Proceedings of a Symposium,* National Research Council Food and Nutrition Board, National Academy Press, Washington, DC, 1986, pp. 126–140.
122. Smiciklas-Wright, H., Krebs-Smith, S., and Krebs-Smith, J., 'Variety in Foods,' in *What Is America Eating?: Proceedings of a Symposium,* National Research Council Food and Nutrition Board, National Academy Press, Washington, DC, 1986, pp. 126–140.
123. Sommer, R. and Steele, J., Social effects on duration in restaurants, *Appetite,* 29, 25–30, 1997.
124. Spiegel, T.A. and Stellar, E., Effects of variety on food intake of underweight, normal-weight and overweight women, *Appetite,* 15, 47–61, 1990.
125. Stroebele, N. and de Castro, J.M., Television viewing is associated with an increase in meal frequency in humans, *Appetite,* 42, 111–113, 2004.

126. Stubbs, R.J., Johnstone, A.M., Mazlan, N., Mbaiwa, S.E., and Ferris, S., Effect of altering the variety of sensorially distinct foods, of the same macronutrient content, on food intake and body weight in men, *Eur. J. Clin. Nutr.,* 55, 19–28, 2001.
127. Telch, C.F. and Agras, W.S., The effects of short-term food deprivation on caloric intake in eating-disordered subjects, *Appetite,* 26, 221–233, 1996.
128. Tsai, A.G. and Wadden, T.A., Systematic review: an evaluation of major commercial weight loss programs in the United States, *Ann. Intern. Med.,* 142, 56–66, 2005.
129. Utter, J., Neumark-Sztainer, D., Jeffery, R., and Story, M., Couch potatoes or french fries: are sedentary behaviors associated with body mass index, physical activity, and dietary behaviors among adolescents? *J. Am. Diet. Assoc.,* 103, 1298–1305, 2003.
130. Valenstein, E.S., Cox, V.C., and Kakolewski, J.W., Reexamination of the role of the hypothalamus in motivation, *Psychol. Rev.,* 77, 16–31, 1970.
131. Vidal-Guevara, M.L., Samper, M., Martinez-Silla, G., Canteras, M., Ros, G., Gil, A., and Abellan, P., Meal replacement as a dietary therapy for weight control: assessment in males and females with different degrees of obesity, *Nutr. Hosp.,* 19, 202–208, 2004.
132. Wansink, B. and Kim, J., Bad popcorn in big buckets: portion size can influence intake as much as taste, *J. Nutr. Educ. Behav.,* 37, 242–245, 2005.
133. Wansink, B., Painter, J.E., and North, J., Bottomless bowls: why visual cues of portion size may influence intake, *Obes. Res.,* 13, 93–100, 2005.
134. Warren, C. and Cooper, P.J., Psychological effects of dieting, *Br. J. Clin. Psychol.,* 27 (Pt 3), 269–270, 1988.
135. Weingarten, H.P., Stimulus control of eating: implications for a two-factor theory of hunger, *Appetite,* 6, 387–401, 1985.
136. Wiecha, J.L., Peterson, K.E., Ludwig, D.S., Kim, J., Sobol, A., and Gortmaker, S.L., When children eat what they watch — impact of television viewing on dietary intake in youth, *Arch. Pediatr. Adolesc. Med.,* 160, 436–442, 2006.
137. Wing, R.R. and Jeffery, R.W., Food provision as a strategy to promote weight loss, *Obes. Res.,* 9 (Suppl. 4), 271S–275S, 2001.
138. Wing, R.R., Jeffery, R.W., Burton, L.R., Thorson, C., Nissinoff, K.S., and Baxter, J.E., Food provision vs structured meal plans in the behavioral treatment of obesity, *Int. J. Obes. Relat. Metab. Disord.,* 20, 56–62, 1996.
139. Wing, R.R., Tate, D.F., Gorin, A.A., Raynor, H.A., and Fava, J.L., A self-regulation program for maintenance of weight loss, *N. Engl. J. Med.,* 355, 1563–1571, 2006.
140. Wooley, S.C. and Garner, D.M., Dietary treatments for obesity are ineffective, *BMJ,* 309, 655–656, 1994.
141. Yao, M., McCrory, M.A., Ma, G., Tucker, K.L., Gao, S., Fuss, P., and Roberts, S.B., Relative influence of diet and physical activity on body composition in urban Chinese adults, *Am. J. Clin. Nutr.,* 77, 1409–1416, 2003.
142. Zandstra, E.H., de Graaf, C., and van Trijp, H.C., Effects of variety and repeated in-home consumption on product acceptance, *Appetite,* 35, 113–119, 2000.
143. Zhang, Q. and Wang, Y., Trends in the association between obesity and socioeconomic status in U.S. adults: 1971 to 2000, *Obes. Res.,* 12, 1622–1632, 2004.

3 Appetitive and Consummatory Aspects of Food Intake in Rodents

Neil E. Rowland and Clare M. Mathes

CONTENTS

3.1 APPETITE AND FEEDING

3.1.1 APPETITIVE BEHAVIORS

The modern dictionary defines *appetite* as the desire to eat food. It is perceived as hunger. This definition is close to that used almost 90 years ago by Craig[1]:

> An appetite is a state of agitation which continues so long as a certain stimulus, which may be called the appeted stimulus, is absent. When the appeted stimulus is at length received it stimulates a consummatory reaction, after which the appetitive behavior ceases and is succeeded by a state of relative rest.

In the case of feeding, the "appeted stimulus" is food and/or its postingestive effects. This definition implicitly includes a preconsummatory or appetitive phase distinct from the consummatory phase. Appetite by either of these definitions does not predict amount eaten. Indeed, the phrase "at length received" suggests that an indeterminate foraging period may occur before a food object is encountered. *A priori,* the amount of food encountered while foraging is uncertain and, depending on the amount, may or may not satisfy or satiate the appetite. For this reason, the term appetite should not be used to imply amount eaten.

The derived adjective, *appetitive*, has been used to describe behaviors such as foraging that either bring organisms into contact with or maintain contact with a food source. It should be emphasized that these two phases of appetitive behavior are distinct and involve quite different mechanisms. The aspect of "coming into contact with" generally implies locomotion through the environment as in Craig's "state of agitation," what we ordinarily think of as foraging or search. It may be random in time and space, but more often is guided by individual or socially transmitted memories of previous successful foraging episode(s) and by the distal sensations (sight, sound, or smell) of the food object.

The second phase of appetitive behavior is that triggered, in addition to sight, sound, and smell, by the proximate senses of touch and taste (the latter, in combination with odor, giving rise to the global sensation of flavor). Thus, taste itself has appetitive qualities, perhaps best encapsulated in a French saying "*L'appetit vient en mangeant*" (appetite comes with eating). The object evaluation afforded by these proximate senses, especially taste and odor, is the primary determinant of whether an object placed in the mouth is swallowed or ejected.

3.1.2 CONSUMMATORY BEHAVIORS

This consideration leads to the position that the defining consummatory act is swallowing, not just placing the object into the mouth. Swallowing, unlike placing food in the mouth, is an irrevocable act: once swallowed, food cannot normally be expelled voluntarily (emesis, whether caused by a toxin or self-induced, does of course occur in some species but goes beyond the scope of this chapter). The taste-reactivity test, developed by Norgren and Grill,[2] specifically isolates the proximate evaluative components of the appetitive phase. In this test, tastant solutions are infused into the mouth of animals, and their oral-motor behaviors are divided most simply into accept (swallowing) or reject (active expulsion) categories. This test has been used to evaluate affective responses to tastants under different physiological conditions, with the underlying assumption that swallowing implies a pleasant sensory experience and expulsion indicates an unpleasant sensory experience. Many of these oral motor responses are organized at a relatively primitive neural level (brain stem) of rodents.

The proximate appetitive and consummatory phases normally occur in temporal alternation: handle and bite/chew, followed by swallowing, and the sequence repeats. If the food object is not particularly large, then locomotion (foraging) may occur within the food patch or locale (e.g., picking berries from a bush, pecking a rotted tree trunk for grubs, or grazing a pasture). This phase or alternation is terminated either (1) when a sufficient amount has been consumed (Craig's appeted stimulus), in which case there is a behavioral satiety sequence, or (2) when there is no more food available at an economically viable cost within the patch, in which case remote foraging or travel to a new patch occurs.

So how do we define *feeding*? Should it refer only to the consummatory act, should it also include the proximate preconsummatory acts of handling and chewing, and should it include both the remote and proximate appetitive phases? In many laboratory studies, the remote appetitive phase is abrogated; animals are simply presented with an edible source, and their only choice is whether to accept or reject the next mouthful. As we will develop later in this chapter, this is an unfortunate omission in our current understanding of feeding behavior.

3.2 MOTIVATION

3.2.1 Characteristics of Motivated Behavior

One of the hallmarks of behavior is motivation, the hypothetical underlying motive force. Early theorists considered concepts of *drive* and *incentive*, which describe the internal need for a commodity and its external or sensory allure, respectively (see Bolles[3] for review). These terms have fallen out of favor, and in the case of feeding have been replaced by the concepts of hunger and palatability, which are arguably more specific.

Epstein[4] considered three defining characteristics to distinguish motivated from instinctive behaviors. The first characteristic of motivated behavior is *individuation*, a concept that learning experiences sculpt the future motivation through the expression of conditioned operants. The second, also a learned characteristic, is the *expectancy* or anticipation of goals. This property gives the behavior goal-directedness. The third characteristic is *affect*. The concept of *palatability* (defined as sufficiently acceptable to be consumed) is implicit in this definition. Epstein further argued that, so defined, motivated behaviors are relatively rare compared with occurrences of instinctive behavior.

Useful though this list may be, the three characteristics do not always coexist, especially in animal models. For example, the taste-reactivity test, while embracing the third characteristic of affect, engages little if any of the first two characteristics of individuation and expectancy. In fact, these first two characteristics could be considered more usually allied with the appetitive-remote foraging phase that we have emphasized, while the affective component is more usually allied with the proximate appetitive cues.

Behavior analysts often use the term establishing operation (EO) or motivating operation (MO) to define the precondition for behavior,[5] for example as 24 hours of food deprivation or 10% weight loss. However, in many real-world applications to feeding, the MO(s) may be difficult to isolate, and so it is parsimonious to use the term motivation to refer to the internal states that underlie emission of a goal-directed behavior. In addition to direct observation as a change in behavior, these states are potentially observable as changes in physiology, such as gene expression, metabolic activity, and hormonal regulators of brain function.

3.3 HOMEOSTASIS

One of the most enduring concepts relating to the organization of motivated behaviors is that of homeostasis, originally used by Cannon[6] in relation to observed constancy or narrow normal range of physiological variables, such as core temperature or blood glucose concentration. The concept as most commonly applied requires that an ideal value or set point be biologically encoded, and that deviations from that set point be detected and used to activate responses, including motivated behavior, that will cause the regulated variable to return to the set point. It should be noted that more elaborate, varied, and flexible types of homeostasis have been proposed.[7,8] For example, a system with a biased error signal could favor energy deposition; such homeostatic models have not been widely considered by the field. The application of the narrower definition to a complex physiological state such as body weight is controversial.[8,9] Nonetheless, many contemporary neural models of feeding, for example the reciprocal activation of hunger-modulating neuropeptide Y (NPY) and agouti-related protein (AgRP) neurons and satiety-modulating proopiomelanocortin (POMC) neurons in the arcuate nucleus (see Irani and Haskell-Luevano[10] for a review) are, at heart, narrow homeostasis.

Inextricably linked to the concept of homeostasis is that of physiological need. This works well for tightly regulated variables such as core temperature. If your set point is 37°C and your actual temperature is 36°C, then need may be quantified, because it is "here and now" and is only satisfied when temperature rises by 1°C, at which point the physiological or behavioral adjustments engaged by being cold cease. However, once one departs from a tightly regulated variable, the concept of need becomes arbitrary from the perspectives of both amount consumed and the temporal urgency of that behavior. As a hypothetical example, suppose that two subjects of identical height/length differ in body weight and fat content, thus body mass index (BMI). If both subjects are now deprived of food for 24 hours (an MO), will their need be identical? From an evolutionary perspective, clearly not — the fatter individual initially has greater corporeal energy stores and so has a temporal buffer against periods of no food, while the leaner individual is less buffered. But if the subjects were asked how hungry they are, they may both give similar reports (or exhibit similar motivated behavior if nonverbal). Likewise, basic homeostasis does not account for eating that occurs in the absence of need, as in eating a second portion of dessert just because it tastes good.

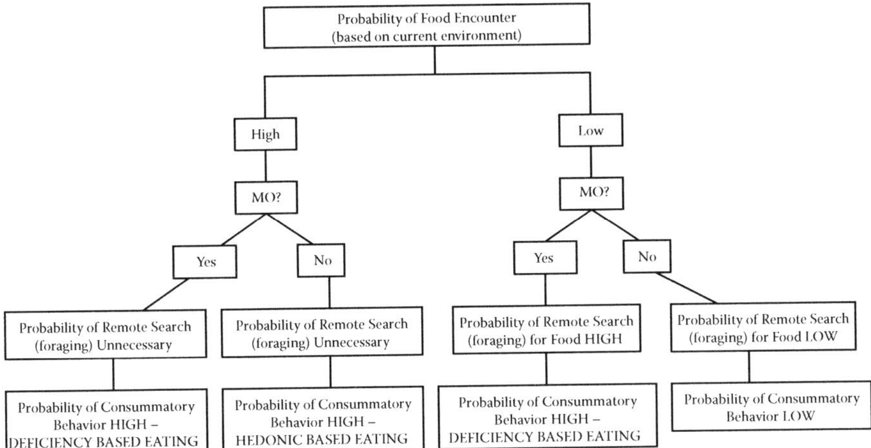

FIGURE 3.1 Schematic of how changes in the probability of encountering food in the environment, and the presence or absence of a motivating operation (MO; functionally, deprivation or weight loss) affects appetitive (i.e., foraging) and consummatory behaviors. Note that we can divide feeding into that based on need and not (assumed here to be driven hedonically).

3.4 OPPORTUNISTIC PERSPECTIVE

Other theorists, especially those coming from an ecological perspective, have argued that energy balance is critically related to the environmental controls of feeding. On an evolutionary timescale these have been issues of food procurement. Optimal foraging theory emphasizes that animals will regulate their food intake in relation to the energy expenditures necessary to procure that food.[11] From that perspective, set point is an unnecessary concept.[12] In unpredictable environments, animals must be opportunists that eat "cheap" food whenever it is encountered, whether or not the result of goal-directed search. Mrosovsky[8] (p. 12) summarized a statement by Cannon as follows: "Homeostasis was for poetry rather than for producing grandchildren." Homeostasis relates to an ideal and perhaps evolutionarily infrequent situation when the commodity itself is not rate-limiting. Our brains have not evolved in ideal environments, and so purely homeostatic models cannot illuminate this ecological aspect.

We may define *opportunistic feeding* in terms of the probability of progressing from the state of initial identification of the food source through telereceptive sensations such as smell or sight to the consummatory phase of swallowing (Figure 3.1). Thus, in the presence of an MO such as low body energy reserves, this probability is high. In the absence of an MO or the presence of satiety signals indicative of recent feeding, this probability will be lower, but may not be zero, in which case "need-free feeding" is observed. Concurrent with this change in probability is a change in food acceptance — the higher the need the more substances are deemed palatable. This latter process is primarily at the proximate appetitive level; the presence or absence of locomotor behaviors evoked in the presence of an EO will of course greatly influence the probability of encounter.

3.5 APPETITIVE BEHAVIOR IN RODENT MODELS

We noted earlier that the vast majority of modern feeding experiments in laboratory animals place little emphasis on the appetitive phase. This is an interesting development because many early (pre-1960) experiments did involve explicit measurement of motivation, for example running an alley or pressing a lever. Indeed, Miller[13] argued that the true measure of motivation was the number of times an animal would surmount an obstacle to obtain a goal object and the vigor of that response. Yet with few exceptions, studies of free-feeding meal patterns and derivatives focus on the controls of meal size that have dominated the more recent literature.

3.5.1 Procurement versus Consummatory Costs in Rats

One such exception has been a long series of illuminating studies by George Collier and his colleagues. In a landmark paper,[14] they compared the effects of imposing two types of foraging cost on meal patterns in rats. The first type of foraging cost, which was termed *consummatory,* is a procedure typical of short-session or open-economy studies of operant schedules of reinforcement. For now we consider only fixed ratio (FR) in which an animal has to emit a certain number of responses to obtain a small amount of food. Note that consummatory as used by Collier differs from our earlier definition — his operational definition includes not only swallowing, but also the proximate appetitive aspects including within-patch foraging. Using a continuous-access closed economy in which all food was earned via the operant, rats were willing to emit thousands of presses but maintained free (or low-cost) feeding patterns in terms of meal size and number of meals per day (Table 3.1). In rats, typical free-feeding patterns are 8 to 12 meals per day averaging 8 to 12 kcal; a typical meal-defining criterion is 20 minutes of rest.

The second type of foraging cost, which Collier termed *procurement,* required the rat to press a lever a fixed number of times to open a door behind which was a large bowl of food. The rat could then eat as much as it wished, but once it left the feeder area for a meal-defining criterion time, the door closed and a new ratio was required when the rat was ready to start a new access period. Under these closed-

TABLE 3.1
Typical Meal Parameters of Rats Subjected to Low or High Consummatory Costs or to Low or High Procurement Costs

Type of Schedule	Consummatory FR = 1 (low)	Consummatory FR = 200 (high)	Procurement FR = 1 (low)	Procurement FR = 300 (high)
Meals per day	27	14	10	3
Meal size (g)	0.9	1.2	2.1	6.5
Presses per day	500	75,000	10	900
Cost/45 mg pellet	1.00	200.0	0.02	2.08

Source: Data are means derived or interpolated from figures in Collier, G.C., Hirsch, E., and Hamlin, P.H., *Physiol. Behav.*, 9, 705, 1972. (With permission.)

economy conditions, as procurement cost increased to only a few hundred presses the number of meals per day decreased to 1–2/day and their size increased reciprocally (Table 3.1). Meal parameters appear to be exquisitely tuned to the environmental contingencies of procurement. Note that in this protocol food was always available, so no deprivation or explicit MO was imposed by the experimenter. This definition of procurement maps fairly closely onto the remote aspects of appetitive behavior. So what appears to be happening is that, as procurement cost increases, the physiological threshold for triggering motivated behavior rises, leading to longer intermeal intervals. Once the food encounter occurs, which in this case has 100% probability following a certain number of presses, the probability of continuing an eating bout in the presence of proximate cues is increased, leading to larger meal sizes.

3.5.2 Other Species

Collier has found similar results in several species other than rats, and we have recently extended the paradigm to mice.[15–17] We found that leptin-deficient obese mice (C57BL lep$^{-/-}$) showed similar changes to lean (wild-type) controls in meal number as procurement cost was varied. However, the meal size of the lep$^{-/-}$ mice was consistently higher than in wild types, leading to a net hyperphagia and maintenance of their obese phenotype.[15]

A different result was found using another obese mouse, the melanocortin type 4 receptor knockout mouse (MC4RKO). These mice showed meal number and size changes identical to wild-type controls; as a result, they lost weight every time they were tested but regained it during experimental holidays of free feeding.[16] One possible reason for this result is that MC4RKO mice are unwilling or unable to emit the large numbers of lever presses that would be required to sustain hyperphagia. To test this, we used a protocol that imposed a within-patch foraging cost in the form of a progressive ratio (PR) schedule; this emulates a patch that is depleting of resources.[17] On the PR that we used, the first pellet in a meal cost one press, the second pellet two presses, and so on. Animals terminate an ongoing meal because they are functionally unwilling to pay the next highest price per pellet; this is termed the break or breaking point.[18] One of the break point and meal termination criteria we employed was 20 minutes elapsed without a pellet, which is comparable to common definitions of a meal in no cost, free-feeding protocols. In the PR, an optimal or cost-minimizing strategy would be to take many small meals with intermeal intervals of just over 20 minutes. Wild-type controls indeed did increase their meal number and decrease meal size (Table 3.2) relative to a low consummatory cost condition (about 7 to 10 meals/day[17]), but the surprise was that the MC4RKO mice took larger meals than wild type. Compared with wild-type controls, the MC4RKO mice were hyperphagic, remained obese, showed a higher breaking point, and performed a higher mean cost per pellet.

This PR result, as well as several other studies of FR consummatory cost,[14,19–20] suggests that within-patch foraging costs have less effect on meal parameters than comparable procurement costs. It should be noted that these costs impact different parts of the appetitive sequence — procurement costs occur during the remote or distal phase, and consummatory costs occur during the proximate phase (cf. Figure 3.1). This distinction

TABLE 3.2
Food Intake and Meal Parameters of Melanocortin-4 Receptor Heterozygous (HET) and Homozygous (KO) Mice Compared with Wild Type (WT) under Progressive Ratio Consummatory Cost

Genotype	Daily Food Intake (g)	Meal Size (mg)	Number of Meals/Day	Lever Presses or Cost per Pellet
WT	4.2	180	23.3	5.6
HET	4.7[a]	220[a]	21.4	6.1[a]
KO	5.7[b]	280[b]	20.4	7.7[b]

Source: Shown are group means from Tables 1 and 2 and Figure 2 for the 20-minute reset criterion to define a meal, from Vaughan, C. et al., *Peptides*, 27, 2829, 2006. (With permission.)

[a] $P < 0.05$ versus WT.

[b] $P < 0.05$ versus WT and HET.

is critical to, but typically has not been made in research in the field of behavioral economics. Conversely, physiological experiments that are devoid of an economic choice are likely to miss most of the motivational aspect. Last, although beyond the present discussion, animals may hoard or cache food rather than or in addition to eating, and this is an important and functionally anticipatory appetitive behavior.[21]

3.6 DEFICIENCY-BASED APPETITE

Because body weight or a correlate of fat content is not tightly regulated, it is difficult to define physiological need in an absolute sense. MOs are the independent variables. It is instructive first to consider behavioral regulation of a physiological parameter that is reasonably tightly regulated — sodium balance. Excursion of plasma or interstitial sodium concentrations beyond ~10% of the mean is essentially incompatible with mammalian life.

3.6.1 Sodium Appetite as a Model to Quantify Need

Sodium appetite has been used as a model drive system.[22] Some (but not all) strains of rodents show a preference for near-isotonic solutions of sodium salts[23,24] under need-free conditions, but avoid strongly hypertonic solutions. Studies of *sodium appetite* have most frequently used such hypertonic solutions so that their consumption can be ascribed to an appetitive state rather than spontaneous or need-free ingestion. Since it appears that concentrated sodium solutions are unpalatable, their consumption is akin to overcoming an obstacle, as in Miller's definition of a motivated behavior. Depletion of body sodium occurs naturally by prolonged dietary sodium insufficiency,[25] but experimentally it is more usually and rapidly produced by administration of a natriuretic agent.[26]

This type of depletion has been documented to increase foraging behavior in both natural[25] and laboratory[27,28] conditions, to increase the consumption of NaCl across the entire concentration range,[24] and to increase the acceptability of concentrated NaCl in taste-reactivity or brief-access tests in which postingestive effects are minimized.[29] In other words, the entire appetitive spectrum from remote foraging to proximate consumption is engaged, although from a theoretical and a practical perspective these can be separated. It should be noted in this regard that the taste of sodium is critical to the phenomenon of salt appetite.[30] Indeed, the conditioning of postingestive events to sensory properties of foods or fluids is overwhelmingly if not exclusively dependent on taste or flavor.[31,32]

When rats are depleted of sodium by administration of a diuretic and subsequently allowed free access to concentrated NaCl solution, the amount they consume is dependent on the time elapsed since the depletion. At its maximum ~24 hours later, rats consume 2 to 4 times as much sodium as their actual physiological deficit.[26,33] When studies are conducted under no-cost, free-access conditions, their consumption is manifestly in excess of need. We[34] recently examined the consequences of imposing a consummatory cost on this overconsumption. Briefly, rats were depleted of sodium by daily injection of the natriuretic agent, furosemide and were allowed to replete themselves either by free access to NaCl or in various PR operant protocols (emulating costs incurred within a salt patch), in each case for about 1 hour/day. The principal result was that, while the rats overconsumed under no-cost conditions, the imposition of a within-patch PR caused the intake to more closely match the estimated physiological need. Animals were willing to "pay" the incremental costs until the true need was satisfied, but not beyond. This takes us back to Craig's definition of appetite; his "appeted stimulus" differs between the operant (~2 milliequivalents of NaCl) and no-cost (~4 milliequivalents) conditions, yet both intakes are engaged by the same defined EO of sodium depletion. What seems to differ between the conditions is that the probability of continuing a bout is dependent on proximate foraging costs coupled with the fact that concentrated NaCl becomes palatable in a physiological state of sodium loss. This in turn implies that palatability or more generally hedonic factors are very influential in determining the probability of continuing, and possibly initiation of ingestive episodes. We turn now to a consideration of these hedonic factors.

3.7 HEDONIC-BASED APPETITE

If appetite and food intake are behaviors that are regulated exclusively by physiological parameters, obesity would be an issue in only those few individuals with genetic anomalies that short-circuit the homeostatic mechanisms of the hypothalamus and other brain regions. This is not the case. Data suggest that 60 to 75% of humans in developed or developing countries have a BMI classifiable as obese or overweight, a proportion that cannot be explained by genetic variables alone. Studies with animals demonstrate that caloric overconsumption and subsequent development of obesity are modulated by environmental factors interacting with need state. An example of the behavioral contingency was described above[16] in the MC4RKO mice that lost weight on a procurement-cost protocol but not on a PR schedule. The sensory properties of food, including how they act within the brain and the associated behavioral contingencies, impact appetite and food intake as much as any genetically proscribed mechanisms underlying energy homeostasis.

Although food is a necessary commodity, it also serves as a stimulus with reinforcing and rewarding components. By definition, a reinforcer increases the probability of the future occurrence of behavior upon which presentation of the commodity is contingent. Thus, the consumption of a pleasant-tasting food may increase intake independent of the presence of discriminative stimuli associated with need. The taste and consumption of food stimulate brain pathways associated with reward and are modulated by dopamine, opioid, and endocannabinoid systems, all of which are associated with the acquisition and perseveration of consummatory behavior.[35,36] With the increase in availability of high-fat, high-sugar, palatable foods and the subsequent increase in consumption of these commodities, it has been proposed that some foods may have reached the status of addicting substances.[37]

3.7.1 Palatability

On the cusp between appetitive and consummatory behaviors, food is put in the mouth and comes into contact with sensory receptors where the sensory characteristics of the food are evaluated and inform a decision concerning ingestion or rejection. This hedonic evaluation of food is referred to as palatability. The definition of palatability sometimes has lead to a circular logic in which increased food intake is attributed to an increase in the pleasantness of the food. Although pleasantness rating in humans may support this, it is not always an available or accurate assessment in animal studies. For example, high-fat diets are often considered palatable, yet rats may actually consume fewer grams of a high-fat diet than a low-fat diet when offered successively. However, given a simultaneous choice, they may consume almost exclusively the high-fat diet. Preference measured via consumption is not a valid marker of palatability, because rats will consume a lower volume of a high-concentration sucrose solution compared to a weaker concentration in a two-bottle preference test, but will choose and lick more avidly for the higher concentration in discrete trials. One reason for the discrepancy is that consumption measures involve short- and long-term postingestive factors, whereas palatability usually is an initial or instantaneous evaluation. Palatability is not an intrinsic property of a food, but rather is a mechanism of the appetitive process in which factors that enhance the hedonic evaluation of the sensory characteristics of food may predict preference and sometimes levels of consumption.

The evaluation of palatability, either by self report in humans or by behavioral means such as taste-reactivity measures in animals, does not exist in isolation. Food pleasantness is rated or decisions to ingest are made in the context of both physiological and environmental factors, such as current satiety level and food availability. The use of palatability as an independent variable in animal studies must take these factors into consideration, but they are experimentally separable. Such separation can be used, for example, to analyze the mechanisms underlying the effect of pharmacological agents on food consumption.

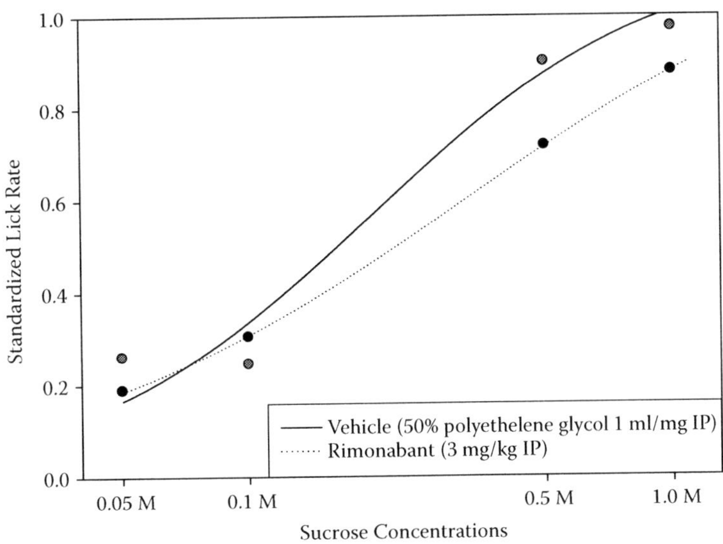

FIGURE 3.2 Effect of Rimonabant administration in male Sprague-Dawley rats on lick rate of sucrose solutions in brief access (6 second) trials. Solutions were presented repeatedly in random order through a 45-minute session. Standardized lick rate is the ratio of number of licks of a commodity compared to the number of licks to water while water deprived; this measure is used to standardize differences in lick rates among rats. Rimonabant shifted the curve to the right, suggesting a decrease in avidity for licking to sweet solutions. (Mathes and Rowland, unpublished data, 2005.) We thank Dr. Alan Spector for use of the "Davis rig" apparatus.

3.7.1.1 Endocannabinoids

Compounds that interfere with normal endocannabinoid function decrease food intake, in particular consumption of sweet and fatty food, and are thought to do so by modulating the evaluation of the palatability of food.[38–40] However, previous work addressing this hypothesis has not excluded postingestional factors or assessed the effect of these agents on food choice.

Brief-access tests assess proclivity toward a range of taste concentrations while excluding satiety factors by keeping actual ingestion at a minimum. Using an apparatus known as the Davis rig,[41] we repeatedly presented rats a range of sucrose solutions (0.05, 0.1, 0.5, and 1.0 *M*), each available in random order in 6-second trials for a total 45-minute session. After baseline performance was evaluated, rats were injected with either the cannabinoid CB1 receptor inverse agonist Rimonabant (SR141716, 3 mg/kg i.p.) or its vehicle. Rimonabant produced a concentration-dependent rightward shift of avidity of licking to the sucrose solutions (Figure 3.2). This suggests that a decrease of central endocannabinoid function reduces the hedonic evaluation of sweet independent of satiety factors and without effect on maximal lick rates. Rats administered Rimonabant treated higher concentrations of sucrose as though they were lower. Whether this occurs at the level of taste transduction or centrally in the context of appetitive motivation remains an important factor to be explored.

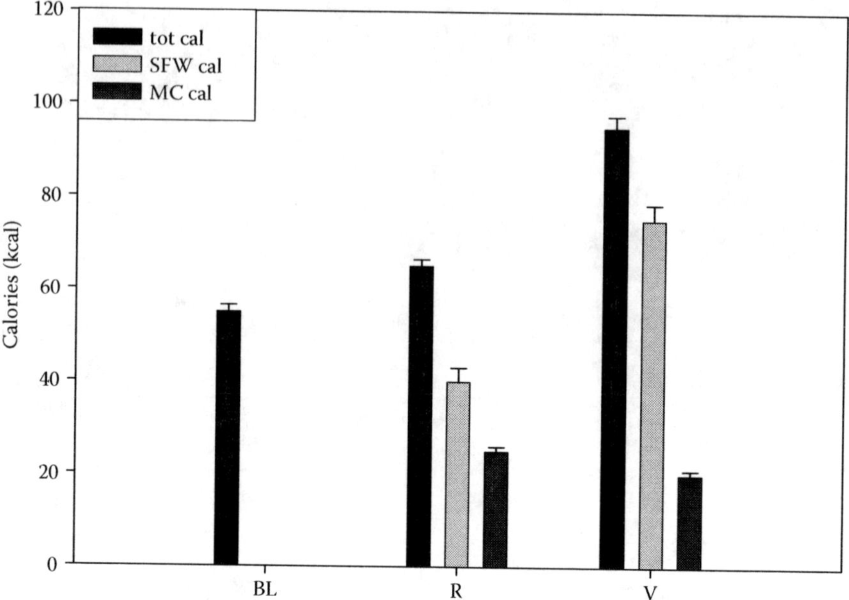

FIGURE 3.3 Mean effect of 1 week Rimonabant (R, 1 mg/kg i.p.) or vehicle (V, 50% polyethylene glycol 1 mg/ml) administration in female rats on 24-h total caloric intake from moist chow (MC) and sugar fat whip (SFW) compared to baseline (BL, MC only). Rimonabant reduced total caloric intake by reducing preference for SFW without affecting MC intake. (Mathes et al., unpublished data, 2006.)

It is also important to assess the palatability-modulating effect of drugs such as Rimonabant within a real-world situation that presents an array of food choices. Administration of Rimonabant has been shown to reduce consumption of high-fat and high-sugar diets,[42] but preference assessments have not been reported previously. Using a dessert protocol that promotes overconsumption and weight gain in rats, we have recently evaluated the effect of Rimonabant on choice between a maintenance diet (moist chow; 1:1 Purina 5001 and tap water; 1.67 kcal/g) and a palatable high-caloric-density dessert (sugar fat whip; 2:1 vegetable shortening and white table sugar; 7.35 kcal/g). Rimonabant (1 mg/kg) or vehicle was administered 30 minutes prior to each daily presentation of fresh chow and sugar fat whip. Total caloric intake was measured for 1 week. Rimonabant treatment produced a transient decrease in total caloric intake (Figure 3.3). This decrease was due entirely to a reduction in intake of sugar fat whip; calories consumed from moist chow were similar between the groups. This result suggests that Rimonabant selectively decreases intake of palatable foods. However, our data also indicate that some tolerance to this effect develops within 1 week, questioning the long-term efficacy of this intake-suppressing agent.

3.7.2 Availability

In the past century, advances in food technology have made a variety of safe foods readily available. This contrasts with the feast or famine environment(s) that humans have endured in evolutionary time that would have promoted higher inclusive fitness of individuals who were able to consume large amounts when available — *viz* opportunists. Opportunism is now a disadvantage in a society that includes ubiquitous vending machines and fast food restaurants with low-cost menus. The economics of access to calorically dense food leading to overconsumption and patterns of restriction and bingeing have been suggested to be primary culprits in the obesity epidemic[43] and are important factors to emulate in animal models.

There are two facets of availability — spatial and temporal — that are ecologically intertwined and yet experimentally separable. Spatial availability is defined as amount of food available per unit area, including number of food patches in a territory as well as the density of food within a patch. Temporal availability refers to the amount of food available per unit time and, in particular, when patches become available only at certain times. The studies to be discussed in the following sections illustrate these factors under free-food *ad libitum* access conditions (cf. Figure 3.1) that we posit lead to hedonic-based eating.

3.7.2.1 Spatial Density

Tordoff[44] used the term *obesity by choice* to describe a protocol in which rats had 24-hour access, in addition to standard chow, to either one or more bottles of sucrose solution and water. Rats given a high ratio of sucrose to water bottles consumed more sucrose than those rats given a low ratio of sucrose to water bottles. This suggests that preference as measured in this protocol was a function of the probability that an encountered drinking spout would contain sucrose rather than water.

We adapted this protocol to solid foods by examining the effect of spatial availability of a high-fat food on total caloric intake. Rats were housed in rectangular polycarbonate cages fitted with a food jar in either one or all four corners. The jars contained either powdered standard chow (Purina 5001; 3.34 kcal/g) or a high-fat diet (2:1 Purina chow and vegetable shortening; 5.23 kcal/g). In contrast to Tordoff's findings with sucrose solutions, all groups consumed equivalent total calories regardless of diet or spatial availability (Figure 3.4), showing that under these conditions caloric homeostasis prevailed over any effect of spatial density. The impact of spatial availability on choice of different diets and/or consumption of an optional high calorie source (i.e., desserts such as sugar fat whip) remains to be evaluated.

3.7.2.2 Temporal Density and Binging

To evaluate the effect of temporal availability, we examined whether repeated introduction of a palatable dessert would stimulate intake to a greater extent than continuous access to the same diet. Rats were presented moist chow (used in lieu of dry chow to minimize spillage). One group additionally received a sweet gel (6% sugar solution solidified with 5% gelatin; 0.34 kcal/g) and another group received the sugar fat whip (7.35 kcal/g) described earlier. The desserts were available either for uninterrupted sessions, consisting of 8 straight nocturnal hours, or for intermittent sessions, consisting of four 30-minute periods every 2 hours over the same 8-hour nocturnal period. The hypothesis was that each introduction of food would signal a new dessert opportunity and so increase total intake. The results refuted this

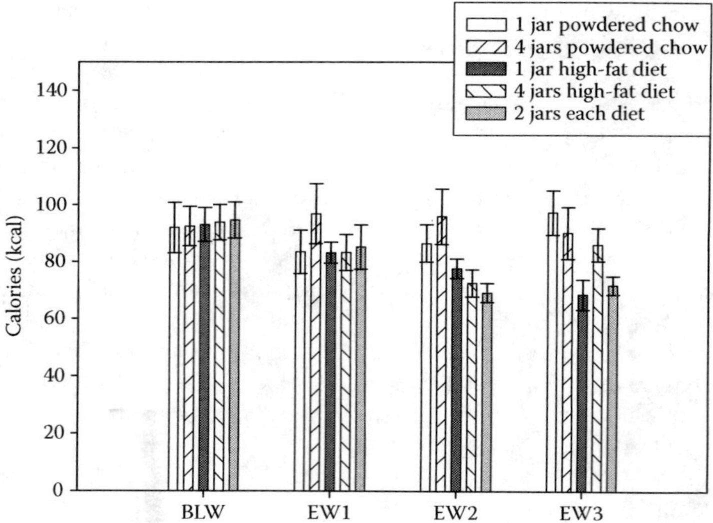

FIGURE 3.4 Mean effect of spatial availability of two diet types on 24-hour caloric intake in rats. Retired breeder Sprague-Dawley female rats were housed in standard cages with either one or four food jars, containing either high-fat diet or powdered chow, present *ad libitum*. One group had two jars of each diet. Mean intakes are averaged for each group over a 1-week baseline (chow only, BLW) period, and three consecutive 1-week test periods (EW1,2,3). There were no significant group differences in caloric intake. (Mathes, unpublished Masters thesis, 2003.)

hypothesis, because rats given uninterrupted access consumed the same or slightly more dessert than those given intermittent access (Figure 3.5). The total caloric intake was higher in those rats given the high-caloric-density sugar fat whip than either the low-calorie gel dessert group or a chow-only control group. However, the total time available for consumption (2 versus 8 hours) did not have an effect on dessert intake in this protocol.

Other protocols of binge-like eating have been successful in showing a short-term effect of availability on food intake. Corwin and colleagues have established a protocol in which presentation of vegetable shortening to young female rats for a 2-hour session every other day increases consumption of shortening compared to rats given 2-hour access to shortening everyday.[45] However, this protocol does not support large increases in daily caloric intake or body weight gain and so does not directly address the issue of overconsumption. To assess the generality of these findings, and whether we can produce overconsumption, we have modified this protocol to use sugar fat whip. Our preliminary results suggest that young female rats show a binge-like pattern, but that older females do not. It is important to evaluate more completely the conditions under which this opportunity-based eating occurs and either does or does not lead to sustained weight gain.

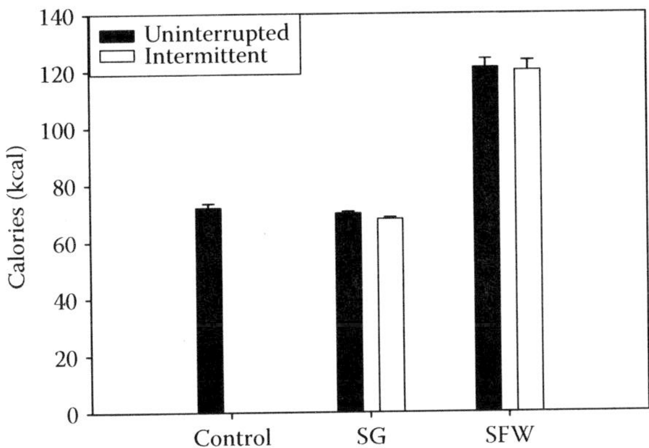

FIGURE 3.5 Mean effect of either uninterrupted (8 hours nocturnally) or intermittent (4 × 30 minutes at 2-hour intervals) presentation of either no dessert (control), sugar gel (SG), or sugar fat whip (SFW) on total 24-hour caloric intake (moist chow plus dessert) in retired breeder female Sprague-Dawley rats across 1 week of study. Intakes of the SFW groups differed from ND and SG, but there was no effect of presentation style (uninterrupted versus intermittent). (Mathes, unpublished data, 2004.)

3.8 CONCLUSIONS

Although feeding is a necessary behavior to sustain life, physiological need is sufficient but not necessary to initiate feeding. The probability of appetitive and consummatory behaviors is based on opportunities presented within the environment interacting with the short- and long-term physiological events that underlie motivation and homeostasis. Experimental protocols involving animals must be aware of the distinctions between deficiency-based and hedonic eating and identify dependent measures appropriate to the part of the appetitive and consummatory behavior sequence that they address. The reductionist approach has led to many animal studies that analyze these aspects in simple environments.

Humans do not live in simple laboratory environments, but do display the same patterns associated with feeding as seen in rodent models. These patterns are experimentally separable. At the level of remote foraging, studies of food shopping patterns, especially in relation to physiological parameters such as BMI and socioeconomic context, would be of relevance. At a more analytical level, studying the impact of economic (price, availability) manipulations on that shopping behavior would be relevant. At the proximate level, how people actually eat at home or in social settings and factors that affect this behavior are of relevance. Studies of effects of portion size on intake, essentially absent in much of the rodent work discussed above, are clearly relevant in humans. Studies of food opportunities and especially snacks on consumption also are amenable to analysis. Since self reports, including food diaries, are not uniformly reliable, residential laboratory work may be the most useful avenue of study. Elements of feeding behavior can be elucidated in rodent models, but the holistic picture must be established in long-term, carefully monitored human studies.

REFERENCES

1. Craig, W., Appetites and aversions as constituents of instincts, *Biol. Bull.*, 34, 91, 1918.
2. Grill, H.J. and Norgren, R., The taste reactivity test. I. Mimetic responses to gustatory stimuli in neurologically normal rats, *Brain Res.*, 143, 263, 1978.
3. Bolles, R.C., *Theory of Motivation,* Harper & Row, New York, 1967.
4. Epstein, A.N., Instinct and motivation as explanations for complex behavior, in *The Physiological Mechanisms of Motivation,* Pfaff, D.W., Ed., Springer-Verlag, New York, 1982, p. 25.
5. Laraway, S. et al., Motivating operations and terms to describe them — some further refinements, *JABA,* 36, 407, 2003.
6. Cannon, W.B., Organization for physiological homeostasis, *Physiol. Rev.*, 9, 399, 1929.
7. Carpenter, R.H., Homeostasis: a plea for a unified approach, *Adv. Physiol. Educ.*, 28, 180, 2004.
8. Mrosovsky, N., *Rheostasis: The Physiology of Change,* Oxford University Press, New York, 1990.
9. Toates, F.M., The control of ingestive behaviour by internal and external stimuli — a theoretical review, *Appetite,* 2, 35, 1981.
10. Irani, B.G. and Haskell-Luevano, C., Feeding effects of melanocortin ligands — a historical perspective, *Peptides,* 26, 1788, 2005.
11. Schoener, T.W., Theory of feeding strategies, *Annu. Rev. Ecol. System,* 2, 307, 1971.
12. Houston, A.I. and McNamara, J.M., The value of food: effects of open and closed economies, *Anim. Behav.,* 37, 546, 1989.
13. Miller, N.E., Experiments on motivation. Studies combining psychological, physiological, and pharmacological techniques, *Science,* 126, 1271, 1957.
14. Collier, G.C., Hirsch, E., and Hamlin, P.H., The ecological determinants of reinforcement in the rat, *Physiol. Behav.,* 9, 705, 1972.
15. Vaughan, C.H. and Rowland, N.E., Meal patterns of lean and leptin-deficient obese mice in a simulated foraging environment, *Physiol. Behav.*, 79, 275, 2003.
16. Vaughan, C.H., et al., Meal patterns and foraging in melanocortin receptor knockout mice, *Physiol. Behav.*, 84, 129, 2005.
17. Vaughan, C., et al., Food motivated behavior of melanocortin-4 receptor knockout mice under a progressive ratio schedule, *Peptides,* 27, 2829, 2006.
18. Stafford, D., LeSage, M.G., and Glowa, J. R., Progressive-ratio schedules of drug delivery in the analysis of drug self-administration, *Psychopharmacolgy (Berl.),* 139, 169, 1998.
19. Bauman, R., An experimental analysis of the cost of food in a closed economy, *J. Exp. Anal. Behav.,* 56, 33, 1991.
20. Hursh, S.R., Economic concepts for the analysis of behavior, *J. Exp. Anal. Behav.*, 34, 219, 1980.
21. Bartness, T.J. and Day, D.E., Food hoarding: a quintessentially anticipatory appetitive behavior, in *Progress in Psychobiology and Physiological Psychology,* Fluharty S.J. and Grill H.J., Eds., Academic Press, New York, 2003, p. 69.
22. Daniels, D. and Fluharty, S.J., Salt appetite: a neurohormonal viewpoint, *Physiol. Behav.,* 81, 319, 2004.
23. Bachmanov, A.A., Beauchamp, G.K., and Tordoff, M.G., Voluntary consumption of NaCl, KCl, and NH_4CL solutions by 28 mouse strains, *Behav. Genet.,* 32, 445, 2002.
24. Fregly, M.J. and Rowland, N.E., Role of renin-angiotensin- aldosterone system in NaCl appetite of rats, *Am. J. Physiol. Regul. Integr. Comp. Physiol.,* 248, R1, 1985.
25. Denton, D.A., *The Hunger for Salt: An Anthropological, Physiological, and Medical Analysis,* Springer-Verlag, New York, 1982.
26. Jalowiec, J.E., Sodium appetite elicited by furosemide: effects of differential dietary maintenance, *Behav. Biol.,* 10, 313, 1974.

27. Colbert, C.L. and Rowland, N.E., Sodium preference and appetite in rats in an operant protocol, *Physiol. Behav.,* 83, 715, 2005.
28. McCutcheon, B. and Levy, C., Relationship between NaCl rewarded bar-pressing and duration of sodium deficiency, *Physiol. Behav.,* 8, 761, 1972.
29. Berridge, K.C., et al., Sodium depletion enhances salt palatability in rats, *Behav. Neurosci.,* 98, 652, 1984.
30. Nachman, M. and Valentino, D., Roles of taste and postingestional factors in the satiation of sodium appetite in rats, *J. Comp. Physiol. Psychol.,* 62, 280, 1966.
31. Garcia, J., Hankins, W.G., and Rusiniak, K.W., Behavioral regulation of the milieu interne in man and rat, *Science,* 185, 824, 1974.
32. Elizade, G. and Sclafani, A., Flavor preferences conditioned by intragastric polycose infusions: a detailed analysis using an electronic esophagus preparation, *Physiol. Behav.,* 47, 63, 1990.
33. Rowland, N.E. and Morian, K.R., Roles of aldosterone and angiotensin in maturation of sodium appetite in furosemide-treated rats, *Am. J. Physiol. Reg. Int. Comp. Physiol.,* 276, R1453, 1999.
34. Starr, L.J. and Rowland, N.E., Characteristics of salt appetite in chronically sodium-depleted rats using a progressive ratio schedule of procurement, *Physiol. Behav.,* 88, 433, 2006.
35. Berridge, K.C., Pleasures of the brain, *Brain Cogn.,* 52, 106, 2003.
36. Cooper, S.J., Endocannabinoids and food consumption: comparisons with benzodiazepine and opioid palatability-dependent appetite, *Eur. J. Pharmacol.,* 500, 37, 2004.
37. Corwin, R.L. and Hajnal, A., Too much of a good thing: neurobiology of non-homeostatic eating and drug abuse, *Physiol. Behav.,* 86, 5, 2005.
38. Miller, C.C. et al., Cannabinoid agonist, CP 55,940, facilitates intake of palatable foods when injected into the hindbrain, *Physiol. Behav.,* 80, 611, 2004.
39. Higgs, S., Williams, C.M., and Kirkham, T.C., Cannabinoid influences on palatability: microstructural analysis of sucrose drinking after delta-9-tetrahydrocanabinol, anadamide, 2-arachidonoyl glycerol, and SR141716, *Psychopharmacology,* 165, 370, 2003.
40. Koch, J.E., Delta(9)-THC stimulates food intake in Lewis rats: effects on chow, high fat, and sweet high fat diets, *Pharmacol. Biochem. Behav.,* 68, 539, 2001.
41. Spector, A.C. and Smith, J.C., A detailed analysis of sucrose drinking in the rat, *Physiol. Behav.,* 33, 127, 1984.
42. Verty, A.N., McGregor, I.S., and Mallet, P.E., Consumption of high carbohydrate, high fat, and normal chow is equally suppressed by a cannabinoid antagonist in non-deprived rats, *Neurosci. Lett.,* 354, 217, 2004.
43. Drewnowski, A., Obesity and the food environment: dietary energy density and diet costs, *Am. J. Prev. Med.,* 27, 154, 2004.
44. Tordoff, M.G., Obesity by choice: the powerful influence of nutrient availability on nutrient intake, *Am. J. Physiol. Regul. Integr. Comp. Physiol.,* 282, R1536, 2002.
45. Dimitriou, S.G., Rice, H.B., and Corwin, R.L., Effects of limited access to a fat option on food intake and body composition in female rats, *Int. J. Eat. Disord.,* 28, 436, 2000.

4 Appetite and Food Intake: A Human Experimental Perspective

Martin R. Yeomans and Emma J. Bertenshaw

CONTENTS

4.1 INTRODUCTION

Our experience of appetite is an essential element of our conscious experience: As humans, we frequently assess our current appetitive state, and feelings of hunger and cravings for food can interfere with our ability to conduct other tasks. However, the relationship between the experience of appetite and our actual eating behavior remains less clear. Although some progress has been made by assessing this relationship based on diary records of people eating in their normal environment,[1] this type of study lacks the degree of control over behavior needed to be able to assess causal relationships. An alternative approach has been to study in detail eating behavior under controlled laboratory conditions, and this chapter reviews what such studies have told us about the relationship between appetite and food intake.

4.2 DEFINING APPETITE

Appetite is defined in terms of a strong urge or desire for something, in the present context a desire to eat food. Appetite can also be used to denote a more specific desire for a set of nutrients (for example, sodium appetite to describe increased acceptance of sodium chloride) and is often associated with the idea of urges and cravings for food. However, the relationship between the terms appetite, hunger, and food craving remains poorly defined, and in order to clarify the use of these terms in this chapter some discussion of the nature of these terms is needed. Most confusion comes from two common uses of the term hunger: on one hand, the subjective experience of hunger (indexed by hunger ratings, discussed later in this chapter) is interpreted as an indication of the current desire to eat. Yet hunger has also been used historically to describe a specific set of physiological processes which increase the likelihood of feeding, most classically with the idea of a specific hunger center in the brain.[2] The term *appetite* is broader than either of these uses of the term *hunger*, and while many researchers use ratings of hunger to assess appetite, there remains sufficient distinction between the meaning of the terms hunger and appetite to warrant their continued use. In this chapter, appetite is used to mean the immediate desire to eat, and hunger state to mean the current subjective experience of appetite.

4.3 ASSESSING SUBJECTIVE APPETITE

Experimental studies which explore the relationship between appetite and eating in humans make widespread use of our ability to introspect and so give some expression of our current motivational state, through the use of appetite ratings. The earliest studies tended to use categorical, or Likert, scales, with discrete numbers representing different levels of the relevant experience (Figure 4.1a). These scales have largely been replaced by visual analogue, or line-scales, (VAS) (Figure 4.1b), where experience is rated on a continuous dimension between two extreme possibilities. A more recent approach (the affective generalized labeled magnitude scale, AgLMS) (Figure 4.1c), developed from the gLMS used widely to assess sensory evaluations,[3] recognizes that such ratings may not be truly linear, and that contrasts of ratings between participants may be confounded by different interpretations of the anchors of unlabeled VAS. To get around this, the AgLMS consists of a forced choice of like or dislike, followed by a rating of the strength of liking/disliking on a continuous scale but with clearer definition of the levels of liking at each level of motivation. Although the gLMS has clear advantages when measuring sensory evaluations,[3] whether the AgLMS approach has true advantages over the VAS scale remains unclear, and the VAS remains the most widely used method for measuring our experience of appetite.

It has been suggested that appetite, hunger, and fullness ratings may all measure a single motivational variable, desire to eat.[4] This approach makes scientific sense unless there are clear experimental findings which dissociate these ratings. Indeed, in the case of hunger and fullness ratings, it is clear that gross patterns of change in hunger and fullness tend to mirror each other. However, there are subtle differences in the way these ratings change within an eating episode that suggest that participants

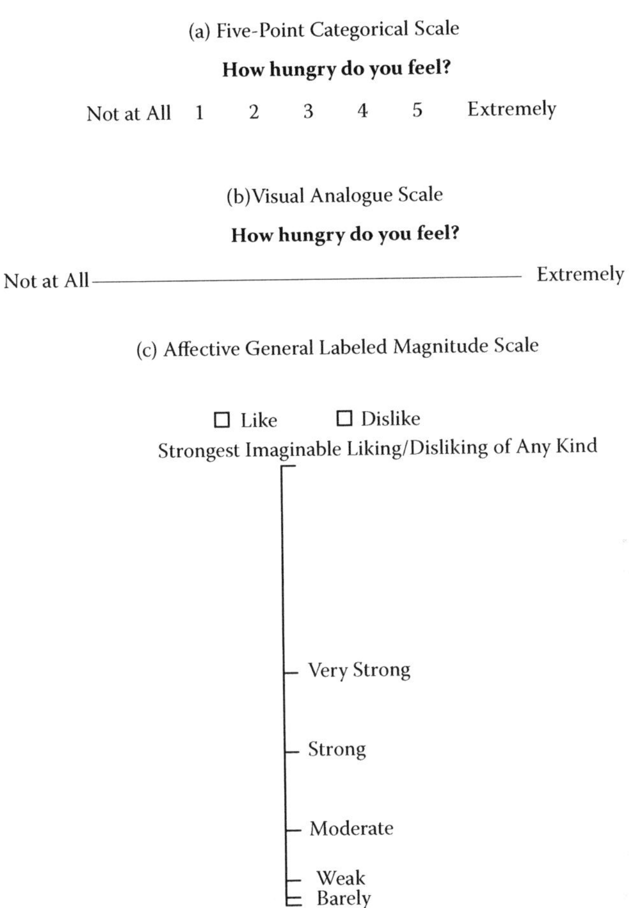

FIGURE 4.1 Different scales used to assess subjective appetite.

can reliably distinguish between feelings of fullness (reflecting the amount of food consumed) and feelings of hunger (the desire to eat more), suggesting that hunger and fullness are to some extent dissociable. Perhaps the clearest dissociation between hunger and fullness comes from studies of the effects of gastric distension. For example, increasing gastric distension using a barostat reliably increased ratings of fullness, but did not impact on ratings of hunger.[5] Likewise, infusion of the gastric hormone cholecystokinin (CCK) reduced rated fullness but did not reliably alter rated hunger,[6] although the combination of CCK and gastric distension reduced both hunger and fullness. Along with other findings, these data suggest that people can distinguish between feelings associated with a full gut (fullness) and a desire to eat (hunger). These findings also invalidate experimental approaches based on rating scales which treat appetite as a linear scale between "extremely full" and "extremely hungry."[7]

The most sensitive way to explore the relationship between appetite and food intake in the human experimental laboratory is to explore changes in the experience of appetite as a function of periods with and without eating. The rate at which hunger is reinstated after a set meal may thus be a useful measure of the degree to which the consumed food generated satiety, and so offers a tool to explore the nature of satiety itself. In contrast, changes in rated appetite within a meal facilitate exploration of how different processes stimulated by the ingested food (sensory effects, learning, and postingestive nutrients) interact to generate appetite and so determine meal size. The approach of collecting appetite ratings within a meal[8] was built on a broader approach to the microstructural analysis of eating as a tool to explore the nature of appetite control in humans,[9] which in turn was developed from pioneering work on analyses of meal patterns in rodents.[10,11] In all studies of eating, the ultimate variable common to studies in humans and other animals is the amount consumed, both in terms of mass and energy. However, when trying to understand the interrelationship between appetite and ingestion, subtle differences in the way food is consumed have proved valuable in experimental studies with animals and humans.[9–14] Thus the rate at which eating progresses, the overall duration of a meal, bite-rate, etc. may all give clues about the nature of appetite associated with that eating episode. Even more information becomes available if ratings of appetite are included progressively across the meal and are then related to the amount consumed. Such analyses have shed light on many aspects of appetite, including the effects of palatability,[15,16] the effects of satiation and satiety on appetite in a meal,[17–20] and disturbances in appetite in anorexia, bulimia, and binge-eating disorder.[21–25] Adding measures beyond simple intake thus provide important insights into the fundamental processes underlying appetite control and how these may be disturbed to allow overeating or anorexic behavior.

4.4 THEORETICAL FRAMEWORK FOR EXPLORING CONTROLS OF MEAL SIZE

Figure 4.2 shows three alternative conceptual models of the relationship between the experience of appetite and food intake within a meal. All three models make a distinction between appetite prior to the onset of eating (classically thought of as the appetitive phase) and appetite within the meal (the consummatory phase). All three models interpret appetite prior to a feeding episode in the same way, with a progressive increase in appetite during the interval between meals, since it is clear that the experience of "hunger" increases progressively during the time since the last time food was ingested, and as the likelihood of eating again increases. Although for simplicity this increase is illustrated as linear, actual changes vary depending on a multitude of both internal and external appetite signals. Thus, although the classic homeostatic interpretation of these changes is in terms of physiological hunger cues arising from internal signals related to the use of ingested nutrients, it is also clear that temporal and social cues may enhance appetite as well. Regardless of the underlying nature of premeal hunger, a clear prediction is that the experience of appetite at the onset of eating should influence meal size.

The main purpose of the models outlined in Figure 4.2 is to illustrate alternative accounts of how appetite might change once eating has started, and it is this feature of appetite which is the primary focus of this chapter. The first two models are based on homeostatic principles that appetite will decline as food in ingested,

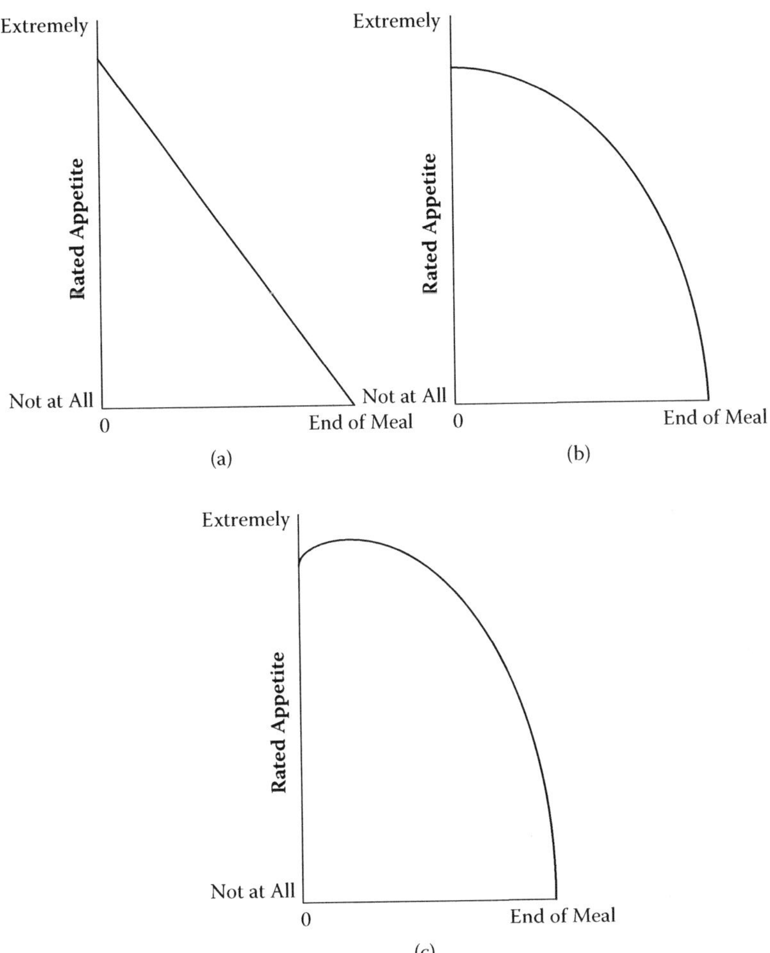

FIGURE 4.2 Three alternative models of appetite change during a meal based on (a) appetite decreasing as a linear function of food consumed, (b) a progressive increase in satiation across the meal, and (c) an integration of orosensory positive feedback and satiation.

with the simplest model suggesting that this decrease will be a linear function of food ingested, and the second model suggesting that the impact of satiation on appetite will be progressive. Thus, just as use of nutrients may lead to the onset of eating, so according to homeostatic principles, the cessation of eating should be predicted by the ingestion of sufficient nutrients to restore nutritional deficit. The predicted relationship between the experience of appetite and food intake is therefore a progressive increase in appetite during the interval between meals, and then a progressive decrease in appetite during a meal as a consequence of satiation based on two negative feedback systems.

The major problem with a purely homeostatic account of meal size is that it offers no explanation for sensory influences. Thus according to the approach outlined in the first two models, provided the nutrient content of the food being ingested is the same, meal size should be the same regardless of whether the food has a pleasant or unpleasant taste. Yet it is clear that hedonic evaluation has a major impact on meal size. The third model offers a conceptual framework through which to understand how this could arise. The key difference is the inclusion of a positive feedback element arising from the hedonic evaluation of the ingested food which interacts with the negative feedback elements of satiation to determine overall meal size.

The framework outlined in Figure 4.2 allows explicit tests of the nature of the relationship between appetite and eating, and laboratory-based studies in humans provide overwhelming evidence in favor of a model integrating positive and negative feedback processes arising from hedonic evaluation of the food on one hand, and satiating effects of the food on the other. The rest of this chapter examines the evidence behind this conclusion, and explores other influences on meal size which help us understand the nature of these feedback mechanisms.

4.5 DOES HUNGER PREDICT INTAKE? RELATIONSHIPS BETWEEN APPETITE AND MEAL SIZE

If the experience of appetite, indexed by hunger ratings, represents motivation to eat, then it is apparent that rated hunger at the start of a meal should predict meal size. In practice this relationship has proved to be less clear. Some data are clearly consistent with the idea that the subjective experience of hunger prior to a meal is a reliable predictor of meal size. For example, analysis of self-reported amount consumed at spontaneous meals recorded using extended diet diaries reported a correlation between rated hunger beforehand and the size of the meal.[26] Not all such studies based on diary-based reports find these effects, however.[27] It may be that the habitual nature of the timing of meals in real life may mask any underlying relationship between the experience of appetite and intake. For example, hunger cued by the expectation of meals at a fixed time, or facilitated by social interaction, may result in people either eating when rated hunger is low, or experiencing transient, cued feelings of hunger when food in unavailable.

One way of exploring the relationship between rated appetite and intake in the laboratory is to examine the relationship between rated appetite and intake in acute tests of intake following manipulations that should enhance or decrease appetite. One of the simplest approaches is to examine effects of presatiation through consumption of a disguised high-energy preload prior to the test meal. This approach does lend some support to the hypothesis that intake can be predicted by rated hunger, since disguised high-energy preloads can reduce both rated hunger at the onset of eating and subsequent test meal intake.[19,28] Moreover, some studies have found significant correlations between pre-*ad libitum* test meal motivational ratings and subsequent intake.[29,30] However, not all studies find such effects. Some preload studies report reduced intake in the absence of changes in hunger after loads differing in energy[31] or nutrient content,[32,33] while others report that higher energy loads[34–36] or higher preload protein content[37–39] reduced hunger without leading to subsequent intake adjustment.

Why then might hunger at the start of a meal be an unreliable predictor of intake in some preload studies? There are many potential explanations for these differences, some relating to methodological shortcomings (for example, use of insensitive rating scales or underpowered studies), but others relating to the nature of the eating experience. For example, it is well known that variety enhances intake.[40–44] Notably, several preload studies which employed a buffet-style meal as the intake test found reduced premeal hunger but no effect on intake.[34,36,37] The explanation could be that preload energy and/or nutrient content reduced appetite, but this effect was then masked by stimulation of appetite by variety. Furthermore, those studies cited above finding differences in subsequent intake, but not hunger, used a homogenous test meal.[32,33] A further issue relates to the degree to which test-meal intake may be influenced by habitual behaviors, such as participants consuming all of a set serving, so masking any effects of the test preload manipulation.

Another crucial factor influencing the relationship between rated appetite and intake may be the timing of the appetite evaluations. It may be that people are unable to truly judge their level of appetite until the appropriate food cues are present, and variability in the timing of ratings and presence of food cues across studies then determine whether a clear relationship is found or not. If our experience of hunger reflects an integration of internal cues predicting energy need derived from homeostatic processes with expectations of food availability or hedonic quality, then ratings of hunger made in the absence of knowledge of available food is likely to be a poor predictor of intake. To test this, we reanalyzed data from studies in our laboratory where hunger ratings were made before food was presented, once food was tasted, and throughout the test meal to test which rating was the best predictor of intake. This reanalysis suggested that the strongest predictor of intake was the hunger rating made immediately after the food to be consumed had been tasted (Table 4.1). This reanalysis confirms that differences in the timing of ratings of appetite relative to food presentation may have contributed to the inconsistency in the literature on whether appetite ratings predict subsequent intake. These data also imply that our experience of appetite requires integration of our appetitive state at the onset of eating with the

TABLE 4.1
Correlations between Rated Hunger at Various Stages of a Meal and Meal Size

	Pearson R[a] for Correlation between Meal Intake and:		
Data Source	**Premeal Hunger[b]**	**Hunger after Tasting[b]**	**Maximum Hunger[b]**
19	0.42	0.57[c]	0.52[c]
20	0.53[c]	0.65[c]	0.58[c]
17	0.27[d]	0.51[c]	0.45[d]
18	0.31[d]	0.48[c]	0.42[d]

[a] The data are partial correlations between rated hunger and intake, accounting for differences in experimental conditions in each study.

[b] "Premeal hunger" was rated in the absence of food cues, "Hunger after tasting" following consumption of a mouthful of the food to be eaten, and "Maximum hunger" was the highest rating made at any stage during the eating episode.

[c] $P < 0.001$.

[d] $p < 0.01$.

immediate sensory experience of the food to be ingested. The next section therefore evaluates how sensory qualities may impact on the expression of hunger.

4.6 UNDERSTANDING POSITIVE FEEDBACK STIMULATION OF EATING

> Appetite comes with eating; the more one has, the more one would have. (French Proverb)

The origins of this classic French proverb remain obscure, but the general implication, that the more you eat the greater your appetite, goes against the basic principle of homeostatic control. However, there is now substantial evidence that eating foods which are palatable, that is those which are rated as pleasant tasting, results in marked increases in meal size. These effects are equally evident in human and animal studies. Giving rats access to a diet which is rich in fat, sugar, or both reliably leads to overeating and consequent obesity.[45,46] Since sweetness is innately preferred and results in positive hedonic responses in rats based on judgments of orofacial responses to the sweet taste,[12] we can infer that the positive hedonic response to sweetness is the primary cause of increased intake. Sated rats also eat little of an unpreferred food (such as their normal laboratory chow) but consume significant quantities of a preferred food such as sucrose or cookies. Manipulated palatability has similar effects on short-term eating in humans.[47,48] The most widely used technique is to modify the flavor of a test food to make it more or less palatable, while leaving the nutritional components unaltered, and then to measure subsequent intake and the experience of appetite. The consistent finding is that volunteers consume more when food is rated as palatable.[15,16,49–60] Analysis of the relationship between the relative difference in liking and consequent change in intake (Figure 4.3) shows a clear linear relationship. This consistency is all the more remarkable considering that these data encompass a wide variety of foods consumed by different participants

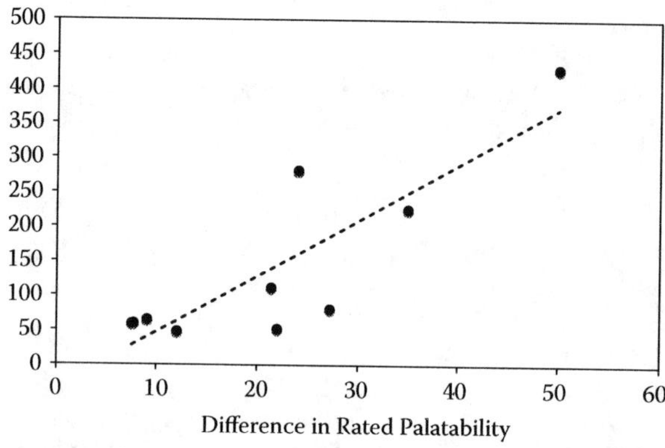

FIGURE 4.3 The relationship between differences in food pleasantness and consequent increases in food intake in humans. (Adapted from Yeomans, M.R., in *Appetite and Body Weight: Integrative systems and the Development of Anti-Obesity Drugs,* Cooper, S.J. and Kirkham, T.C., Eds., Elsevier, London, 2007, pp. 247–269. With permission.)

in a number of laboratories. Effects of palatability on meal size are also evident in diary-based data where, even though people generally do not self-select items they rate as unpalatable, hedonic ratings of the meal they consumed are a consistent predictor of meal size and operate independently of hunger.[61,62] The implication of the predictability of the effects of palatability on intake is that these effects reflect a set of processes that are sensitive to hedonic evaluation of the sensory qualities of food but are relatively insensitive to the actual sensory qualities or nutritional composition of the ingested food.

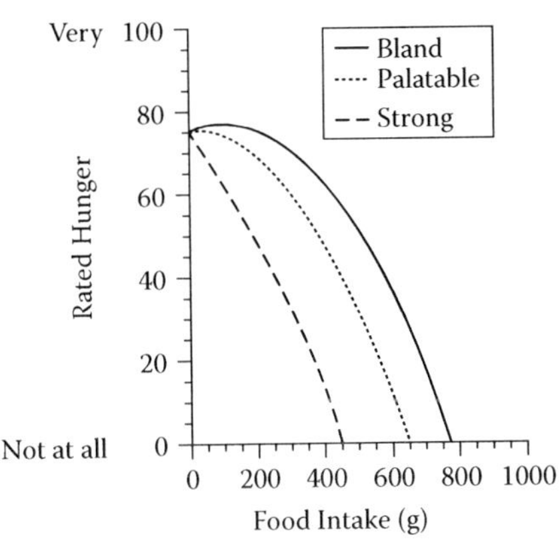

FIGURE 4.4 Effects of manipulated palatability on the experience of appetite during a meal. (Adapted from Yeomans, M.R., *Appetite,* 1996, 27, 119–133. With permission.)

What then are the processes underlying hedonic stimulation of appetite? The most widely accepted interpretation of the effects of palatability on meal size is that this reflects stimulation of a positive feedback motivational system associated with orosensory reward.[48,63] Several lines of experimental evidence support the idea that palatability stimulates appetite in this way in humans; thus people eat faster,[52,64–66] chew faster,[13,67,68] and eat for longer[15,64,69] when presented with a more palatable food option. Moreover, rated appetite increases in the early stages of meals with a flavored, palatable food relative to a nutrient-matched bland version of the same food (Figure 4.4). All of these data are consistent with the actions of a positive feedback reward system driven by the hedonic evaluation of the sensory qualities of the food being consumed.

As well as clear behavioral evidence that palatability stimulates appetite, laboratory-based experimental studies in humans provide some insights into the neurochemical basis for this effect. Extensive research in animals provides overwhelming evidence for an important role of opioid peptides in hedonic aspects of eating.[70,71] Blockade of opioid receptors using specific receptor antagonists in humans also has effects consistent with the idea that these neurochemicals play a critical role in determining the hedonic response to foods and consequent stimulation of appetite.[72] Thus opioid receptor antagonists reduce the rated pleasantness of a wide variety of foods, while having minimal impact on sensory evaluation, and cause a consistent reduction in short-term food intake. Perhaps the clearest evidence that opioids are involved in the stimulation of appetite by palatability was the finding that opioid blockade reversed the normal increase in rated appetite during the initial phase of a test meal.[73]

More recent attention on the neurobiology of sensory hedonics has examined the role of the cannabinoid system,[71,74,75] where there is now overwhelming evidence that cannabinoids interact with opioid systems in relation to the rewarding effects of food in animals. In humans, despite an anecdotal literature suggesting that marijuana increases appetite, effects of smoked marijuana on appetite in laboratory studies have been variable,[76] with typically only 50% of participants showing enhanced appetite after marijuana. A more detailed evaluation[77] of effects of the active compound in marijuana, tetrahydracannabinol (THC), on appetite found little evidence of acute appetite stimulation, but did find increased daily energy intake following chronic dosing with THC, while an earlier study found consistent increases in intake following oral THC.[78] There is also evidence that dronabinol, an artificial analogue of THC, increases appetite in patients suffering from weight loss and impaired appetite associated with wasting diseases.[79,80] It has also been suggested that the endocannabinoid system may be upregulated in people who are obese,[81] consistent with the idea that overeating and obesity may both represent some degree of heightened sensitivity to palatability.

4.7 NEGATIVE FEEDBACK: THE BASIS OF SATIATION AND SATIETY

If positive feedback stimulated by liked sensory qualities serves to enhance meal size, what factors are involved in the cessation of feeding? It is now recognized that the processes underlying meal termination (satiation) and subsequent suppression of appetite (satiety) are multifaceted and involve a complex integration of cognitive, sensory, postingestive and postabsorptive cues. The sequence of cues remains to be fully clarified, but the satiety cascade model (Figure 4.5)[82] provides a framework through which these effects can be explored. Although a simple model of meal control might suggest that feeding terminates when sufficient nutrients have been ingested to meet nutritional needs, it is clear that the normal rate of eating means that meal termination occurs too early to reflect absorption of the ingested nutrients. This is clear from analysis of meals in experimental studies. Thus, artificially lengthening the duration of a meal should increase postingestive feedback and so lead to reduced meal size. However, artificially lengthening meal duration by introducing pauses in eating was found to increase rather than decrease overall intake in humans,[16] in contradiction to the idea that slowing eating rate may be a useful component of behavioral treatments for overeating.[83] There is some evidence that increasing meal duration can reduce meal size in rats,[84,85] but meal duration has to be doubled before intake is reduced reliably. Further evidence that immediate ingested nutrients

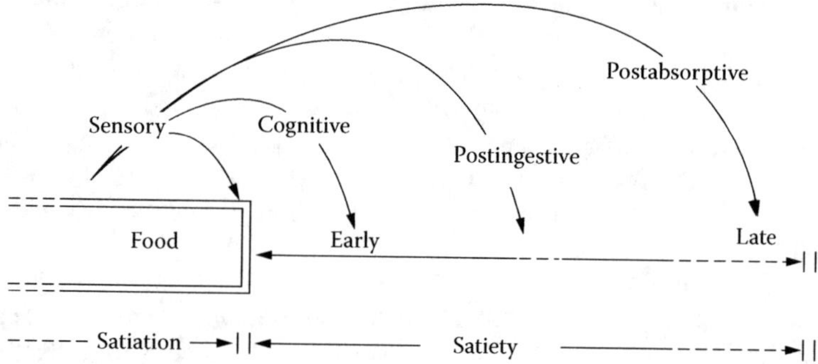

FIGURE 4.5 The satiety cascade. (From Blundell, J.E. and Tremblay, A., *Nutr. Res. Rev.*, 1995, 8, 225–242. With permission.)

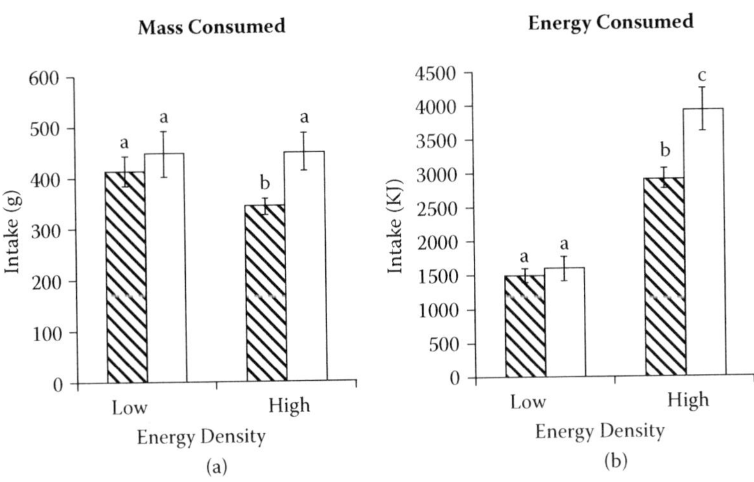

FIGURE 4.6 Total mass (a) and energy (b) consumed of both high- and low-energy-density porridge cereal served both in a bland (\\\) and palatable form (▭). Bars marked by different letters differ significantly ($p < 0.05$ or greater). (Adapted from Yeomans, M.R., Weinberg, L., and James, S., *Physiol. Behav.*, 2005, 86, 487–499. With permission.)

have minimal impact on meal size comes from a study where energy density was increased in a disguised manner.[55] Thus, when presented with a breakfast food (porridge) in bland or palatable form and either with high or low energy density, energy density had no effect on amount consumed, whereas palatability increased meal size (Figure 4.6). Most strikingly, infusion of high or low volumes of a nutritive soup while people were eating had minimal impact on the mass consumed, meaning that energy consumption was nearly doubled when voluntary intake was combined with intragastric infusion of a high volume (450 ml) of an energy-dense soup (Figure 4.7). Thus actual nutrient content of the ingested food appears to have minimal impact on meal termination under laboratory conditions.

So what then determines meal termination? As discussed earlier, reduced appetite at the start of eating tends to reduce meal size. However, a combination of cognitive and sensory factors probably determine the amount consumed once eating has started. It is clear that energy density and portion size are both important determinants of short-term energy intake, and Figure 4.7 is a dramatic indication of how differences in energy density which are hidden from the consumer can greatly affect short-term energy intake. In the majority of laboratory studies discussed so far, portion size was effectively irrelevant, since participants were unable to use the completion of a portion to determine when to stop eating (the protocol ensured either that the amount presented was far in excess of what could be consumed or that food was topped up whenever the portion available fell below a certain level). In real life, however, the amount consumed may be better determined by the amount served rather than how much of that serving is consumed. Larger portion sizes have been shown to result in greater intake,[35,86–89] while other studies confirm that hidden energy can lead to passive overconsumption.[90,91] However, while these data further confirm the lack of physiological control of short-term intake in humans by ingested nutrients,

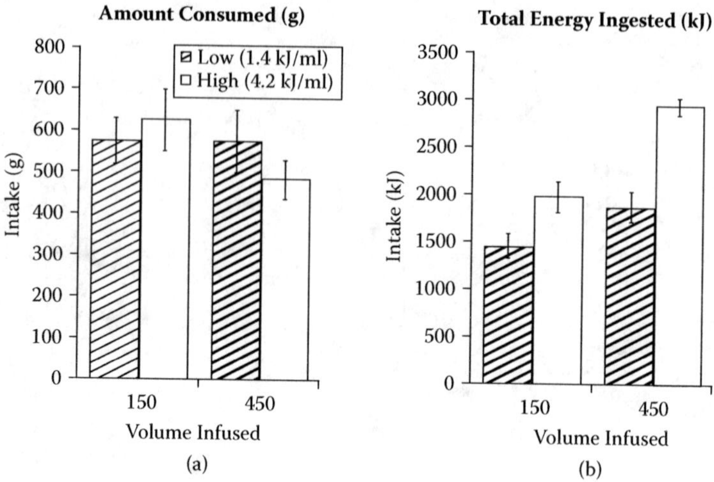

FIGURE 4.7 Total mass (a) and energy (b) consumed of a pasta lunch consumed while receiving an intragastric load of 150 or 450 ml of soup in low- or high-energy-density form. (Robinson, French, Gray, and Yeomans, unpublished data.)

we are far from understanding the nature of the cognitive factors that do determine meal size.

4.8 HOW POSITIVE AND NEGATIVE FEEDBACK INTERACT

As can be seen in Figure 4.6, increasing positive feedback leads to greater intake regardless of the energy content of the food consumed. Indeed, the combined effects of increased palatability and energy density resulted in participants consuming 2.5 times as much in a palatable/high-energy condition than they did in the bland/low-energy condition. The ability of satiety cues generated by high-energy preloads to reduce intake is further compromised by the palatability of the food offered afterwards. Thus participants came close to compensating for the energy in a disguised soup preload when the test lunch was bland, but only reduced intake marginally when the food was more palatable.[20] Similar findings were seen when the premeal preload was infused intragastrically rather than ingested,[57] in line with studies showing that preloads are most effective when ingested orally.[92] These data together imply that positive feedback systems override the negative feedback effects of satiety and satiation and so promote short-term overeating. This has clear implications for understanding the causes of overeating associated with obesity. If, as has been widely suggested,[93–97] our modern diet is more energy dense and palatable, our understanding of control of meal size in humans based on these laboratory studies provides clear evidence that increased availability of palatable foods in our diet will promote overconsumption.

4.9 LEARNING, SENSORY HEDONICS, AND SATIETY

Understanding how differences in palatability enhance intake is important, but begs the question about why some foods are experienced as more palatable than others.

A full discussion of innate and acquired components of hedonic evaluation of flavors is beyond the scope of this chapter and has been the subject of several recent reviews.[98–100] However, some of the key arguments relating to acquired flavor liking are relevant to understanding the relationship between appetite and intake. It is generally accepted that, with the notable exceptions of innate preferences for sweet and salty tastes, the majority of human flavor preferences are acquired. Two learning models highlight important mechanisms by which we acquire liking for novel flavors. The first model suggests that the contingent association between the flavor of a food and the resulting postingestive effects leads to appropriate changes in flavor liking: flavors that predict illness become disliked, while those that predict some form of benefit become liked (flavor-consequence learning). The second model suggests that once a flavor component is liked or disliked, coexperience of a novel flavor component and the liked or disliked flavor results in hedonic transfer between these elements (flavor–flavor learning). These two processes may operate alongside each other; thus consumption of a novel flavored drink sweetened with sucrose could promote an increase in liking by association with sweetness and to associate the flavor with the energy provided by the sucrose. However, recent data[101] suggest that these two types of association differ in terms of their sensitivity to manipulated appetite: pairing a drink flavor with a noncaloric sweetener increases liking for the flavor regardless of whether the association is acquired when hungry or sated. However, increased liking for a sucrose-sweetened drink is greater when trained hungry than sated. The implication is that acquired liking which is reinforced by energy may be controlled by current hunger state, whereas those driven by flavor-based associations may not. This has implications for the overall relationship between appetite, palatability, and intake: the prediction would be that appetitive state will be better able to control meal size where liking has been acquired by flavor-nutrient associations than when based on flavor–flavor associations.

Another learning paradigm that has significance for the relationship between appetite and intake is the concept of learned satiety.[4] According to this idea, associations between the flavor of a food and postingestive effects not only modify liking, but also lead to an acquired ability to control intake in anticipation of the predicted level of postingestive satiety. There is clear evidence for this acquired control of meal size in animal studies,[102,103] but evidence in humans is less convincing.[99] In particular, the widespread finding that increased energy density, which should lead to greater opportunity for learned satiety to develop, leads to increased energy intake[88,90,91,104,105] argues against any strong role of learned satiety in control of normal food intake in humans.

4.10 CONCLUSIONS

Laboratory-based studies of normal eating in humans have greatly increased our understanding of the basic motivational controls of eating in general and the complexity of the relationship between appetite and intake in particular. The idea that our experience of appetite can be used as a proxy measure of intake is clearly an oversimplification, but the detailed analysis of appetite changes in relation to intake has allowed us to start to dissociate the positive and negative feedback systems that control short-term food intake. Future research can build on these findings to better understand the neural processes subserving these motivational systems and thereby gain greater insight into appetite control in general.

4.11 IMPLICATIONS FOR THE DIRECTION OF FUTURE ANIMAL RESEARCH

The current understanding of human appetite outlined in the previous discussion raises many questions, particularly in relation to the interaction of environment, food availability, and motivational state. As outlined in the accompanying chapter by Rowland and Mathes (Chapter 3), the vast majority of studies of feeding in animals concentrate on short-term measures of food intake for rodents in environments with access to a single nutritious but hedonically uninteresting food, and in the absence of more detailed analysis of either appetitive behaviors or the overall pattern of ingestion. However, the current human environment offers unrestricted access to an almost limitless variety of palatable foods, and faced with this diet the incidence of obesity and overweight has increased dramatically. To help understand how the current human environment promotes overconsumption, and to develop treatments that may effectively counter human obesity, there needs to be a shift in emphasis in animal work away from the study of the neural basis of homeostatic controls of feeding to a better understanding of the processes underlying stimulation of appetite through palatability and variety. There have been significant shifts in some recent animal work that have started to address these issues: for example, studies that evaluate how environment-specific associations with food may potentiate short-term feeding,[106,107] the specific development of animal-models of binge-like behavior,[108,109] and the increased cross-talk between animal models of feeding and drug-addiction.[110,111] However, some of these approaches tend to see the effects of reward and pleasure in eating as separate from the traditional homeostatic models that have been the main focus of most recent research on control of ingestion. What perhaps is now needed is greater integration of these approaches to develop a better understanding of, for example, how palatability-induced eating overrides short-term satiety cues, and how specific food-related cues can both initiate and potentiate food intake. Such integration will in turn allow greater substantiation of the sorts of approaches to understanding human appetite outlined in this chapter and will help to bring together human and nonhuman animal research on appetite.

REFERENCES

1. de Castro, J.M., Eating behaviour: lessons from the real world of humans. *Nutrition*, 2000, 16, 800–813.
2. Stellar, E., The physiology of motivation, *Psychol. Rev.*, 1954, 61, 5–22.
3. Bartoshuk, L.M., Duffy, V.B., Fast, K., Green, B.G., Prutkin, J., and Snyder, D.J., Labelled scales (e.g., category, Likert, VAS) and invalid cross-group comparisons: what we have learned from genetic variation in taste, *Food Qual. Pref.*, 2002, 14, 1125–1138.
4. Booth, D.A., Cognitive experimental psychology of appetite, in *Eating Habits*, Boakes, R.A., Burton, M.J., and Popplewell, D.A., Eds., Wiley, Chichester, England, 1987, pp. 175–209.

5. Carmagnola, S., Cantu, P., and Penagini, R., Mechanoreceptors of the proximal stomach and perception of gastric distension, *Am. J. Gastroenterol.*, 2005, 100, 1704–1710.
6. Melton, P.M., Kissileff, H.R., and Pi-Sunyer, F.X., Cholecystokinin (CCK-8) affects gastric pressure and ratings of hunger and fullness in women, *Am. J. Physiol.*, 1992, 263, R452–R456.
7. Cardello, A.V., Schutz, H.G., Lesher, L.L., and Merrill, E., Development and testing of a labeled magnitude scale of perceived satiety, *Appetite*, 2005, 44, 1–13.
8. Yeomans, M.R., Rating changes over the course of meals: what do they tell us about motivation to eat? *Neurosci. Biobehav. Rev.*, 2000, 24, 249–259.
9. Kissileff, H. and Guss, J., Microstructure of eating behavior in humans, *Appetite*, 2001, 36, 70–78.
10. Clifton, P.G., Meal patterning in rodents: psychopharmacological and neuroanatomical studies, *Neurosci. Biobehav. Rev.*, 2000, 24, 213–222.
11. Davis, J.D., The microstructure of ingestive behavior, *Ann. N.Y. Acad. Sci.*, 1989, 575, 106–121.
12. Berridge, K.C., Measuring hedonic impact in animals and infants: microstructure of affective taste reactivity patterns, *Neurosci. Biobehav. Rev.*, 2000, 24, 173–198.
13. Bellisle, F., Guy-Grand, B., and Le Magnen, J., Chewing and swallowing as indices of the stimulation to eat during meals in humans: effects revealed by the edogram method and video recordings, *Neurosci. Biobehav. Rev.*, 2000, 24, 223–228.
14. Westerterp-Plantenga, M.S., Eating behavior in humans, characterized by cumulative food intake curves — a review, *Neurosci. Biobehav. Rev.*, 2000, 24, 239–248.
15. Yeomans, M.R., Palatability and the microstructure of eating in humans: the appetiser effect, *Appetite*, 1996, 27, 119–133.
16. Yeomans, M.R., Gray, R.W., Mitchell, C.J., and True, S., Independent effects of palatability and within-meal pauses on intake and subjective appetite in human volunteers, *Appetite*, 1997, 29, 61–76.
17. Gray, R.W., French, S.J., Robinson, T.M., and Yeomans, M.R., Dissociation of the effects of preload volume and energy content on subjective appetite and food intake, *Physiol. Behav.*, 2002, 76, 57–64.
18. Gray, R.W., French, S.J., Robinson, T.E., and Yeomans, M.R., Increasing preload volume with water alters rated appetite but not food intake even with minimal delay between the preload and test meal, *Nutr. Neurosci.*, 2003, 6, 29–37.
19. Yeomans, M.R., Gray, R.W., and Conyers, T., Maltodextrin preloads reduce intake without altering the appetiser effect, *Physiol. Behav.*, 1998, 64, 501–506.
20. Yeomans, M.R., Lee, M.D., Gray, R.W., and French, S.J., Effects of test-meal palatability on compensatory eating following disguised fat and carbohydrate preloads, *Int. J. Obes.*, 2001, 25, 1215–1224.
21. Halmi, K.A., Sunday, S., Puglisi, A., and Marchi, P., Hunger and satiety in anorexia and bulimia-nervosa, *Ann. N.Y. Acad. Sci.*, 1989, 575, 431–445.
22. Halmi, K.A. and Sunday, S.R., Temporal patterns of hunger and fullness ratings and related cognitions in anorexia and bulimia, *Appetite*, 1991, 16, 219–237.
23. Sunday, S.R. and Halmi, K.A., Microanalyses and macroanalyses of patterns within a meal in anorexia and bulimia-nervosa, *Appetite*, 1996, 26, 21–36.
24. Guss, J., Kissileff, H.R., Walsh, B.T., and Devlin, M.J., Binge eating behaviour in patients with eating disorders, *Obes. Res.*, 1994, 2, 355–363.
25. Goldfein, J.A., Walsh, B.T., Lachaussee, J.L., Kissileff, H.R., and Devlin, M.J., Eating behavior in binge eating disorder, *Int. J. Eat. Disord.*, 1993, 14, 427–431.
26. de Castro, J.M. and Elmore, D.K., Subjective hunger relationships with meal patterns in the spontaneous feeding behaviour of humans: evidence for a causal connection, *Physiol. Behav.*, 1988, 43, 159–165.

27. Mattes, R.D., Hunger ratings are not a valid proxy measure of reported food intake in humans, *Appetite,* 1990, 15, 103–113.
28. Yeomans, M.R., Lartamo, S., Procter, E.L., Lee, M.D., and Gray, R.W., The actual, but not labelled, fat content of a soup preload alters short-term appetite in healthy men, *Physiol. Behav.,* 2001, 73, 533–540.
29. Rolls, B.J., Kim, S., McNelis, A.L., Fischman, M.W., Foltin, R.W., and Moran, T.H., Time course of effects of preloads high in fat or carbohydrate on food-intake and hunger ratings in humans, *Am. J. Physiol.,* 1991, 260, R 756–R 763.
30. Hulshof, T., de Graaf, C., and Weststrate, J.A., The effects of preloads varying in physical state and fat content on satiety and energy intake, *Appetite,* 1993, 21, 273–286.
31. Bertenshaw, E.J., Lluch, A., and Yeomans, M.R., Satiating effects of protein but not carbohydrate consumed in a beverage context, *Physiol. Behav.,* 2007, in press.
32. Borzoei, S., Neovius, M., Barkeling, B., Teixeira-Pinto, A., and Rossner, S., A comparison of effects of fish and beef protein on satiety in normal weight men, *Eur. J. Clin. Nutr.,* 2006, 60, 897–902.
33. Williamson, D.A., Geiselman, P.J., Lovejoy, J., Greenway, F., Volaufova, J., Martin, C.K., Arnett, C., and Ortego, L., Effects of consuming mycoprotein, tofu or chicken upon subsequent eating behaviour, hunger and safety, *Appetite,* 2006, 46, 41–48.
34. Almiron-Roig, E. and Drewnowski, A., Hunger, thirst and energy intakes following consumption of caloric beverages, *Physiol. Behav.,* 2003, 79, 767–773.
35. Rolls, B.J., Roe, L.S., Kral, T.V., Meengs, J.S., and Wall, D.E., Increasing the portion size of a packaged snack increases energy intake in men and women, *Appetite,* 2004, 42, 63–69.
36. Tsuchiya, A., Almiron-Roig, E., Lluch, A., Guyonnet, D., and Drewnowski, A., Higher satiety ratings following yogurt consumption relative to fruit drink or dairy fruit drink, *J. Am. Diet. Assoc.,* 2006, 106, 550–557.
37. Fischer, K., Colombani, P.C., and Wenk, C., Metabolic and cognitive coefficients in the development of hunger sensations after pure macronutrient ingestion in the morning, *Appetite,* 2004, 42, 49–61.
38. Harper, A., James, A., Flint, A., and Astrup, A., Increased satiety after intake of a chocolate milk drink compared with a carbonated beverage, but no difference in subsequent ad libitum lunch intake, *Br. J. Nutr.,* 2007, 97, 579–583.
39. Westerterp-Plantenga, M.S. and Verwegen, C.R.T., The appetizing effect of an aperitif in overweight and normal-weight humans, *Am. J. Clin. Nutr.,* 1999, 69, 205–212.
40. Spiegel, T.A. and Stellar, E., Effects of variety on food intake of underweight, normal-weight and overweight women, *Appetite,* 1990, 15, 47–61.
41. Meiselman, H.L., de Graaf, C., and Lesher, L.L., The effects of variety and monotony on food acceptance and intake at a midday meal, *Physiol. Behav.,* 2000, 70, 119–125.
42. Wansink, B., Environmental factors that increase the food intake and consumption volume of unknowing consumers, *Annu. Rev. Nutr.,* 2004, 24, 455–479.
43. Guerrieri, R., Nederkoorn, C., and Jansen, A., How impulsiveness and variety influence food intake in a sample of healthy women, *Appetite,* 2007, 48, 119–122.
44. Norton, G.N., Anderson, A.S., and Hetherington, M.M., Volume and variety: relative effects on food intake, *Physiol. Behav.,* 2006, 87, 714–722.
45. Sclafani, A., Dietary obesity, in *Obesity: Theory and Therapy,* Stunkard, A.J. and Wadden, T.A., Eds., Raven Press, New York, 1993, pp. 125–136.
46. Warwick, Z.S. and Schiffman, S.S., Role of dietary fat in calorie intake and weight gain, *Neurosci. Biobehav. Rev.,* 1992, 16, 585–596.
47. Sorensen, L.B., Moller, P., Flint, A., Martens, M., and Raben, A., Effect of sensory perception of foods on appetite and food intake: a review of studies on humans, *Int. J. Obes.,* 2003, 27, 1152–1166.

48. Yeomans, M.R., Blundell, J.E., and Lesham, M., Palatability: response to nutritional need or need-free stimulation of appetite? *Br. J. Nutr.*, 2004, 92, S3–S14.
49. Kissileff, H.R., Quantitative relationship between palatability and food intake in man, in *The Chemical Senses and Nutrition*, Vol. 3, Kare, M. and Brands, J., Eds., Academic Press, New York, 1986, pp. 293–317.
50. Bobroff, E.M. and Kissileff, H., Effects of changes in palatability on food intake and the cumulative food intake curve of man, *Appetite*, 1986, 7, 85–96.
51. Guy-Grand, B., Lehner, V., and Doassans, M., Effects of palatability and meal type on food intake in normal weight males, *Appetite*, 1989, 12, 213–214.
52. Bellisle, F., Lucas, F., Amrani, R., and Le Magnen, J., Deprivation, palatability and the micro-structure of meals in human subjects, *Appetite*, 1984, 5, 85–94.
53. Sawaya, A.L., Fuss, P.J., Dallal, G.E., Tsay, R., McCrory, M.A., Young, V., and Roberts, S.B., Meal palatability, substrate oxidation and blood glucose in young and older men, *Physiol. Behav.*, 2001, 72, 5–12.
54. Helleman, U. and Tuorila, H., Pleasantness ratings and consumption of open sandwiches with varying NaCl and acid contents, *Appetite*, 1991, 17, 229–238.
55. Yeomans, M.R., Weinberg, L., and James, S., Effects of palatability and learned satiety on energy density influences on breakfast intake in humans, *Physiol. Behav.*, 2005, 86, 487–499.
56. Yeomans, M.R., Tovey, H.M., Tinley, E.M., and Haynes, C.L., Effects of manipulated palatability on appetite depend on restraint and disinhibition scores from the Three Factor Eating Questionnaire, *Int. J. Obes.*, 2004, 28, 144–151.
57. Robinson, T.M., Gray, R.W., Yeomans, M.R., and French, S.J., Test-meal palatability alters the effects of intragastric fat but not carbohydrate preloads on intake and rated appetite in healthy volunteers, *Physiol. Behav.*, 2005, 84, 193–203.
58. Kauffman, N.A., Herman, C.P., and Polivy, J., Hunger-induced finickiness in humans, *Appetite*, 1995, 24, 203–218.
59. Zandstra, E.H., de Graaf, C., Mela, D.J., and Van Staveren, W., Short- and long-term effects of changes in pleasantness on food intake, *Appetite*, 2000, 34, 253–260.
60. Vickers, Z., Holton, E., and Wang, J., Effect of ideal-relative sweetness on yoghurt consumption, *Food Qual. Pref.*, 2001, 12, 521–526.
61. de Castro, J.M., Bellisle, F., and Dalix, A.-M., Palatability and intake relationships in free-living humans: measurement and characterisation in the French, *Physiol. Behav.*, 2000, 68, 271–277.
62. de Castro, J.M., Bellisle, F., Dalix, A.-M., and Pearcey, S.M., Palatability and intake relationships in free-living humans: characterization and independence of influence in North Americans, *Physiol. Behav.*, 2000, 70, 343–350.
63. Smith, G.P., The controls of eating: a shift from nutritional homeostasis to behavioral neuroscience, *Nutrition*, 2000, 16, 814–820.
64. Bellisle, F. and Le Magnen, J., The analysis of human feeding patterns: the edogram, *Appetite*, 1980, 1, 141–150.
65. Spiegel, T.A., Shrager, E.E., and Stellar, E., Responses of lean and obese subjects to preloads, deprivation and palatability, *Appetite*, 1989, 13, 46–69.
66. Spiegel, T.A., Kaplan, J.M., Tomassini, A., and Stella, E., Bite size, ingestion rate and meal size in lean and obese women, *Appetite*, 1993, 21, 131–145.
67. Pierson, A. and Le Magnen, J., Etude quantificaiton du processus de regulation des reponses alimentaires chez hommes, *Physiol. Behav.*, 1969, 4, 61–67.
68. Spiegel, T.A., Rate of intake, bites and chews: the interpretation of obese-lean differences, *Neurosci. Biobehav. Rev.*, 2000, 24, 229–237.
69. Hill, S.W., Eating responses of humans during dinner meals, *J. Comp. Physiol. Psychol.*, 1974, 86, 652–657.

70. Bodnar, R.J., Endogenous opioids and feeding behavior: a 30-year historical perspective, *Peptides,* 2004, 25, 697–725.
71. Cota, D., Tschop, M.H., Horvath, T.L., Levine, A.S., Cannabinoids, opioids and eating behavior: the molecular face of hedonism? *Brain Res. Brain Res. Rev.,* 2006, 51, 85–107.
72. Yeomans, M.R., Opioids and human ingestive behaviour, in *Food Cravings and Addiction,* Hetherington, M.M., Leatherhead Publishing, Leatherhead, UK, 2001, pp. 147–168.
73. Yeomans, M.R. and Gray, R.W., Effects of naltrexone on food intake and changes in subjective appetite during eating: evidence for opioid involvement in the appetiser effect, *Physiol. Behav.,* 1997, 62, 15–21.
74. Cooper, S.J., Endocannabinoids and food consumption: comparisons with benzodiazepine and opioid palatability-dependent appetite, *Eur. J. Pharmacol.,* 2004, 500, 37–49.
75. Kirkham, T.C., Endocannabinoids in the regulation of appetite and body weight, *Behav. Pharmacol.,* 2005, 16, 297–313.
76. Sallan, S.E., Cronin, C., Zelen, M., and Zinberg, N.E., Antiemetics in patients receiving chemotherapy for cancer: a randomized comparison of delta-9-tetrahydrocannabinol and prochlorperazine, *N. Engl. J. Med.,* 1980, 302, 135–138.
77. Mattes, R.D., Engelman, K., Shaw, L.M., and Elsohly, M.A., Cannabinoids and appetite stimulation. *Pharmacol. Biochem. Behav.,* 1994, 49, 187–195.
78. Hollister, L., Hunger and appetite after single doses of marijuana, alcohol and dextroamphetamine, *Clin. Pharmacol. Ther.,* 1971, 12, 45–49.
79. Haney, M., Rabkin, J., Gunderson, E., and Foltin, R.W., Dronabinol and marijuana in HIV(+) marijuana smokers: acute effects on caloric intake and mood, *Psychopharmacology (Berl.),* 2005, 181, 170–178.
80. Beal, J.E., Olson, R., Lefkowitz, L., Laubenstein, L., Bellman, P., Yangco, B., Morales, J.O., Murphy, R., Powderly, W., Plasse, T.F., Mosdell, K.W., and Shepard, K.V., Long-term efficacy and safety of dronabinol for acquired immunodeficiency syndrome-associated anorexia, *J. Pain Symptom Manage.,* 1997, 14, 7–14.
81. Engeli, S., Bohnke, J., Feldpausch, M., Gorzelniak, K., Janke, J., Batkai, S., Pacher, P., Harvey-White, J., Luft, F.C., Sharma, A.M., and Jordan, J., Activation of the peripheral endocannabinoid system in human obesity, *Diabetes,* 2005, 54, 2838–2843.
82. Blundell, J.E. and Tremblay, A., Appetite control and energy (fuel) balance, *Nutr. Res. Rev.,* 1995, 8, 225–242.
83. Jordan, H.A., Levitz, L.S., and Kimbrell, G.M., *Eating is Okay!* Rawson Associates, New York, 1976.
84. Clifton, P.G., Popplewell, D.A., and Burton, M.J., Feeding rate and meal patterns in the laboratory rat, *Physiol. Behav.,* 1984, 32, 369–374.
85. Lucas, G.A. and Timberlake, W., Interpellet delay and meal patterns in the rat, *Physiol. Behav.,* 1988, 43, 259–264.
86. Rolls, B.J., Morris, E.L., and Roe, L.S., Portion size of food affects energy intake in normal-weight and overweight men and women, *Am. J. Clin. Nutr.,* 2002, 76, 1207–1213.
87. Flood, J.E., Roe, L.S., and Rolls, B.J., The effect of increased beverage portion size on energy intake at a meal, *J. Am. Diet. Assoc.,* 2006, 106, 1984–1990; discussion 1990–1991.
88. Rolls, B.J., Roe, L.S., and Meengs, J.S., Salad and satiety: energy density and portion size of a first-course salad affect energy intake at lunch, *J. Am. Diet. Assoc.,* 2004, 104, 1570–1576.
89. Diliberti, N., Bordi, P.L., Conklin, M.T., Roe, L.S., and Rolls, B.J., Increased portion size leads to increased energy intake in a restaurant meal, *Obes. Res.,* 2004, 12, 562–568.

90. Rolls, B.J., Bell, E.A., Castellanos, V.H., Chow, M., Pelkman, C.L., and Thorwart, M.L., Energy density but not fat content of foods affected energy intake in lean and obese women, *Am. J. Clin. Nutr.,* 1999, 69, 863–871.
91. Westerterp-Plantenga, M.S., Effects of energy density of daily food intake on long-term energy intake, *Physiol. Behav.,* 2004, 81, 765–771.
92. Cecil, J.E., Francis, J., and Read, N.W., Relative contributions of intestinal, gastric, oro-sensory influences and information to changes in appetite induced by the same liquid meal, *Appetite,* 1998, 31, 377–390.
93. Blundell, J.E. and Cooling, J., Routes to obesity: phenotypes, food choices and activity, *Br. J. Nutr.,* 2000, 83 (Suppl. 1), S33–38.
94. Drewnowski, A., Energy density, palatability and satiety: implications for weight control, *Nutr. Rev.,* 1998, 56, 347–353.
95. Westerterp, K.R., Perception, passive overfeeding and energy metabolism, *Physiol. Behav.,* 2006, 89, 62–65.
96. Drewnowski, A. and Specter, S.E., Poverty and obesity: the role of energy density and energy costs, *Am. J. Clin. Nutr.,* 2004, 79, 6–16.
97. Hill, J.O. and Peters, J.C., Environmental contributions to the obesity epidemic, *Science,* 1998, 280, 1371–1374.
98. Yeomans, M.R., The role of learning in development of food preferences, in *Psychology of Food Choice,* Shepherd, R. and Raats, M., Eds., CABI Publishing, Wallingford, UK, 2006, pp. 93–112.
99. Brunstrom, J.M., Dietary learning in humans: directions for future research, *Physiol. Behav.,* 2005, 85, 57–65.
100. Gibson, E.L. and Brunstrom, J.M., Learned influences on appetite, food choice and intake, in *Appetite and Body Weight: Integrative Systems and the Development of Anti-Obesity Drugs,* Kirkham, T.C. and Cooper, S.J., Eds. Elsevier, London, 2007, pp. 271–300.
101. Mobini, S., Chambers, L.C., and Yeomans, M.R., Interactive effects of flavour-flavour and flavour-consequence learning in development of liking for sweet-paired flavours in humans, *Appetite,* 2007, 48, 20–28.
102. Booth, D.A., Conditioned satiety in the rat, *J. Comp. Physiol. Psychol.,* 1972, 81, 457–471.
103. Booth, D.A. and Grinker, J.A., Learned control of meal size in spontaneously obese and nonobese bonnet macaque monkeys, *Physiol. Behav.,* 1993, 53, 51–57.
104. Kral, T.V. and Rolls, B.J., Energy density and portion size: their independent and combined effects on energy intake, *Physiol. Behav.,* 2004, 82, 131–138.
105. Mendoza, J.A., Drewnowski, A., and Christakis, D.A., Dietary energy density is associated with obesity and the metabolic syndrome in U.S. adults, *Diabetes Care,* 2007, 30, 974–979.
106. Petrovich, G.D., Ross, C.A., Gallagher, M., and Holland, P.C., Learned contextual cue potentiates eating in rats, *Physiol. Behav.,* 2007, 90, 362–367.
107. Le Merrer, J. and Stephens, D.N., Food-induced behavioral sensitization, its cross-sensitization to cocaine and morphine, pharmacological blockade, and effect on food intake, *J. Neurosci.,* 2006, 26, 7163–7171.
108. Corwin, R.L., Bingeing rats: a model of intermittent excessive behavior? *Appetite,* 2006, 46, 11–15.
109. Rada, P., Avena, N.M., and Hoebel, B.G., Daily bingeing on sugar repeatedly releases dopamine in the accumbens shell, *Neuroscience,* 2005, 134, 737–744.
110. Kelley, A.E., Schiltz, C.A., and Landry, C.F., Neural systems recruited by drug- and food-related cues: studies of gene activation in corticolimbic regions, *Physiol. Behav.,* 2005, 86, 11–14.

111. Corwin, R.L. and Hajnal, A., Too much of a good thing: neurobiology of non-homeostatic eating and drug abuse, *Physiol. Behav.,* 2005, 86, 5–8.
112. Yeomans, M.R., The role of palatability in control of food intake: implications for understanding and treating obesity, in *Appetite and Body Weight: Integrative Systems and the Development of Anti-Obesity Drugs,* Cooper, S.J. and Kirkham, T.C., Eds., Elsevier, London, 2007, pp. 247–269.

5 Motivation to Eat: Neural Control and Modulation

Dianne Figlewicz Lattemann

CONTENTS

5.1 INTRODUCTION

A dramatic increase in obesity incidence in Westernized societies has been observed over the past 15 years. Because obesity is recognized as a significant risk factor for diabetes, cardiovascular disease, several cancers, and shortened life span,[1,2] there is a new focus on environmental and psychological factors that contribute to overeating and perturbed energy homeostasis. A major psychological factor which modulates food intake is the hedonic evaluation of food (i.e., food reward). The study of food reward has expanded over the past several years as details of the functional neurocircuitry are becoming known; and as an appreciation has developed for the role of energy regulatory factors — both intrinsic and extrinsic to the central nervous system (CNS) — in modulating food reward. The goal of this chapter is to provide an overview of current knowledge regarding CNS mediation of food reward/motivation and the evidence in support of its potential regulation or modulation.

Historically, studies of food reward and studies of energy homeostasis have focused upon different CNS subcircuitries and different signals. Studies evaluating the physiological defense of caloric intake by the CNS have focused upon the medial hypothalamus (including the arcuate [ARC], ventromedial nucleus, and paraventricular nucleus [PVN]) as a major anatomical site of integration[3,4] and have evaluated the actions of hormones and neurotransmitters. Prior to this focus, research identified a potential role of circulating glucose, fat, or amino acids (i.e., the glucostatic, lipostatic, and aminostatic controls); current research validates and extends the valid contributions of nutrients to energy homeostasis. In addition, in 1979, Woods and colleagues[5] proposed a model of a negative feedback loop between the brain and endocrine energy regulatory signals (circulating factors such as insulin and leptin, whose concentrations reflect the size of adipose stores, and that convey this information to the CNS), which has received substantial experimental support.[6] Whereas earlier studies focused on factors which reflect a positive energy balance, ongoing study of the neuroendocrine peptide ghrelin[7,8] emphasizes that there are also signals which reflect negative energy balance.

Anatomical studies of motivation and reward have focused on the lateral hypothalamic area (LHA) and midbrain dopaminergic (DA) cell bodies and their projection sites, and functional studies have focused on paradigms such as brain self-stimulation or self-administration of various neurally active substances.[9,10] Not surprisingly, it has become appreciated that additional CNS sites have a role in mediating the rewarding aspects of stimuli. As an anatomical basis for potential crosstalk between energy regulatory circuitry and reward circuitry, it must be appreciated that the medial hypothalamic nuclei are extensively connected with the CNS regions that mediate reward and motivation: the LHA, amygdala, select regions of the cerebral cortex, the ventral tegmental area (VTA), and ventral striatum or nucleus accumbens (NAc). For detailed discussion, the reader is referred to recent reviews of the relevant anatomy and behavioral pharmacology by Berthoud or Kelley.[11,12] In addition to anatomical links between the reward circuitry and energy regulatory circuitry, there are functional links. This is reflected in the observation that fasting or food restriction activates, or enhances the activation of, motivational circuitry as evaluated in several different behavioral paradigms.[13–15]

5.2 MESOCORTICOLIMBIC CIRCUITRY

Within the reward circuitry, the mesocorticolimbic (VTA; ventral tegmental area) dopamine neurons, which project to the ventral striatum or NAc, and to the prefrontal cortex, have been viewed as a central neuroanatomical substrate for reward and motivation.[16] Activation of VTA dopamine neurons, and release of dopamine within the NAc in association with environmental stimuli including food, have long been viewed as indicative of reward enhancement. The relevance of this dopaminergic activation remains a topic of discussion.[17–20] Recent measurements of DA release kinetics with better time resolution are beginning to shed some light on this, as new measurements allow for differentiation between approach behavior, consummatory, and postconsummatory behaviors.[21,22] Specific components of dopamine signaling, i.e., the D1 receptor[23,24] and the reuptake transporter (DAT)[25,26] have been implicated in food reward. Berridge and colleagues have proposed that mesocorticolimbic dopamine activity reflects an increase in the "incentive salience" of a stimulus, including food.[27]

DA neuronal activation can be modulated by the experience or nutritional status of an animal. Thus, with repeated access to a diet in a defined physical environment, initial exposure leads to increased release of dopamine in the NAc shell, whereas subsequent exposure leads to either no increase of dopamine,[28] or an increase of dopamine in anticipation of the presentation of food,[29] increased release of dopamine within a different part of the NAc,[30] and sustained release of dopamine in the prefrontal cortex.[30,31] Further, Wilson and colleagues demonstrated that food-restricted rats trained to drink a palatable liquid food had greater dopamine release in the NAc than free-feeding rats.[32] One question, then, is whether these dopamine neurons are a target for neural or endocrine factors that change in association with fasting and food restriction. Indeed, a neuroendocrine milieu exists in fasted animals that would bias them toward enhanced dopaminergic function. Adrenal glucocorticoid levels are elevated with fasting, and Piazza and colleagues have provided evidence that glucocorticoids can facilitate dopamine release and dopamine-mediated behaviors.[33] Additionally, both insulin and leptin levels rapidly decrease in association with food restriction or fasting,[34] and both inhibit performance in food-reward behavioral tasks that are dopamine dependent.[35–37] Work from a number of investigators has demonstrated the presence of insulin and leptin receptors on VTA neurons,[38,39] functional coupling of these receptors to intracellular signaling pathways,[37,39] and *in vitro* and *in vivo* modulation of synaptic mechanisms to decrease dopamine signaling.[40–42] Conversely, new studies demonstrate that ghrelin — which is increased in association with food deprivation — can increase NAc dopamine levels[43] and, acting at the VTA, can stimulate feeding[44,45] and increase dopamine neuronal activity.[45]

5.3 BRAIN OPIOID NETWORKS

Endogenous opioid neural networks appear to play a role in the regulation of food intake, food hedonics, and food choice in animals[46,47] and in human subjects.[48–50] Although experimental evidence demonstrates that DA and the opioids play somewhat different roles in the mediation of food reward, the neuroanatomical circuitry that is implicated in opioid effects overlaps significantly with the VTA/NAc reward circuitry. Opioids injected into either the VTA or the NAc stimulate food intake,[51–53] and food-induced DA release in the NAc is dependent upon opioid action in the VTA.[54] Thus, in the mesolimbic reward pathway there is functional crosstalk between opioids and dopamine.

An enormous literature documents that endogenous opioids and synthetic opiate peptides enhance food intake.[55–70] One ongoing question is whether opioids are responsible for intake of food in general or only of pleasurable food intake. The opioid antagonist naloxone has been shown to decrease preferentially motivation for, and consumption of, a palatable food (compared to rat chow) in nondeprived rats.[71–73] Thus, opioids appear to signal hedonic value of a food independent from nutritional needs. However, in a study where animals were deprived of food for 24 hours, then given a choice between a preferred diet and a nonpreferred diet, the general opioid antagonist, naltrexone, injected into the PVN decreased intake of both diets, but naltrexone injected into the amygdala decreased intake only of each animal's preferred diet.[74] Since the PVN plays a larger role in energy homeostasis, and the amygdala mediates portions of the emotional response to feeding, the study concluded that opioids affect different aspects of food intake in different CNS sites.

Some have argued that opioids specifically enhance intake of fat. Indeed, many studies support a role for opioids in fat appetite.[64,75–79] Other studies, however, suggest that opioids modulate intake of an animal's preferred food, regardless of nutrient content.[46,47,75,80–83] The conclusion so far can only be that macronutrient content, individual preference, and source of macronutrient all contribute to the food choice an animal (or person) makes. (See Chapter 15 for a discussion of the regulation of macronutrient intake.)

An animal's energy state can impact activity of the opioid system and the behaviors mediated by opioids.[84,85] With regard to CNS-intrinsic energy regulatory signals, as reviewed by Olszewski and Levine,[86] the opioid nociceptin may enhance or sustain feeding by interacting with feeding-termination neuropeptide pathways such as alpha melanocyte stimulating hormone (α-MSH), oxytocin, or corticotropin releasing hormone (CRH). Anatomical evidence supports this interaction as well. Food-restricted rats show significant reductions in μ- and increases in κ-opioid receptor binding in several forebrain areas related to food reward and in the hindbrain parabrachial nucleus.[87–89] Conversely, μ-opioid receptor binding is increased in reward-related sites in animals made obese on a high-fat diet.[90] The adiposity signals, insulin and leptin, decrease intake of sucrose in nondeprived rats and modulate opioid effects on sucrose intake. For example, intraventricular insulin decreases sucrose pellet intake stimulated by a κ opioid agonist and acts cooperatively with a subthreshold dose of a κ opioid antagonist to decrease baseline intake of sucrose pellets.[91] Similarly, sucrose pellet intake stimulated by direct intra-VTA injection of the μ-opioid agonist D-Ala2-NMePhe4-Gly-ol-enkephalin (DAMGO) can be inhibited by concurrent injection of insulin or leptin into the same site.[37]

5.4 ENDOGENOUS CANNABINOIDS

Recent evidence supports the role of CNS endogenous cannabinoids (endocannabinoids, or ECs) anandamide and 2-arachidonoyl glycerol (2-AG) in food intake. Please see recent reviews for detailed discussion of this system; evidence supports both forebrain and hindbrain sites of efficacy to enhance palatable food intake.[92–96] Important for this chapter, current knowledge supports the concept that the ECs may be at the interface of CNS energy-regulatory systems and the reward system (see discussion by Ravinet Trioulli et al.[97]). There is some evidence demonstrating interaction of ECs with CNS leptin effects and also interaction with the mesocorticolimbic dopamine system.[98–100] Protocols evaluating motivation or reward certainly implicate ECs in feeding. Thus the CB1 antagonist SR141716 (rimonabant) decreases place preference conditioned by food,[101] as well as self-administration of food.[102] Duarte et al.[103] demonstrated that relapse to food intake is enhanced by a dopamine D3 agonist, and this effect is blocked by a CB1 receptor antagonist. "Progressive ratios" performance for sucrose self-administration is decreased in CB1 knockout mice.[104] Finally, LHA-stimulation-induced feeding is increased by (exogenous) tetrahydrocannabinol[105] and decreased by CB1 antagonism.[106] Together these studies argue for a role of the ECs in the motivational aspect(s) of feeding. Other than the limited studies examining possible leptin-EC interaction, little is known regarding the impact of (extrinsic) energy regulatory signals on EC function, or vice versa. Clearly this is an area that warrants additional study. A recent study has examined EC interaction with the orexigen, ghrelin; Tucci et al.[107] show that a dose of CB1 antagonist, which does not decrease food intake on its own, will reverse feeding induced by ghrelin administration into the PVN. This finding supports a role of the ECs in ghrelin feeding effects within the medial hypothalamus.

5.5 LATERAL HYPOTHALAMIC AREA (LHA) CIRCUITRY

As discussed above, a central neuroanatomical substrate for coordinating both reward inputs and energy circuitry inputs may be the LHA. The LHA receives direct and indirect limbic inputs and direct projections from the ARC (which is a major target for candidate adiposity signals) as well as numerous intrahypothalamic and neuro-endocrine inputs.[108] Lesion experiments conducted over 50 years ago by Anand and Brobeck revealed a critical role for the lateral hypothalamus (LHA) in the regulation of ingestive behavior. LHA lesions reduce food intake and body weight and reduce motivation for pleasurable stimuli.[109] On the other hand, electrical stimulation[110] or glutamate receptor stimulation within the LHA[111,112] potently stimulate food intake. Additional research confirms that the LHA is an important neural substrate in the control of food intake (for review see Bernardis and Bellinger[113]). The LHA is also an important hypothalamic site mediating reward.[114] Rats robustly self-stimulate electrical current delivered within the LHA. The LHA sites that elicit self-stimulation overlap with sites that also stimulate food intake in response to electrical stimulation.[115] Those studies demonstrate that the majority of animals self-stimulate in response to a lower level of current after 24 hours of food deprivation; thus nutritional status influences the reinforcing and rewarding effect of lateral hypothalamic self-stimulation. This has been replicated and evaluated by other investigators.[116,117]

The neuropeptide melanin-concentrating hormone (MCH), uniquely expressed in the LHA,[118] has emerged as a potentially critical neuropeptide at the interface of both feeding behavior and reward/motivation mechanisms. The majority of MCH neurons are localized to the perifornical region of the LHA (a site from which self-stimulation can be robustly elicited[14,114]). Administered centrally, MCH potently stimulates food intake in satiated animals,[119] and overexpression of MCH increases fat intake and body weight,[120] whereas MCH knockout mice are hypophagic and lean,[121] reminiscent of LHA-lesioned animals. LHA MCH mRNA expression is sensitive to changes in energy balance and energy status.[122,123] MCH neurons receive dense projections from chemically defined cell groups within the ARC that receive both leptin and insulin signals,[108,124] and MCH neurons express the leptin receptor.[125]

5.6 ADDITIONAL SITES IN CENTRAL NERVOUS SYSTEM (CNS) MOTIVATIONAL CIRCUITRY

The nucleus accumbens shell (NAcSh), long appreciated for its involvement in motivated behaviors and reward,[126–128] is also critical to feeding behavior via its connectivity with the LHA. MCH receptors are heavily expressed within the NAcbSh,[129] and the LHA exhibits a reciprocal functional projection to the NAcbSh,[130–132] in which both MCH and the neuropeptide orexin/hypocretin[133] are implicated. MCH signaling between the LHA and AcbSh may play an important role in enhancing the rewarding aspects of food intake. In support of this hypothesis, it was recently demonstrated that MCH, delivered directly into the AcbSh, potently stimulates food intake in satiated rats.[134] Stimulation of $GABA_A$ or $GABA_B$ receptors[135,136] or excitatory amino acid receptor antagonism there[137] potently stimulates food intake, a response that is blocked by LHA inactivation.[137] The reader is referred to the excellent recent review and discussion on this topic by Kelley.[138]

Other forebrain structures are implicated in both limbic function and food reward/motivation. Studies from Baunez and colleagues have demonstrated that the subthalamic nucleus plays a critical role in food-related motivation.[139] This nucleus is a component of the basal ganglia circuitry, within a functional loop that includes the NAc and ventral pallidum. Baunez and colleagues observed that bilateral lesion of the subthalamic nucleus results in an increased rate of eating food pellets, an increase in performance in the "progressive ratios" paradigm, and increased reinforcing properties of food-associated stimuli. These effects were situation dependent and not due to a nonspecific enhancement of motor responding.[140] Additionally, specific subcomponents of the cerebral cortex are integrally involved in taste recognition, taste memory and valuation, and executive function in initiating ingestive decisions based on visual and olfactory cues.[141] Primary taste cortex (i.e., agranular insular cortex) has efferent connections to the orbitofrontal cortex (OFC) and the other major limbic areas and autonomic motor CNS structures. The OFC receives multimodal inputs including gustatory, olfactory, visual, and somatosensory information. For example, some OFC neurons respond to the oral texture of fat.[142] Outputs from this region of the cortex project to the striatum, the ventral midbrain, and the sympathetic nervous system.[11] In rats, electrical stimulation of the OFC initiates feeding,[143] and infusion of various neuropeptides or neurotransmitters into the OFC can alter respiratory quotient and energy expenditure as thermogenesis.[144–146]

5.7 MERGING HUMAN AND ANIMAL STUDIES: AT THE FRONTIER

The study of motivation to eat (and its regulation or modulation) from the physiological perspective is clearly a field that is still in its infancy. The potential clinical and public health significance underlying this basic knowledge is sufficient to warrant future animal studies as well as clinical investigations. However, the understanding of integration of peripheral adiposity signals and psychological controls of feeding in humans is likewise an emerging field. At this point, the approach of functional imaging (fMRI) is beginning to yield insights into the relationship between physiological and psychological factors in human appetite and feeding. Such studies are investigating the localization of food reward in the CNS under normal and energy-challenged conditions and the overlap of these sites with loci involved in drug reward. In humans, the medial prefrontal cortex, thalamus, and hypothalamus appear to be central to the rewarding and motivating aspects of food stimuli, whereas the amygdala and OFC respond to food cues without regard to caloric value.[147–149] In a study of brain activity in response to glucose taste, Frank et al.[147] observed increased right medial OFC activation in healthy normal-weight adult women. The marked OFC activation suggests that tastes with hedonic or emotional value are represented preferentially in this brain region. Gottfried et al.[148] used fMRI to study hungry volunteers who were first presented with picture–odor pairings and then fed a meal specific to the presented odor until sated, simultaneously lessening the subject's reported value of the picture. This devaluation was associated with strikingly decreased neural responses to the picture, in the left dorsomedial amygdala and OFC, after the meal in comparison to just before the meal, with modest decreases in the ventral striatum, insula and cingulate. A speculative interpretation of this study is that satiety signals generated during feeding contribute to the decrease in the value of a food-related sensory cue, whether the cue is primary or secondary to a learned association. OFC activation has been observed to be low in obese (relative to lean) men in response to a satiating meal.[149] This latter study strongly suggests a role of the OFC in human energy balance, in addition to hedonic valuation of food.[150,151]

Studies investigating localization of neurotransmitter signaling during meal consumption are also yielding noteworthy insights concerning food reward and reinforcement. Small et al.[152] used labeled raclopride (a dopamine receptor ligand) positron emission tomography (PET) scanning following a 16-h fast and a favorite meal in normal volunteers to measure regional dopamine (DA) binding. Reduced raclopride binding was observed in the full vs. hungry state in the dorsal striatum, indicating DA release upon food consumption. This was correlated with meal pleasantness, but not with hunger or satiety, indicating that the amount of dorsal striatal DA released correlates with pleasure. Using similar imaging methodology, Volkow et al.[153] correlated DA release with eating behavior survey results and food stimulation (smell and taste) in normal volunteers. Eating restraint scores were positively correlated with DA release to food stimulation, and emotionality scores were negatively correlated with baseline D_2 receptors — all in the dorsal, not ventral, striatum. Volkow et al.[154] also found an increase in dorsal striatal extracellular DA following nonconsumed food display in normal-weight fasting subjects, further implicating the dorsal striatum as the neural substrate in the incentive properties of ingestion. Finally, in a study using PET scanning to investigate brain DA involvement in pathologically obese individuals, Wang et al.[155] found that D_2 receptor availability in these subjects was inversely correlated with body weight (in contrast to normal-weight controls), suggesting that decreased brain DA activity in the obese may well predispose them to excessive food intake.

The collective point of these studies is that the multisensory experience of feeding and food choice in humans strongly activates the limbic forebrain, and activation patterns differ depending upon the nutritional status (physiology) and degree of obesity (pathophysiology) of human subjects. The value of information from the human studies is that they can confirm and extend findings in animal studies and provide new information on perceptions, feelings, and sensations associated with temporal and functional components of the feeding experience. Obviously these can at best be inferred from observing animal behaviors. The combined animal and human findings are powerful because they will yield a convergence of information about the functional anatomy of motivation to eat, which may provide the basis for new therapeutic approaches to diet-induced obesity or eating disorders.

ACKNOWLEDGMENT

Dianne Figlewicz Lattemann is supported by the Merit Review Program of the Department of Veterans Affairs and NIH Grant RO1-DK40963.

REFERENCES

1. Mokdad, A. et al., The continuing epidemics of obesity and diabetes in the United States, *JAMA,* 286, 1195, 2001.
2. Pi-Sunyer, X., A clinical view of the obesity problem, *Science,* 299, 859, 2003.
3. Saper, C.B., Chou, T.C., and Elmquist, J.K., The need to feed: homeostatic and hedonic control of eating, *Neuron,* 36, 199, 2002.
4. Williams, G. et al., The hypothalamus and the control of energy homeostasis: different circuits, different purposes, *Physiol. Behav.,* 74, 683, 2001.
5. Woods, S.C. et al., Chronic intracerebroventricular infusion of insulin reduces food intake and body weight of baboons, *Nature,* 282, 503, 1979.
6. Baskin, D.G. et al., Insulin and leptin: dual adiposity signals to the brain for the regulation of food intake and body weight, *Brain Res.,* 848, 114, 1999.
7. Bhatti, S.F. et al., Ghrelin, an endogenous growth hormone secretagogue with diverse endocrine and nonendocrine effects, *Am. J. Vet. Res.,* 67, 180, 2006.
8. Cummings, D.E. and Shannon, M.H., Roles for ghrelin in the regulation of appetite and body weight, *Arch. Surg.,* 138, 389, 2003.
9. Olds, J., Hypothalamic substrate of reward, *Physiol. Rev.,* 42, 554, 1962.
10. Wise, R.A., Psychomotor stimulant properties of addictive drugs, *Ann. N.Y. Acad. Sci.,* 537, 228, 1988.
11. Berthoud, H.R., Multiple neural systems controlling food intake and body weight, *Neurosci. Biobehav. Rev.*, 26, 393, 2002.
12. Kelley, A.E., Ventral striatal control of appetitive motivation: role in ingestive behavior and reward-related learning, *Neurosci. Biobehav. Rev.*, 27, 765, 2004.
13. Carr, K.D., Augmentation of drug reward by chronic food restriction: behavioral evidence and underlying mechanisms, *Physiol. Behav.,* 76, 353, 2002.
14. Fulton, S., Woodside, B., and Shizgal, P., Potentiation of brain stimulation reward by weight loss: evidence for functional heterogeneity in brain reward circuitry, *Behav. Brain Res.*, 174, 56, 2006.
15. Carroll, M.E. and Meisch, R.A., Increased drug-reinforced behavior due to food deprivation, *Adv. Behav. Pharmacol.,* 4, 47, 1984.
16. Ikemoto, S. and Panksepp, J., Dissociations between appetitive and consummatory responses by pharmacological manipulations of reward-relevant brain regions, *Behav. Neurosci.,* 100, 331, 1996.
17. Hoebel, B. et al., Microdialysis studies of brain norepinephine, serotonin, and dopamine release during ingestive behavior. Theoretical and clinical implications, *Ann. N.Y. Acad. Sci.,* 575, 171, 1989.
18. Salamone, J.D. et al., Nucleus accumbens dopamine and the regulation of effort in food-seeking behavior: implications for studies of natural motivation, psychiatry, and drug abuse, *J. Pharm. Exp. Ther.,* 305, 1, 2003.
19. Schultz, W., Getting formal with dopamine and reward, *Neuron,* 36, 241, 2002.
20. Schultz, W., Neural coding of basic reward terms of animal learning theory, game theory, microeconomics and behavioural ecology, *Curr. Opin. Neurobiol.*, 14, 139, 2004.
21. Phillips, P.E. et al., Subsecond dopamine release promotes cocaine seeking, *Nature,* 422, 614, 2003.
22. Roitman, M.F. et al., Dopamine operates as a subsecond modulator of food seeking, *J. Neurosci.*, 24, 1265, 2004.
23. Cooper, S.J. and Al-Naser, H.A., Dopaminergic control of food choice: contrasting effects of SKF38393 and quinpirole on high-palatability food preference in the rat, *Neuropharmacology,* 50, 953, 2006.
24. El-Ghundi, M. et al., Attenuation of sucrose reinforcement in dopamine D1 receptor deficient mice, *Eur. J. Neurosci.*, 17, 851, 2003.

25. Pecina, S. et al., Hyperdopaminergic mutant mice have higher "wanting" but not "liking" for sweet rewards, *J. Neurosci.*, 23, 9395, 2003.
26. Cagniard, B. et al., Mice with chronically elevated dopamine exhibit enhanced motivation, but not learning, for a food reward, *Neuropharmacology*, 31, 1362, 2006.
27. Berridge, K.C., Food reward: brain substrates of wanting and liking, *Neurosci. Biobehav. Rev.*, 28, 309, 1996.
28. Richardson, N.R. and Gratton, A., Behavior-relevant changes in nucleus accumbens dopamine transmission elicited by food reinforcement: an electrochemical study in rat, *J. Neurosci.*, 24, 8160, 1996.
29. Kiyatkin, A.E., Functional significance of mesolimbic dopamine, *Neurosci. Biobehav. Rev.*, 19, 573, 1995.
30. Bassareo, V. and DiChiara, G., Differential influence of associative and nonassociative learning mechanisms on the responsiveness of prefrontal and accumbal dopamine transmission to food stimuli in rats fed ad libitum, *J. Neurosci.*, 17, 851, 1997.
31. Bassareo, V. and DiChiara, G., Modulation of feeding-induced activation of mesolimbic dopamine transmission by appetitive stimuli and its relation to motivational state, *Eur. J. Neurosci.*, 11, 4389, 1999.
32. Wilson, C. et al., Dopaminergic correlates of motivated behavior: importance of drive, *J. Neurosci.*, 15, 5169, 1995.
33. Marinelli, M. and Piazza, P.V., Interaction between glucocorticoid hormones, stress, and psychostimulant drugs, *Eur. J. Neurosci.*, 16, 387, 2002.
34. Havel, P.J., Role of adipose tissue in body-weight regulation: mechanisms regulating leptin production and energy balance, *Proc. Nutr. Soc.*, 59, 359, 2000.
35. Figlewicz, D.P. et al., Leptin reverses sucrose-conditioned place preference in food-restricted rats, *Physiol. Behav.*, 73, 229, 2001.
36. Figlewicz, D.P. et al., Intraventricular insulin and leptin reverse place preference conditioned with high-fat diet in rats, *Behav. Neurosci.*, 118, 479, 2004.
37. Figlewicz, D.P., Naleid, A.M., and Sipols, A.J., Modulation of food reward by adiposity signals, *Physiol. Behav.*, 91, 473, 2007.
38. Figlewicz, D.P. et al., Expression of receptors for insulin and leptin in the ventral tegmental area/substantia nigra (VTA/SN) of the rat, *Brain Res.*, 964, 107, 2003.
39. Hommel, J.D. et al., Leptin receptor signaling in midbrain dopamine neurons regulates feeding, *Neuron*, 51, 801, 2000.
40. Figlewicz, D.P., Adiposity signals and food reward: expanding the CNS roles of insulin and leptin, *Am. J. Physiol.*, 284, R882, 2003.
41. Garcia, B.G. et al., Akt is essential for insulin modulation of amphetamine-induced human dopamine transporter cell-surface distribution, *Mol. Pharm.*, 68, 102, 2005.
42. Krugel, U. et al., Basal and feeding-evoked dopamine release in the rat nucleus accumbens is depressed by leptin, *Eur. J. Pharmacol.*, 482, 185, 2003.
43. Jerlhag, E. et al., Ghrelin stimulates locomotor activity and accumbal dopamine-overflow via central cholinergic systems in mice: implications for its involvement in brain reward, *Addict. Biol.*, 11, 45, 2006.
44. Naleid, A.M. et al., Ghrelin induces feeding in the mesolimbic reward pathway between the ventral tegmental area and the nucleus accumbens, *Peptides*, 26, 2274, 2005.
45. Abizaid, A. et al., Ghrelin modulates the activity and synaptic input organization of midbrain dopamine neurons while promoting appetite, *J. Clin. Invest.*, 116, 3229, 2006.
46. Glass, M.J., Billington, C.J., and Levine, A.S., Role of lipid type on morphine-stimulated diet selection in rats, *Am. J. Physiol.*, 277, R1345, 1999.
47. Levine, A.S., Kotz, C.M., and Gosnell, B.A., Sugars and fats: the neurobiology of preference, *J. Nutr.*, 133, 831S, 2003.

48. Yeomans, M.R. et al., Effect of nalmefene on feeding in humans. Dissociation of hunger and palatability, *Psychopharmacology,* 100, 426, 1990.
49. Drewnowski, A. et al., Taste responses and preferences for sweet high fat foods: evidence of opioid involvement, *Physiol. Behav.,* 51, 371, 1992.
50. Drewnowski, A. et al., Naloxone, an opiate blocker, reduces the consumption of sweet high fat foods in obese and lean female binge eaters, *Am. J. Clin. Nutr.,* 61, 1206, 1995.
51. Badiani, A. et al., Ventral tegmental area opioid mechanisms and modulation of ingestive behavior, *Brain Res.*, 670, 264, 1995.
52. Noel, M.B. and Wise, R.A., Ventral tegmental injections of a selective mu or delta opioid enhance feeding in food-deprived rats, *Brain Res.*, 673, 304, 1995.
53. Lamonte, N. et al., Analysis of opioid receptor subtype antagonist effects upon mu opioid agonist-induced feeding elicited from the ventral tegmental area of rats, *Brain Res.*, 929, 96, 2002.
54. Tanda, G. and DiChiara, G., A dopamine-mu 1 opioid link in the rat ventral tegmentum shared by palatable food (Fonzies) and non-psychostimulant drugs of abuse, *Eur. J. Neurosci.*, 10, 1179, 1998.
55. Martin, W.R. et al., Tolerance to and physical dependence on morphine in rats, *Psychopharmacologia,* 65, 247, 1963.
56. Lang, I.M. et al., Effects of chronic administration of naltrexone on appetitive behaviors of rats, *Prog. Clin. Biol. Res.*, 68, 197, 1981.
57. Marks-Kaufman, R., Balmagiya, T., and Gross, E., Modifications in food intake and energy metabolism in rats as a function of chronic naltrexone infusions, *Pharm. Biochem. Behav.*, 20, 911, 1984.
58. Kirkham, T.C. and Blundell, J.E., Effect of naloxone and naltrexone on the development of satiation measured in the runway: comparisons with d-amphetamine and d-fenfluramine, *Pharm. Biochem. Behav.*, 25, 123, 1986.
59. Yu, W.Z., Ruegg, H., and Bodnar, R.J., Delta and kappa opioid receptor subtypes and ingestion: antagonist and glucoprivic effects, *Pharm. Biochem. Behav.*, 56, 353, 1997.
60. Yu, W.Z. et al., Pharmacology of flavor preference conditioning in sham-feeding rats: effects of naltrexone, *Pharm. Biochem. Behav.*, 64, 573, 1999.
61. Frisina, P.G. and Sclafani, A., Naltrexone suppresses the late but not early licking response to a palatable sweet solution: opioid hedonic hypothesis reconsidered, *Pharm. Biochem. Behav.*, 74, 163, 2002.
62. Jarosz, P.A. and Metzger, B.L., The effect of opioid antagonism on food intake behavior and body weight in a biobehavioral model of obese binge eating, *Biol. Res. Nurs.*, 3, 198, 2002.
63. Arjune, D. et al., Reduction by central beta-funaltrexamine of food intake in rats under freely-feeding, deprivation and glucoprivic conditions, *Brain Res.*, 535, 101, 1990.
64. Islam, A.K. and Bodnar, R.J., Selective opioid receptor antagonist effects upon intake of a high-fat diet in rats, *Brain Res.*, 508, 293, 1990.
65. Levine, A.S. et al., Nor-binaltorphimine decreases deprivation and opioid-induced feeding, *Brain Res.*, 534, 60, 1990.
66. Arjune, D., Bowen, W.D., and Bodnar, R.J., Ingestive behavior following central [D-Ala2,Leu5,Cys6]-enkephalin (DALCE), a short-acting agonist and long-acting antagonist at the delta opioid receptor, *Pharm. Biochem. Behav.*, 39, 429, 1991.
67. Carr, K.D. et al., Effects of parabrachial opioid antagonism on stimulation-induced feeding, *Brain Res.*, 545, 283, 1991.
68. Levine, A.S., Grace, M., and Billington, C.J., Beta-funaltrexamine (beta-FNA) decreases deprivation and opioid-induced feeding, *Brain Res.*, 562, 281, 1991.
69. Kirkham, T.C. and Cooper, S.J., Attenuation of sham feeding by naloxone is stereospecific: evidence for opioid mediation of orosensory reward, *Physiol. Behav.*, 43, 845, 1988.

70. Kirkham, T.C. and Cooper, S.J., Naloxone attenuation of sham feeding is modified by manipulation of sucrose concentration, *Physiol. Behav.*, 44, 491, 1988.
71. Cleary, J. et al., Naloxone effects on sucrose-motivated behavior, *Psychopharmacology,* 126, 110, 1996.
72. Giraudo, S.Q. et al., Naloxone's anorectic effect is dependent upon the relative palatability of food, *Pharm. Biochem. Behav.*, 46, 917, 1993.
73. Barbano, M.F. and Cador, M., Differential regulation of the consummatory, motivational, and anticipatory aspects of feeding behavior by dopaminergic and opioidergic drugs, *Neuropsychopharmacology,* 31, 1371, 2006.
74. Glass, M.J., Billington, C.J., and Levine, A.S., Naltrexone administered to central nucleus of amygdala or PVN: neural dissociation of diet and energy, *Am. J. Physiol.*, 279, R86, 2000.
75. Glass, M.J. et al., Potency of naloxone's anorectic effect in rats is dependent on diet preference, *Am. J. Physiol.*, 271, R217, 1996.
76. Weldon, D.T. et al., Effect of naloxone on intake of cornstarch, sucrose, and polycose diets in restricted and non-restricted rats, *Am. J. Physiol.*, 270, R1183, 1996.
77. Zhang, M., Gosnell, B.A., and Kelley, A.E., Intake of high-fat food is selectively enhanced by mu opioid receptor stimulation within the nucleus accumbens, *J. Pharm. Exp. Ther.*, 285, 908, 1998.
78. Kelley, A.E. et al., Opioid modulation of taste hedonics within the ventral striatum, *Physiol. Behav.,* 76, 365, 2002.
79. Yanovski, S.Z. and Yanovski, J.A., Obesity, *N. Engl. J. Med.*, 346, 591, 2002.
80. Marks-Kaufman, R., Plager, A., and Kanarek, R.B., Central and peripheral contributions of endogenous opioid systems to nutrient selection in rats, *Psychopharmacology,* 85, 414, 1985.
81. Gosnell, B.A. and Krahn, D.D., The effects of continuous naltrexone infusions on diet preferences are modulated by adaption to the diets, *Physiol. Behav.*, 51, 239, 1992.
82. Glass, M.J. et al., Role of carbohydrate type on diet selection in neuropeptide Y-stimulated rats, *Am. J. Physiol.*, 273, R2040, 1997.
83. Pomonis, J.D., Levine, A.S., and Billington, C.J., Interaction of the hypothalamic paraventricular nucleus and central nucleus of the amygdala in naloxone blockade of neuropeptide Y-induced feeding revealed by c-fos expression, *J. Neurosci.*, 17, 5175, 1997.
84. Rudski, J.M., Billington, C.J., and Levine, A.S., Naloxone's effects on operant responding depend upon level of deprivation, *Pharm. Biochem. Behav.*, 49, 377, 1994.
85. Levine, A.S. et al., Naloxone blocks that portion of feeding driven by sweet taste in food-restricted rats, *Am. J. Physiol.*, 268, R248, 1995.
86. Olszewski, P.K. and Levine, A.S., Minireview: characterization of influence of central nociceptin/orphanin FQ on consummatory behavior, *Endocrinology,* 145, 2627, 2004.
87. Wolinsky, T.D. et al., Effects of chronic food restriction on mu and kappa opioid binding in rat forebrain: a quantitative autoradiographic study, *Brain Res.,* 656, 274, 1994.
88. Wolinsky, T.D., Abrahamsen, G.C., and Carr, K.D., Diabetes alters mu and kappa opioid binding in rat brain regions: comparison with effects of food restriction, *Brain Res.,* 738, 167, 1996.
89. Wolinsky, T.D. et al., Chronic food restriction alters mu and kappa opioid receptor binding in the parabrachial nucleus of the rat: a quantitative autoradiographic study, *Brain Res.*, 706, 333, 1996.
90. Smith, S.L., Harrold, J.A., and Williams, G., Diet-induced obesity increases mu opioid receptor binding in specific regions of the rat brain, *Brain Res.*, 953, 215, 2002.
91. Sipols, A.J. et al., Intraventricular insulin decreases kappa opioid-mediated sucrose intake in rats, *Peptides,* 23, 2181, 2002.
92. Berry, E.M. and Mechoulam, R., Tetrahydrocannabinol and endocannabinoids in feeding and appetite, *Pharmacol. Ther.,* 95, 185, 2002.

93. Fride, E., Endocannabinoids in the central nervous system — an overview, *Prostaglandins Leukot. Essent. Fatty Acids,* 66, 221, 2002.
94. Harrold, J.A. and Williams, G., The cannabinoid system: a role in both the homeostatic and hedonic control of eating? *Br. J. Nutr.*, 90, 729, 2003.
95. Kirkham, T.C. and Williams, C.M., Endocannabinoid receptor antagonists, *Treat. Endocrinol.,* 3, 1, 2004.
96. Miller, C.C. et al., Cannabinoid agonist, CP55,940, facilitates intake of palatable foods when injected into the hindbrain, *Physiol. Behav.,* 80, 611, 2004.
97. Ravinet Trillou, C. et al., Anti-obesity effect of SR141716, a CB1 receptor antagonist, in diet-induced obese mice, *Am. J. Physiol.*, 284, R345, 2003.
98. Kirkham, T.C. et al., Endocannabinoid levels in rat limbic forebrain and hypothalamus in relation to fasting, feeding and satiation: stimulation of eating by 2-arachidonoyl glycerol, *Br. J. Pharmacol.,* 136, 550, 2002.
99. DiMarzo, V. et al., Leptin-regulated endocannabinoids are involved in maintaining food intake, *Nature,* 410, 822, 2001.
100. Harrold, J.A. et al., Down-regulation of cannabinoid-1 (CB-1) receptors in specific extrahypothalamic regions of rats with dietary obesity: a role for endogenous cannabinoids in driving appetite for palatable food? *Brain Res.,* 952, 232, 2002.
101. Chaperon, F. et al., Involvement of central cannabinoid (CB1) receptors in the establishment of place conditioning in rats, *Psychopharmacology,* 135, 324, 1998.
102. Arnone, M. et al., Selective inhibition of sucrose and ethanol intake by SR141716, an antagonist of central cannabinoid (CB1) receptors, *Psychopharmacology,* 132, 104, 1997.
103. Duarte, C. et al., Blockade by the cannabinoid CB1 receptor antagonist, Rimonabant (SR141716), of the potentiation by quinelorane of food-primed reinstatement of food-seeking behavior, *Neuropsychopharmacology,* 29, 911, 2004.
104. Sanchis-Segura, et al., Reduced sensitivity to reward in CB1 knockout mice, *Psychopharmacology,* 176, 223, 2004.
105. Trojniar, W. and Wise, R.A., Facilitory effect of delta 9-tetrahydrocannabinol on hypothalamically induced feeding, *Psychopharmacology,* 103, 172, 1991.
106. Deroche-Gamonet, V. et al., SR141716, a CB1 receptor antagonist, decreases the sensitivity to the reinforcing effects of electrical brain stimulation in rats, *Psychopharmacology,* 157, 254, 2001.
107. Tucci, S.A. et al., The cannabinoid CB1 receptor antagonist SR141716 blocks the orexigenic effects of intrahypothalamic ghrelin, *Br. J. Pharmacol.,* 143, 520, 2004.
108. Elias, C.F. et al., Chemically defined projections linking the mediobasal hypothalamus and the lateral hypothalamic area, *J. Comp. Neurol.,* 402, 442, 1998.
109. Anand, B.K. and Brobeck, J.R., Hypothalamic control of food intake in rats and cats, *Yale J. Biol. Med.,* 24, 123, 1951.
110. Delgado, J. and Anand, B.K., Increase of food intake induced by electrical stimulation of the lateral hypothalamus, *J. Comp. Physiol. Psychol.*, 172, 162, 1953.
111. Stanley, B.G. et al., The lateral hypothalamus: a primary site mediating excitatory amino acid-elicited eating, *Brain Res.,* 630, 41, 1993.
112. Khan, A.M. et al., Lateral hypothalamic signaling mechanisms underlying feeding stimulation: differential contributions of Src family tyrosine kinases to feeding triggered either by NMDA injection or by food deprivation, *J. Neurosci.*, 24, 10603, 2004.
113. Bernardis, L.L. and Bellinger, L.L., The lateral hypothalamic area revisited: neuroanatomy, body weight regulation, neuroendocrinology and metabolism, *Neurosci. Biobehav. Rev.*, 17, 141, 1993.
114. Olds, J., Self-stimulation of the brain, *Science,* 127, 315, 1958.
115. Margules, D.L. and Olds, J., Identical "Feeding" and "Rewarding" systems in the lateral hypothalamus of rats, *Science,* 135, 374, 1962.

116. Blundell, J.E. and Herberg, L.J., Effectiveness of lateral hypothalamic stimulation, arousal, and food deprivation in the initiation of hoarding behavior in naïve rats, *Physiol. Behav.*, 4, 763, 1973.
117. Carr, K.D., Streptozotocin-induced diabetes produces a naltrexone-reversible lowering of threshold for lateral hypothalamic self-stimulation, *Brain Res.*, 664, 211, 1994.
118. Bittencourt, J.C. et al., The melanin-concentrating hormone system of the rat brain: an immuno- and hybridization histochemical characterization, *J. Comp. Neurol.*, 319, 218, 92.
119. Qu, D. et al., A role for melanin-concentrating hormone in the central regulation of feeding behavior, *Nature*, 380, 243, 1996.
120. Ludwig, D.S. et al., Melanin-concentrating hormone overexpression in transgenic mice leads to obesity and insulin resistance, *J. Clin. Invest.*, 107, 379, 2001.
121. Shimada, M. et al., Mice lacking melanin-concentrating hormone are hypophagic and lean, *Nature*, 396, 670, 1998.
122. Sergeyev, V. et al., Effect of 2-mercaptoacetate and 2-deoxy-D-glucose administration on the expression of NPY, AGRP, POMC, MCH and hypocretin/orexin in the rat hypothalamus, *NeuroReport*, 11, 117, 2000.
123. Presse, F. et al., Melanin-concentrating hormone is a potent anorectic peptide regulated by food-deprivation and glucopenia in the rat, *Neuroscience*, 71, 735, 1996.
124. Broberger, C. et al., Hypocretin/orexin- and melanin-concentrating hormone-expressing cells form distinct populations in the rodent lateral hypothalamus: relationship to the neuropeptide Y and agouti gene-related protein systems, *J. Comp. Neurol.*, 402, 460, 1998.
125. Hakansson, M.L. et al., Leptin receptor immunoreactivity in chemically defined target neurons of the hypothalamus, *J. Neurosci.*, 18, 559, 1998.
126. Robbins, T.W. and Koob, G.F., Selective disruption of displacement behavior by lesions of the mesolimbic dopamine system, *Nature*, 285, 409, 1980.
127. Koob, G.F. and Bloom, F., Cellular and molecular mechanisms of drug dependence, *Science*, 242, 715, 1988.
128. Robbins, T.W. et al., Limbic-striatal interactions in reward-related processes, *Neurosci. Biobehav. Rev.*, 13, 155, 1989.
129. Saito, Y. et al., Expression of the melanin-concentrating hormone (MCH) receptor mRNA in the rat brain, *J. Comp. Neurol.*, 435, 26, 2001.
130. Phillipson, O.T. and Griffiths, A.C., The topographic order of inputs to nucleus accumbens in the rat, *Neuroscience*, 16, 275, 1985.
131. Heimer, L. et al., Specificity in the projection patterns of accumbal core and shell in the rat, *Neuroscience*, 41, 89, 1991.
132. Kirouac, G.J. and Ganguly, P.K., Topographical organization in the nucleus accumbens afferents from the basolateral amygdala and efferents to the lateral hypothalamus, *Neuroscience*, 67, 625, 1995.
133. Zheng, H. et al., Appetite-inducing accumbens manipulation activates hypothalamic orexin neurons and inhibits POMC neurons, *Am. J. Physiol.*, 284, R1436, 2003.
134. Georgescu, D. et al., The hypothalamic neuropeptide melanin-concentrating hormone acts in the nucleus accumbens to modulate feeding behavior and forced-swim performance, *J. Neurosci.*, 25, 2933, 2005.
135. Stratford, T.R. and Kelley, A.E., GABA in the nucleus accumbens shell participates in the central regulation of feeding behavior, *J. Neurosci.*, 17, 4434, 1997.
136. Basso, A.M. and Kelley, A.E., Feeding induced by GABA (A) receptor stimulation within the nucleus accumbens shell: regional mapping and characterization of macronutrient and taste preference, *Behav. Neurosci.*, 113, 324, 1999.

137. Maldonado-Irizarry, C.S., Swanson, C.J., and Kelley, A.E., Glutamate receptors in the nucleus accumbens shell control feeding behavior via the lateral hypothalamus, *J. Neurosci.*, 15, 6779, 1995.
138. Kelley, A.E. et al., Corticostriatal-hypothalamic circuitry and food motivation: integration of energy, action, and reward, *Physiol. Behav.,* 86, 773, 2005.
139. Baunez, C., Amalric, M., and Robbins, T.W., Enhanced food-related motivation after bilateral lesions of the subthalamic nucleus, *J. Neurosci.,* 22, 562, 2002.
140. Baunez, C. et al., The subthalamic nucleus exerts opposite control on cocaine and 'natural' rewards, *Nat. Neurosci.*, 8, 484, 2005.
141. Rolls, E.T., The functions of the orbitofrontal cortex, *Brain Cogn.,* 55, 11, 2004.
142. Rolls, E.T. et al., Responses to the sensory properties of fat of neurons in the primate orbitofrontal cortex, *J. Neurosci.,* 19, 1532, 1999.
143. Bielajew, C. and Trzcinska, M., Characteristics of stimulation-induced feeding sites in the sulcal prefrontal cortex, *Behav. Brain Res.*, 61, 29, 1994.
144. McGregor, I.S., Menendez, J.A., and Atrens, D.M., Metabolic effects obtained from excitatory amino acid stimulation of the sulcal prefrontal cortex, *Brain Res.*, 529, 1, 1990.
145. McGregor, I.S., Menendez, J.A., and Atrens, D.M., Metabolic effects of neuropeptide Y injected into the sulcal prefrontal cortex, *Brain Res. Bull.*, 24, 363, 1990.
146. Westerhaus, M.J. and Loewy, A.D., Central representation of the sympathetic nervous system in the cerebral cortex, *Brain Res.*, 903, 117, 2001.
147. Frank, G.K. et al., The evaluation of brain activity in response to taste stimuli – a pilot study and method for central taste activation as assessed by event-related fMRI, *J. Neurosci. Methods,* 131, 99, 2003.
148. Gottfried, J.A., O'Doherty, J., and Dolan, R.J., Encoding predictive reward value in human amygdala and orbitofrontal cortex, *Science,* 301, 1104, 2003.
149. Gautier, J.F. et al., Differential brain responses to satiation in obese and lean men, *Diabetes,* 49, 838, 2000.
150. Kringelbach, M.L., O'Doherty, J., Rolls, E.T., and Andrews, C., Activation of the human orbitofrontal cortex to a liquid food stimulus is correlated with its subjective pleasantness, *Cereb. Cortex,* 13, 1064, 2003.
151. Kringelbach, M.L., Food for thought: hedonic experience beyond homeostasis in the human brain, *Neuroscience,* 126, 807, 2004.
152. Small, D.M., Jones-Gotman, M., and Dagher, A., Feeding-induced dopamine release in dorsal striatum correlates with meal pleasantness ratings in healthy human volunteers, *NeuroImage,* 19, 1709, 2003.
153. Volkow, N.D. et al., Brain dopamine is associated with eating behaviors in humans, *Int. J. Eat. Disord.,* 33, 136, 2003.
154. Volkow, N.D. et al., 'Nonhedonic' food motivation in humans involves dopamine in the dorsal striatum and methylphenidate amplifies this effect, *Synapse,* 44, 175, 2002.
155. Wang, G-J. et al., Brain dopamine and obesity, *Lancet,* 357, 354, 2001.

6 Human Eating Motivation in Times of Plenty: Biological, Environmental, and Psychosocial Influences

Michael R. Lowe, Miriam E. Bocarsly, and Angelo Del Parigi

CONTENTS

6.1 INTRODUCTION

With thousands of studies published on topics relevant to human eating motivation, one feels immediately daunted by the prospect of writing a relatively brief chapter on the topic. We knew we would have to limit the range of topics to be covered. We began with the underappreciated observation that, for the vast majority of the existence of our species, our motivational challenge has been to continuously find enough to eat to survive. Today nearly all people in developed countries consume sufficient calories to maintain health and functioning, and most people in the world obtain sufficient calories to avoid starvation. Although malnutrition remains a very significant problem in some countries, the problem is of course not one of motivation but of access to sufficient food. In addition, the opposite problem — being motivated to eat when no energy deficit exists — has contributed to an epidemic of overweight and obesity that has arisen almost *de novo* during the past century. Historically, much more research has been conducted on the mechanisms governing the maintenance of energy balance in normal-weight organisms[1,2] than on the mechanisms governing excessive energy consumption and weight gain. For all these reasons, the primary focus of this chapter will be on human eating motivation in times of plenty.

Two other caveats are needed. First, the purpose of this chapter is to provide a macro-level perspective (i.e., of the "forest"), not a comprehensive review of particular studies (i.e., the "trees"). The latter goal is not only impossible in a brief chapter, but a number of reviews of particular subareas of human eating motivation are already available. Second, although we agree with many other investigators that human food intake is influenced by a wide array of genetic, biological, psychological, environmental, and cultural variables, we believe that a "macro" perspective that is largely missing from the field is an attempt to order the relative importance of these multiple determinants of food intake. To take a noncontroversial example, most appetite researchers would presumably agree that the food environment is much more influential in determining food intake (and body mass) than are beliefs about the healthfulness of foods. Attempting to make such differentiations more broadly, though likely to be controversial, is necessary if clinical and population-level interventions are to be designed in the most rational and cost-effective manner.

The chapter is organized into sections considering biological, environmental, and psychosocial influences on food intake. In each of these sections we evaluate the relative influence of each of these domains. Finally, in keeping with the structure of all the chapters in this book, we conclude with several hypotheses generated by human research that might profitably be tested in animal models.

6.2 BIOLOGICAL INFLUENCES

The vast majority of research that has been conducted on biological underpinnings of human eating motivation has been based on the dual notions of metabolic need emanating from within a person and caloric repletion emanating from foodstuffs. It has long been assumed that people are motivated to eat because they are in a state of energy deficit (or are anticipating the impending development of an energy deficit)[3] and learn that food delivers energy that will reverse (or prevent) such a state. From this traditional perspective there is little reason to expect that people would be motivated to eat when not food deprived — or, conversely, that they would have much motivation to consume foods with few or no calories (because doing so would do little to satisfy energetic needs).

However, there are vast differences between the environment that shaped our appetitive motivations over evolutionary time and modern, food-abundant environments. These differences involve dramatic changes in the widespread availability of highly palatable foods and the greatly reduced level of energy expenditure required to obtain food and to survive in hostile environments. Many other investigators have documented the contrasting demands of ancient and modern environments,[4,5] wherein prehistorical environments involved frequent periods of food scarcity and the resulting development of a "thrifty" genotype.[5] As a result of agriculture and other aspects of the modern environment in developed countries, the challenge for most people has changed from acquiring sufficient calories for survival to avoiding excessive consumption of calories to prevent chronic disease.

6.2.1 Biological Underpinnings of Hedonic Eating

Until recently the vast majority of research in humans and animals has been based on an energy depletion/repletion model of eating motivation.[1,2,6] However, with the emergence of the global obesity epidemic and evidence of the resistance of the obese state to long-term modification, research on hedonically driven eating has rapidly accelerated during the past decade. Nonetheless, we are only just beginning to understand the neurobiological underpinnings of such eating.[7,8]

Many observers have noted that human weight regulation is asymmetrical, meaning that there are vigorous psychological and biological reactions that resist downward deflections in body weight but few if any reactions to counteract upward deflections. This asymmetry presumably helped our ancestors survive fluctuating environmental conditions by slowing metabolism and increasing appetitive drive in times of scarcity while maximizing capacity to eat and store calories in the (relatively infrequent) times of plenty. A significant part of the asymmetry that exists in relation to body weight regulation appears to stem from a similar asymmetry that exists with regard to eating regulation. Regulatory pressures counteracting reductions in energy intake below energy needs appear to be powerful and relentless.[9–11] When energy intake exceeds energy needs, however, there appear to be few countervailing pressures that help individuals compensate for overconsumption. Many studies have found, for instance, that most people do not compensate well for energy intake that supersedes energy needs.[12] Thus, if energy intake exceeds energy requirements by even a small amount, over a period of months and years such small imbalances can produce substantial weight gain.

In the past 15 years, animal and human researchers have made progress in distinguishing between homeostatic and hedonically motivated eating.[13–15] Most of the research examining these motives has so far been conducted with nonhuman animals. We therefore next summarize animal research on hedonic eating (above and beyond that covered in Chapter 5).

6.2.2 Animal Models of Hedonically Motivated Eating

In animals, it has been determined that neurological systems regulating both energy homeostasis and reward-motivated eating are critical in food consumption. While these systems can be functionally dissociated, they both overlap and interact in the brain. However, by dissociating the energy homeostasis and reward-motivated aspects of eating, one can further explore the hedonic eating motives that are so prevalent in today's society. Neurological pathways involved in the processing of hedonic value have been linked to the opioid peptides. Research has indicated that, when opioid receptors are blocked using an antagonist such as naloxone, consumption of a palatable diet is diminished, while consumption of a bland diet is not affected.[16] Additionally, administration of naloxone has been shown to diminish the hedonic effects of a palatable food, based on frequency of facial expressions suggestive of pleasure.[17]

It has also been found that animals that had been fed a diet high in fat and sucrose for 7 days displayed elevated expression of opioid mRNA as compared to bland diet-fed counterparts. This finding indicates an increase in endogenous opioid synthesis as a result of overconsumption of highly palatable stimulus,[16] further demonstrating the role of opioid peptides in hedonic eating. When the amount of the sugar/fat-rich diet the animals were allowed to consume was limited in order to calorie-match the energy consumed by those animals maintained on the bland diet, decreased expression of the same opioid mRNA was observed in the animals fed the bland diet.[16] This change in opioid expression is attributed to the reward deprivation effect, in that the animals that had access to the sugar/fat diet would consume more of the diet, if allowed. By restricting the daily intake, in order to calorie-match the control-fed animals, a state of reward deprivation may have been produced. This could possibly be likened to a human model in which a person might feel sated after consuming 200 kcal of an unflavored hot cereal but still feel hungry after consuming 200 kcal of a more palatable, artificially flavored and sweetened hot cereal. This phenomenon could be the result of palatability-induced changes in the opioid circuitry and other reward-related neurochemicals. A similar phenomenon, labeled "hedonic hunger," may represent the motive underlying an increasing percentage of food intake in humans.[14]

Based on a shared neural network, the hedonic values of palatable foods can be likened to the hedonic value of drugs of abuse.[18–20] One accepted measure of drug abuse is the precipitation of an aversive state when the abused substance is unavailable, removed, or when its effects are blocked. It has been shown that somatic signs of withdrawal can be precipitated by naloxone in animals that had been maintained on a highly palatable cafeteria-style diet.[21] Similarly, animals maintained on a sugar-bingeing diet demonstrated signs of withdrawal, similar to the behaviors seen in morphine-dependent animals, when injected with naloxone, as compared to their saline-injected counterparts or sugar-naive, *ad libitum* chow-fed controls.[20]

Further studies have demonstrated that this withdrawal-like behavior can be precipitated by simply removing all food access (both sugar and chow) in sugar-bingeing rats and does not require the presence of an opioid antagonist.[20] Further, behavioral withdrawal can also be observed in nonenergy-deprived animals that were maintained on a sugar-binging diet and then deprived of sugar.[20] In this model, animals were allowed continuous access to rodent chow during the sugar-deprivation phase and still demonstrated behavioral indicators of increased anxiety, which is indicative of behavioral withdrawal in animal models.[20] Sugar-bingeing animals that had been subsequently deprived of sugar were also willing to work harder when a sugar solution was reintroduced (as measured by a bar-pressing paradigm) than nonbinging, sugar-fed counterparts.[20] This deprivation effect is similar to the behavior seen in drug-deprived, addicted animals.[21] All of these studies lend more support to the similarities in the hedonic nature — and potential for addictive-like responses — between drugs of abuse and palatable foods.

A recent study explored the effects of the introduction and removal of highly palatable foods on neurophysiological and behavioral indicators of anxiety. Teegarden and Bale[22] maintained mice on two highly palatable diets for 4 weeks. The animals were then withdrawn from their palatable diets and placed on a normal rodent-chow diet. This change, from a palatable diet to a bland diet, caused an increase in anxiety-related behavior (which is a well-accepted indicator of "withdrawal" in animal models), as well as changes in the release of corticotrophin-releasing factor (related to stress), and in the expression of reward-related signaling molecules. All of these indicators point to a negative state, similar to the state of withdrawal which is seen when drug-dependent animals are deprived of their addictive substance. When the palatable food was again made available, those animals previously maintained on a palatable, high-fat diet were more willing to endure adverse conditions in order to regain access to the food than control animals, demonstrating that this subgroup of animals desired the deprived substance more than their counterparts who were maintained on chow throughout the study.

Other studies have explored the behavioral effects of highly palatable food. Barbano and Cador[23] provided food-deprived and sated rats with access to chow or palatable chocolate cereal and measured how fast the animals ran to obtain the foods. Food-sated rats ran as fast for the palatable food as food-deprived rats did for chow. Similarly, Corwin[24] determined that even in nondeprived rats, limiting access to a preferred fatty food can induce a binge-type behavior. In this study, all animals were allowed *ad libitum* access to standard rodent chow, while some animals additionally had access to shortening for either (1) 2 hours, 3 days a week, (2) 2 hours everyday, (3) *ad libitum* access to shortening, (4) or no shortening access. As the shortening accessibility decreased, intake for the 2-hour access period increased, while total daily energy intake did not differ across groups. This indicates that limiting access to a preferred, palatable food can induce binge-type eating.

6.2.3 Human Research on Hedonically Motivated Eating

There are two domains of recent human research that hold particular promise for increasing our understanding of hedonically motivated eating. These involve neuroimaging studies (which mostly involve comparisons of obese and normal-weight individuals) and research on restrained eating (which usually involves comparisons among normal-weight individuals differing in restraint).

6.2.4 Neuroimaging Studies (*See Also* Chapter 14)

Independently of a primarily genetic or environmental etiology of overweight and obesity, the chronic dysregulation of eating behavior resulting in positive energy balance and weight gain points to the central nervous system (CNS) as the principal organ of interest. In fact, decades of research in animals[25] and sporadic cases of CNS lesions in humans associated with obesity[26] support the notion that weight gain and the consequent obesity are associated with neurofunctional aberrations.[26] However, direct access to the CNS, and especially to the brain, for the investigation of the biology of the central control of eating behavior has obvious limitations in humans. Among the available options, functional neuroimaging (FN) — essentially positron emission tomography (PET) and functional magnetic resonance imaging (fMRI) — offer the opportunity to explore noninvasively the *in vivo* physiology of the brain by measuring variables indicative of neurotransmitter binding or local neuronal activity.

Depending on the specific techniques applied, FN is instrumental in mapping the regional brain response to a stimulus, or in identifying a specific neurochemical network. Furthermore, FN provides the opportunity to explore the whole brain at once, without the shortcomings of *a priori* assumptions of regions or pathways of interest. On the other hand, several shortcomings need to be considered: first and foremost, the temporal and spatial scale of neuronal events which challenge the resolution capabilities of FN, stimulating continuous technical improvement. Second, the association between a stimulus and its associated functional neuroanatomy is not necessarily indicative of a causative role of one for the other; the study design is of the essence in this respect. In general, the investigation with FN of the pathogenesis of complex diseases, such as obesity, encounters substantial limitations of sensitivity and specificity in the identification of its neurofunctional markers.

Possibly as a result of these and other limitations, FN has not been able, thus far, to translate to humans the overwhelming evidence of neurobiological alterations, mainly reported in the hypothalamus and brain stem of animal models of obesity. It is not within the scope of this chapter to review the few FN studies reporting hypothalamic responses to energy intake in humans.[27,28] In a large scheme, this limited evidence of hypothalamic aberrations in human obesity emphasizes the complexity of the neurophysiologic phenomena underpinning the brain control of eating behavior in humans. The brain stem and hypothalamus, in fact, operate at a nonconscious level, mainly processing homeostatic signals that provide information on shorter- and longer-term energy imbalances. However, what mostly motivates humans to start eating is not the simple need to compensate for an energy deficit. More often the driving force is the pleasure of consuming palatable food and/or cultural norms governing food intake. This suggests that hedonic and cognitive processing associated with other brain regions might play an important role in controlling eating behavior, including limbic and paralimbic areas (processing reward, emotions, and complex sensory stimulations) as well as the prefrontal cortex and other neocortical areas processing and integrating cognition.

Therefore, it is not surprising that FN studies have consistently indicated that the ingestion of liquid[29] or solid food,[30] as well as the sight of food,[31] elicits activation and deactivation of different brain regions, such as the prefrontal cortex and a group of limbic/paralimbic areas (orbitofrontal, insula, cingulate, hippocampus, striatum), respectively. Although the salience of food stimulation differed in these studies from mainly homeostatic to mainly hedonic to sensory, the consistency of these responses and the overlap with reward-associated brain domains is remarkable.

Abnormal activation and deactivation of several of these areas were also demonstrated in obese individuals.[32] Is dopamine, a neurotransmitter involved in reward processing, responsible for the differences between obese and normal-weight individuals? Using a radioligand of the dopamine type 2 receptor (DRD2) and PET, Wang et al. found that the availability of DRD2 is abnormally low in the dorsal striatum of obese individuals, suggesting that obesity might be a reward deficiency syndrome.[33]

Observing a difference between obese and normal-weight individuals does not indicate, however, whether that difference is a consequence or a cause of obesity. The ideal study would require a longitudinal design with assessments in the same individuals before the start of weight gain, during weight gain, and after reaching the steady state. In a cross-sectional comparison between obese, normal-weight, and formerly obese individuals, Del Parigi et al. reported that in formerly obese individuals two paralimbic regions, the middle insula and posterior hippocampus, exhibit an obese-like abnormality in response to tasting and ingesting a satiating meal, respectively, suggesting that they might represent markers for the risk of obesity.[34] If confirmed, the findings suggest that predisposition to obesity may be reflected in functional alterations in brain regions involved in anticipation and reward, food craving, sensory perception, and autonomic control of digestion (middle insula), as well as food craving, and learning/memory (hippocampus).

Taken together, these results show that FN, although admittedly still in its infancy, is a powerful and versatile technology for the investigation of the biology of human eating behavior and its abnormalities. The constant improvement of the technical capabilities, combined with new hypothesis-testing study designs, promise to deliver fundamental insights into the pathophysiology of CNS disorders such as obesity.

6.2.5 Restrained Eating as Resistance to an Obesogenic Environment

During the past 30 years, one of the most widely used frameworks for understanding susceptibility to overeating has been the restrained eating model.[35] This model suggests that dieting "sows the seeds of its own destruction" by making dieters' diets susceptible to disinhibiting influences such as eating forbidden foods or becoming emotionally distressed. This model typically assumes that dieting is motivated by a desire to lose weight to attain a socially desirable level of thinness and attractiveness.[36] (We review this topic under the biological rather than the psychosocial domain because we believe that restraint is notable primarily because it is a proxy for a behavioral and biological susceptibility toward weight gain.)

However, a number of research findings during the past 10 years have begun to paint a different picture of restrained eaters and the reasons for their susceptibility to overeating. This research has been reviewed in several papers,[15,37–39] and space prevents a full exposition here. Essentially, research has shown that most restrained eaters are not dieting to lose weight and do not eat any less in the natural environment than unrestrained eaters. Indeed, several studies have found that measures of restrained eating and dieting prospectively predict weight gain rather than weight loss. In addition, metabolic characteristics of restrained eaters (e.g., low leptin levels, high insulin sensitivity) suggest that they are physiologically prone to weight gain (suggesting that they could be vulnerable to weight gain even if their energy intake is no greater than unrestrained eaters of comparable lean tissue mass). Furthermore, recent evidence suggests that normal-weight restrained eaters are more concerned with not becoming overweight than they are about becoming skinny.[40,41] Thus it appears that restrained eating is better viewed as a response to, rather than as a cause of, overeating and weight gain.

6.2.6 Eating "Beyond Need": Psychological or Biological?

Although behavioral and biological scientists agree that brain responses mediate all behavior, most researchers still divide eating motives into those that are biological and psychological in nature. Eating for reasons "other than biological need" is usually assumed to be caused psychologically. This terminology does not reflect the belief that psychological motives are not grounded in biology (which would be an endorsement of dualism) but that biology plays an essentially passive role in psychologically motivated intake. For instance, in a recent paper reviewing normative factors causing excessive food intake, Herman and Polivy[42] suggested that "people are eating bigger meals not because their hypothalami have been altered, but in spite of the fact that their physiology remains unchanged"[42] (p. 763). There are two problems with this perspective. First, there is evidence that both consumption of palatable foods[22,43] and weight gain[25,44] do, in fact, alter aspects of hypothalamic and other brain circuitry. Second, it seems highly unlikely that an aspect of the environment that was presumably key to our survival for eons (the motivation to find and consume energy when it was available, even in the absence of an immediate energy need) would have no systematic impact on our biology. After all, we appear to be biologically prepared to both defend a normal weight from weight reductions (via homeostatic mechanisms) and to find and consume highly palatable food even if doing so supersedes energy needs and produces weight gain. In this regard, we agree with the position taken by Berthoud[8] in a recent paper describing how brain-based reward mechanisms may overwhelm the homeostatic control of body weight. Berthoud noted that "these neural mechanisms depend no less on physiological processes than metabolic mechanisms do. It is regrettable that these processes are often dubbed 'psychological' or 'behavioral' and ranked lower or treated differently than 'biology' and 'physiology' by leading scientists in the field."

6.3 ENVIRONMENTAL INFLUENCES

Although biological factors certainly contribute to weight gain, the rapid increase in rates of obesity and overweight over a period of relative genetic stability indicates that environmental changes have been largely responsible for triggering the increased weight gain over the past three decades in the United States.[45] Of course, the environmental changes exert their effects through biological mechanisms, but in this case the biological reactions (e.g., to the sight or taste of food) play a more passive role in response to the constant availability of highly palatable foods. The biological diathesis that predisposes most people to gain weight in an obesogenic environment appears to be a latent potentiality that is only activated when "times of plenty" occur not just sporadically (as presumably occurred over evolutionary time) but continuously. This latent potentiality appears to be a prominent but not an omnipresent one, so some individuals are biologically protected and remain lean even in an obesogenic environment.

Through the provision of easily available, varied, good-tasting, inexpensive, energy-dense foods in increasingly larger portion sizes, the immediate food environment is presumed to play a great role in the generation of energy consumption beyond energy needs. Such environmental forces can even work to usurp biological hunger and satiety signals. For example, when participants were given a placebo pill that, they were told, made other subjects hungry or full, those participants classified as restrained eaters subsequently ate more when they received the "hunger" pill and less when they received the "fullness" pill.[46] In addition, when people are given larger portion sizes, they tend to eat more, but do not report higher levels of fullness.[47]

Environment in itself is a complex entity, and though the impact on weight gain of particular features of the food environment have not been identified, research has pointed to several facets of the food environment that prompt people to eat beyond their energy needs.

6.3.1 Portion Size

A great deal of evidence indicates that increased portion size causes increased food intake. The past few decades have shown a dramatic increase in portion and packaging sizes in developed countries generally and in the United States in particular. This size increase is pervasive in nature and has been noted not only in package sizes, but also in restaurant portion sizes, supermarket items, and even cookbook recipe sizes.[48] Doubling a portion size leads to up to a 25% increase in consumption of main staple foods (such as pasta), while a similar increase in packaging can lead to a 45% increase in intake of snack foods.[49]

Portioning and packaging provide consumers with an idea of what unit is appropriate or optimal to eat.[50] In a series of studies, M&Ms were left on the table with either a larger or smaller serving spoon, and instructions to "take your fill." Participants given the larger scoop ate more M&Ms than those given the smaller scoop. In another study, 85 nutrition experts were given either small or large bowls and either small or large ice cream scoops, and told to serve themselves as much ice cream as they like.[51] Despite being nutrition experts, both the larger bowls and the larger scoops caused participants to unknowingly serve themselves more ice cream.

Package size seems to hold great influence on the amount of food people consume, exacting equal or greater influence over food consumption than other identified environmental factors, such as taste or palatability. In one study, moviegoers were either given a medium- or a large-sized bucket of stale popcorn. Those individuals who were given the larger bucket ate appreciably more popcorn, despite its stale texture and undesirable taste.[49] Portion size also has been shown to act independently of energy density, remaining influential even as energy density changes.[52] Interestingly, when portion size and energy density are simultaneously manipulated, additive effects can be seen on overall energy intake. Conversely, reduction in portion sizes and reduction in energy density have been shown to be additive, leading to sustained decrease in energy intake without significantly reducing feelings of satiety.[53]

6.3.2 Energy Density

Energy density, or the amount of energy in a given weight of food (kcal/g), influences overall energy intake. Different food constituents add to energy density differently. For example, fat greatly increases energy density, while water decreases energy density by adding weight and no calories. Studies that examine satiety have demonstrated that it is food volume, rather than energy intake *per se,* that determines satiety.[52] In one study, participants reduced their energy intake during lunch after consuming 600 ml (about 600 kcal) of a preload as compared to those individuals that consumed 300 ml (700 kcal) of a preload higher in energy density. This indicates that the preload with fewer calories and more volume (or, the less energy-dense preload) led to more of a feeling of fullness than the preload with a higher energy content and energy density, but a smaller, volume. Using these paradigms, and other similar experiments, it is apparent that the body utilizes volume, more than total energy or energy density, as a determinant of satiety. By extension, as energy density increases, intake volume does not naturally decrease in order to compensate for the added calories, which can lead to "passive overconsumption" when individuals consume a lot of high-energy-density foods.

6.3.3 Availability

Energy-dense, palatable foods are omnipresent in the current environment. From fast food restaurants on every corner, to elaborate cafeteria buffets, to snack stands at sporting events, palatable food has become an unavoidable stimulus in our day-to-day environment. Simply increasing food visibility increases consumption. For example, when Hershey Kisses are placed in a clear container on an office worker's desk, more of them are consumed than when the same candies are placed in an opaque container.[49]

6.3.4 Variety

In humans, meals that are composed of a variety of foods lead to greater energy intake when compared to calorie-matched meals that are only composed of one food type.[54] Similarly, participants that were given the same meal for several days ate less than those individuals that were given a variety of meals across the same set of days.[55,56] It has been suggested that this observation can be attributed to a "sensory-specific satiety."[57] With repeated exposure to a food, hedonic ratings have been shown to decrease, leading to a decreased intake of the food.[58] Conversely, the vast array of food choices in supermarkets and restaurants suggests that food variety is ultimately leading to higher energy intake.

This variety-driven increase has been shown time and again, using both meal and snack foods; for example, increasing the available flavors and colors of jellybeans increases intake.[59] These studies have taken a step further to suggest that greater variety, even in a characteristic unrelated to food taste or energy, can increase intake. When Kahn and Wansink provided people with M&Ms in either seven or ten colors, those that had the increased color variety consumed more candies in 1 hour than the individuals given less color variety.[59]

6.3.5 Palatability

In today's society, where food consumption is often driven by pleasure, rather than a need for calories, palatability of food is an important factor in food intake. There are many indications that regular exposure to palatable food in and of itself stimulates hunger including the following:

1. Relative to a bland food, consumption of a palatable food actually produces a small increase in hunger early in a meal, as well as a delay in the rate of decline of palatability as the meal progresses.
2. Self-rated appetite is increased by merely seeing a preferred food.
3. Consumption of an equicaloric palatable as opposed to a bland preload produces less reduction in hunger in the former condition.
4. Consumption of palatable foods produces a more rapid recovery of hunger than less palatable foods up to 3 hours following their consumption.[60]

In this section we decomposed environmental influences into discrete categories, addressing each one individually. However, in reality many of these environmental influences occur in conjunction. For example, eating a meal at a restaurant means being bombarded by a variety of delicious, high-energy-density foods, served in large portion sizes. These factors probably combine synergistically to drive excessive consumption. For instance, if a bland food (a plain baked potato) were supersized, it probably would not lead to as much additional intake as supersizing French fries. Although there are not sufficient long-term studies of people's ability to compensate for overconsumption, it is plausible that the combined effect of these food-related stimuli in the environment may repeatedly motivate eating "beyond hunger" and produce weight gain.

6.4 PSYCHOSOCIAL INFLUENCES

There is a very broad range of psychosocial variables that have been associated with qualitative and quantitative aspects of food intake (e.g., cultural norms, food attitudes and beliefs, goal-setting, decision-making, self-efficacy, mother–child interactions, etc.). Given the large number of relevant topics and studies, we will simplify the task of addressing them by dividing them into two broad categories. These categories reflect two fundamentally different levels of analysis: the cultural and the individual levels. It is also important to point out that psychosocial influences on eating motivation, even more than the other influences we have discussed (such as avoiding food intake because of dieting or for religious reasons), are relevant to both the promotion of eating and to its inhibition.

6.4.1 Cultural Influences on Food Intake

Cultural influences on food intake are so pervasive and obvious that documenting them seems almost unnecessary. Such influences are evident both within individual countries (e.g., differences between Caucasian, African American, and Asian American communities within the United States) and between countries (e.g., the

United States and France). There is broad agreement that, while the motivation to meet energy needs is instinctive, the particular manner in which individuals learn to satisfy these needs depends mostly on the familial and cultural context in which they develop and live.[61] One question of particular relevance to this chapter is the extent to which these conclusions apply equally to food intake that satisfies energy needs (the satisfaction of homeostatic hunger) and food intake that surpasses energy needs (the satisfaction of hedonic hunger).

Several studies have compared eating-related habits and customs in France with those in either the United States or England. Such comparisons are thought to be instructive in understanding the possible role of cultural differences in food intake, because all three of these countries are highly developed and modern and their populations have ready access to a variety of palatable foods, making overconsumption more likely. Yet rates of overweight and obesity are far lower in France than in the United States and England. Available research suggests that French culture inculcates norms for food intake that help explain these differences. Rozin et al.[62] interviewed 6000 individuals in the United States and France, among other countries. They asked respondents whether they would prefer being given a choice between 10 or 50 ice cream flavors. The 50-choice option was preferred only by respondents in the United States. U.S. respondents also expected there to be more menu choice options in a restaurant compared to respondents in other countries. Pettinger et al.[63] studied approximately 800 individuals in France and southern England. They found that the French differed from the English in using raw ingredients in cooking more often, ate together as a household more often, and were more likely to follow a regular meal pattern of three meals per day. The English more often relied on ready-prepared and take-away meals, as well as on energy-dense snack foods.

It should also be noted that although French cultural norms appear to help protect the French from the epidemic levels of obesity seen in other developed countries, there is evidence that aspects of the French food environment also help prevent the level of overconsumption seen in other countries. For instance, Rozin et al.[48] found that, relative to the situation in the United States, restaurant portion sizes and portion sizes included in cookbooks are smaller in France. Taken together, the preceding findings suggest that both normative and environmental aspects of a country's culture can help prevent overconsumption and weight gain that might otherwise occur. Indeed, it is plausible that these two factors can combine synergistically to facilitate weight control (e.g., even if people are taught to eat appropriate portion sizes, this cultural practice may have little effect if oversized portions are regularly served in restaurants and cafeterias).

6.4.2 Cognitive Models of Individual Differences in Eating Motivation

Psychosocial variables have been used not only to account for differences in eating behavior between ethnic, racial, national, or cultural groups (as reviewed above), but also to account for individual differences between people within a given cultural context. A wide array of cognitively based theories have been applied to understand, for instance, how to prevent obesity,[64] why some obese people are vulnerable to binge eating,[65] why eating disorders are so persistent,[66] or how attempts to cognitively restrain food intake can produce disinhibitory eating.[67] A sampling of theories that have been applied to understand — and sometimes to treat — aberrant eating behaviors includes self-efficacy theory, the theory of planned behavior, the transtheoretical model, the theory of reasoned action, and self-determination theory. Although these models have sometimes been successfully used to predict various health-related behaviors, for the most part they have not led to advances in the treatment of eating or weight control problems.[64] Similarly, although cognitive therapy techniques have been added to behavioral weight loss programs over the past 20 years, there is little evidence that they have contributed to improved outcomes.[68] In addition, evidence suggests that the direct modification of eating behavior accounts for improvement in bulimia nervosa more than the cognitive modification components of treatment.[69] The cognitive model of restrained eating[67] has also not held up well to experimental tests.[15,37] Part of the reason that cognitive approaches do not have substantial support for their efficacy in eating or weight control may be that cognitively based self-control strategies are overmatched by the combination of an obesogenic environment and the biobehavioral predispositions that make certain individuals susceptible to overconsume in such an environment.[70] Alternatively, the reviewed evidence suggests that biological, environmental, and cultural norms all have powerful effects in determining the eating patterns of individuals. Given this, it may simply be the case that much of the variance in eating behavior and body weight is accounted for by these domains, leaving little room for individual differences in cognitive functioning to yield much influence.

6.5 IDEAS FOR FUTURE ANIMAL RESEARCH

With today's eating environment, increased food consumption is being driven by a number of factors. Not only are people consuming an increased number of calories in each sitting, but they are presumably also eating more times each day. Given the omnipresence of food in today's society, it is hard to avoid situations in which highly palatable food is present or readily available. This relatively new form of exposure to — and frequent consumption of — palatable foods generates many testable research questions. For example, what are the effects of this frequent and persistent consumption, and the subsequent repeated activation of the associated reward brain circuitry? What are the effects of being constantly exposed to and tempted by palatable food without eating it (a situation that restrained eaters may often encounter)? Some of these questions, such as inquiring into the neuronal effects of palatable eating or food exposure, can best be addressed in animal models.

Most previous research on restrained eating and dieting in humans has assumed that dieters are susceptible to overeating because they are frequently or chronically energy deprived. However, much of the current research suggests that most restrained eaters are not energy deprived, in an absolute sense, but are trying to refrain from engaging in hedonic eating (i.e., they appear to be eating less than wanted, not less than needed).[15] Exploring eating behaviors (and their neurophysiological mediators) in animals that are in differing levels of energy balance (negative, neutral, positive) will allow distinctions to be made between drivers of homeostatically and hedonically motivated eating.

Animal models can be used to specifically address the hedonic properties of palatable foods, while controlling for the gustatory sensations and caloric benefits that play obvious roles in the overall eating process. For example, sham feeding (where the stomach is drained of all food through a fistula in the stomach, before caloric absorption) could be used to examine the pleasurable aspects of eating. Not only would this hedonically driven model allow for an examination of the neurological effects of frequent access to palatable foods on the brain, outside of the context of calories, but it would also permit the exploration of behaviors associated with repeated exposure to highly palatable foods. Noncaloric palatable foods, such as saccharin-water, could also be used to address the effects of palatability in animals without adding the confounding stimulus of energy.

From the perspective of homeostatic regulation, or of a set point for fat mass, it makes sense that the more one eats, and the higher body weight rises, the weaker hedonic eating motivation should become. Alternatively, the more positive reinforcement is experienced, perhaps the more one needs to be further reinforced in order to reach the same level of hedonic reward. Animal models could be used to determine if a homeostatic set point perspective is most appropriate here, or if an ever-increasing hedonic tolerance model is more likely. Further, it could be determined how many of the consequences of hedonically motivated eating are due to the gustatory, as opposed to the caloric and energy balance consequences of such eating. It is possible, for instance, that weight gain due to overconsumption of palatable food increases, rather than decreases, the strength of hedonic motivations to eat.

Further experiments should also expand the context of animal analogues to increase their potential relevance to human appetite. For example, it would be desirable to develop an animal analogue of restrained, normal-weight individuals that employs rats that are "hedonically deprived" (that is, like human restrained eaters, they are exposed frequently to highly palatable foods, but only sometimes eat them). Also, studying animals early in life, before they have experienced high-fat diets and the accompanying weight gain, would give insight into whether responses to food exposure predict degree of future weight gain when palatable foods become more regularly available. This would allow for the determination of any interactions between developmental stages and the obesogenic tendencies of animals.

Finally, it has been found in population studies that increases in BMI over time have not been linear, in that a higher percentage of Americans have shifted from overweight to obese than from normal weight to overweight.[71] Could this mean that being overweight makes an obesogenic environment even more irresistible?

REFERENCES

1. Friedman, M.I. and Stricker, E.M., The physiological psychology of hunger: a physiological perspective, *Psychol. Rev.,* 83(6), 409–431, 1976.
2. Keesey, R., A set-point theory of obesity, in *Handbook of Eating Disorders,* Brownell, K., Foreyt, J., Eds., Basic Books, New York, 1986.
3. Woods, S.C., The eating paradox: how we tolerate food, *Psychol. Rev.,* 98(4), 488–505, 1991.
4. Konner, M., *The Tangled Wing: Biological Constraints on the Human Spirit,* W.H. Freeman and Company, New York, 1982.

5. Wells, J.C., The evolution of human fatness and susceptibility to obesity: an ethological approach, *Biol. Rev. Camb. Philos. Soc.,* 81(2), 183–205, 2006.
6. Cabanac, M., Ed., Palatability of food and the ponderostat, in *The Psychobiology of Human Eating Disorders: Preclinical and Clinical Perspectives,* Schneider, L.H., Cooper, S.J., and Halmi, K.A., Eds., New York Academy of Sciences, New York, 1989, pp. 340–352.
7. Levine, A.S., The animal model in food intake regulation: examples from the opioid literature, *Physiol. Behav.,* 89(1), 92–96, 2006.
8. Berthoud, H., Interactions between the "cognitive" and "metabolic" brain in the control of food intake, *Physiol. Behav.,* 91(5), 486–498, 2007.
9. Butryn, M.L., Lowe, M.R., Safer, D.L., and Agras, W.S., Weight suppression is a robust predictor of outcome in the cognitive-behavioral treatment of bulimia nervosa, *J. Abnorm. Psychol.,* 115(1), 62–67, 2006.
10. Keys, A., Brozek, K., Henschel, A., Mickelsen, O., and Taylor, H.L., *The Biology of Human Starvation,* University of Minnesota Press, Minneapolis, 1950.
11. Lowe, M.R., Davis, W., Lucks, D., Annunziato, R., and Butryn, M., Weight suppression predicts weight gain during inpatient treatment of bulimia nervosa, *Physiol. Behav.,* 87(3), 487–492, 2006.
12. Levitsky, D.A., The non-regulation of food intake in humans: hope for reversing the epidemic of obesity, *Physiol. Behav.,* 86(5), 623–632, 2005.
13. Levine, A.S. and Billington, C.J., Why do we eat? A neural systems approach. *Annu. Rev. Nutr.,* 17, 597–619, 1997.
14. Lowe, M.R. and Butryn, M.L., Hedonic hunger: a new dimension of appetite? *Physiol. Behav.,* 91(4), 432–439, 2007.
15. Lowe, M.R. and Levine, A.S., Eating motives and the controversy over dieting: eating less than needed versus less than wanted, *Obes. Res.,* 13, 797–805, 2005.
16. Glass, M.J., Grace, M., Cleary, J.P., Billington, C.J., and Levine, A.S., Potency of naloxone's anorectic effect in rats is dependent on diet preference, *Am. J. Physiol.,* 271(40), R217–R221, 1996.
17. Parker, L.A., Maier, S., Rennie, M., and Crebolder, J., Morphine- and naltrexone-induced modification of palatability: analysis by the taste reactivity test, *Behav. Neurosci.,* 106(6), 999–1010, 1992.
18. Volkow, N.D. and Wise, R.A., How can drug addiction help us understand obesity? *Nat. Neurosci.,* 8(5), 555–560, 2005.
19. Trinko, R., Sears, R.M., Guarnieri, D.J., and Dileone, R.J., Neural mechanisms underlying obesity and drug addiction, *Physiol. Behav.,* 91(5), 499–505, 2007.
20. Colantuoni, C., Rada, P., McCarthy, J., et al., Evidence that intermittent, excessive sugar intake causes endogenous opioid dependence, *Obes. Res.,* 10(6), 478–488, 2002.
21. Le Magnen, J., A role of opiates in food reward and food addiction, in *Taste, Experience, and Feeding,* Capaldi, E.D. and Powley, T.L., Eds., American Psychological Association, Washington, DC, 1990, pp. 241–252.
22. Teegarden, S. and Bale, T., Decreases in dietary preference produce increased emotionality and risk for dietary relapse, *Biol. Psychiatry,* 61, 1021–1029, 2007.
23. Barbano, M.F. and Cador, M., Various aspects of feeding behavior can be partially dissociated in the rat by the incentive properties of food and the physiological state [see comment], *Behav. Neurosci.,* 119(5), 1244–1253, 2005.
24. Dimitriou, S.G., Rice, H.B., and Corwin, R.L., Effects of limited access to a fat option on food intake and body composition in female rats, *Int. J. Eat. Disord.,* 28, 436–445, 2000.
25. Morton, G.J., Cummings, D.E., Baskin, D.G., Barsh, G.S., and Schwartz, M.W., Central nervous system control of food intake and body weight, *Nature,* 443(7109), 289–295, 2006.
26. Bray, G.A., Obesity is a chronic, relapsing neurochemical disease, *Int. J. Obes. Relat. Metab. Disord.,* 28(1), 34–38, 2004.

27. DelParigi, A., Pannacciulli, N., Le, D.N., and Tataranni, P.A., In pursuit of neural risk factors for weight gain in humans, *Neurobiol. Aging,* 26 (Suppl. 1), 50–55, 2005.
28. Tataranni, P.A. and DelParigi, A., Functional neuroimaging: a new generation of human brain studies in obesity research, *Obes. Rev.,* 4(4), 229–238, 2003.
29. Tataranni, P.A., Gautier, J.F., Chen, K., et al., Neuroanatomical correlates of hunger and satiation in humans using positron emission tomography, *Proc. Natl. Acad. Sci. USA,* 96(8), 4569–4574, 1999.
30. Small, D.M., Zatorre, R.J., Dagher, A., Evans, A.C., and Jones-Gotman, M., Changes in brain activity related to eating chocolate: from pleasure to aversion, *Brain,* 124(9), 1720–1733, 2001.
31. Hinton, E.C., Parkinson, J.A., Holland, A.J., Arana, F.S., Roberts, A.C., and Owen, A.M., Neural contributions to the motivational control of appetite in humans, *Eur. J. Neurosci.,* 20(5), 1411–1418, 2004.
32. Del Parigi, A., Gautier, J.F., Chen, K., Salbe, A.D., Ravussin, E., and Tataranni, P.A., Neuroimaging and obesity: mapping the brain responses to hunger and satiation in humans using positron emission tomography, *Ann. N.Y. Acad. Sci.,* 967, 389–397, 2002.
33. Wang, G.J., Volkow, N.D., Logan, J., et al., Brain dopamine and obesity, *Lancet,* 357(9253), 354–357, 2001.
34. DelParigi, A., Chen, K., Salbe, A.D., et al., Persistence of abnormal neural responses to a meal in postobese individuals, *Int. J. Obes. Relat. Metab. Disord.,* 28(3), 370–377, 2004.
35. Herman, C.P. and Polivy, J., Restrained eating, in *Obesity,* Stunkard, A.J., Ed., Saunders, Philadelphia, PA, 1980, 208–225.
36. Polivy, J. and Herman, C.P., Diagnosis and treatment of normal eating. *J. Consult. Clin. Psychol.,* 55(5), 635–644, 1987.
37. Lowe, M.R., The effects of dieting on eating behavior: a three-factor model. *Psychol. Bull.,* 114, 100–121, 1993.
38. Lowe, M.R. and Kral, T.V.E., Stress-induced eating in restrained eaters may not be caused by stress or restraint, *Appetite,* 46, 16–21, 2006.
39. Stice, E., Fisher, M., and Lowe, M.R., Are dietary restraint scales valid measures of dietary restriction? Unobtrusive observational data suggest not, *Psychol. Assess.,* 16(1), 51–59, 2004.
40. Chernyak, Y. and Lowe, M.R., Fear of fatness of drive to be thin: motivations for dieting in normal weight women, in preparation.
41. Thomas, J.G., Wallaert, M., and Lowe, M.R., What motivates restrained eating in normal weight women? *Beh. Res. Ther.,* under review.
42. Herman, C.P. and Polivy, J., Normative influences on food intake, *Physiol. Behav.,* 86(5), 762–772, 2005.
43. Cota, D., Tschop, M.H., Horvath, T.L., and Levine, A.S., Cannabinoids, opioids and eating behavior: the molecular face of hedonism? *Brain Res. Rev.,* 51(1), 85–107, 2006.
44. Irani, B.G., Dunn-Meynell, A.A., and Levin, B.E., Altered hypothalamic leptin, insulin, and melanocortin binding associated with moderate-fat diet and predisposition to obesity, *Endocrinology,* 148(1), 310–316, 2007.
45. Hill, J.O., Wyatt, H.R., Reed, G.W., and Peters, J.C., Obesity and the environment: where do we go from here? [see comment], *Science,* 299(5608), 853–855, 2003.
46. Heatherton, T.F., Polivy, J., and Herman, C.P., Restraint and internal responsiveness: effects of placebo manipulations of hunger state on eating, *J. Abnorm. Psychol.,* 98(1), 89–92, 1989.
47. Ello-Martin, J.A., Ledikwe, J.H., and Rolls, B.J., The influence of food portion size and energy density on energy intake: implications for weight management, *Am. J. Clin. Nutr.,* 82 (Suppl. 1), 236S–241S, 2005.

48. Rozin, P., Kabnick, K., Pete, E., Fischler, C., and Shields, C., The ecology of eating: smaller portion sizes in France than in the United States help explain the French paradox, *Psychol. Sci.,* 14(5), 450–454, 2003.
49. Wansink, B., Environmental factors that increase the food intake and consumption volume of unknowing consumers, *Annu. Rev. Nutr.,* 24, 455–479, 2004.
50. Geier, A.B., Rozin, P., and Doros, G., Unit bias. A new heuristic that helps explain the effect of portion size on food intake, *Psychol. Sci.,* 17(6), 521–525, 2006.
51. Wansink, B., van Ittersum, K., and Painter, J.E., Ice cream illusions bowls, spoons, and self-served portion sizes, *Am. J. Prev. Med.,* 31(3), 240–243, 2006.
52. Kral, T.V., Roe, L.S., and Rolls, B.J., Combined effects of energy density and portion size on energy intake in women, *Am. J. Clin. Nutr.,* 79(6), 962–968, 2004.
53. Rolls, B.J., Roe, L.S., and Meengs, J.S., Reductions in portion size and energy density of foods are additive and lead to sustained decreases in energy intake, *Am. J. Clin. Nutr.,* 83(1), 11–17, 2006.
54. Raynor, H.A. and Epstein, L.H., Dietary variety, energy regulation, and obesity, *Psychol. Bull.,* 127(3), 325–341, 2001.
55. Meiselman, H.L., deGraaf, C., and Lesher, L.L., The effects of variety and monotony on food acceptance and intake at a midday meal, *Physiol. Behav.,* 70(1–2), 119–125, 2000.
56. Zandstra, E.H., De Graaf, C., and Van Trijp, H.C.M., Effects of variety and repeated in-home consumption on product acceptance, *Appetite,* 35(2), 113–119, 2000.
57. Rolls, B.J., Rolls, E.T., Rowe, E.A., and Sweeney, K., Sensory specific satiety in man, *Physiol. Behav.,* 27(1), 137–142, 1981.
58. Rolls, B.J., Experimental analyses of the effects of variety in a meal on human feeding, *Am. J. Clin. Nutr.,* 42 (Suppl. 5), 932–939, 1985.
59. Kahn, B.E. and Wansink, B., The influence of assortment structure on perceived variety and consumption quantities, *J. Consum. Res.,* 30(4), 519–533, 2004.
60. Yeomans, M.R., Blundell, J.E., and Leshem, M., Palatability: response to nutritional need or need-free stimulation of appetite, *Br. J. Nutr.,* 92(1S), S3–14, 2004.
61. Capaldi, E.D. and Powley, T.L., Eds., *Taste, Experience, and Feeding,* American Psychological Association, Washington, DC, 1990.
62. Rozin, P., Fischler, C., Shields, C., and Masson, E., Attitudes towards large numbers of choices in the food domain: a cross-cultural study of five countries in Europe and the USA, *Appetite,* 46(3), 304–308, 2006.
63. Pettinger, C., Holdsworth, M., and Gerber, M., Meal patterns and cooking practices in Southern France and Central England, *Public Health Nutr.,* 9(8), 1020–1026, 2006.
64. Baranowski, T., Cullen, K.W., Nicklas, T., Thompson, D., and Baranowski, J., Are current health behavioral change models helpful in guiding prevention of weight gain efforts? *Obes. Res.,* 11 (Suppl.), 23S–43S, 2003.
65. Wonderlich, S.A., de Zwaan, M., Mitchell, J.E., Peterson, C., and Crow, S., Psychological and dietary treatments of binge eating disorder: conceptual implications, *Int. J. Eat. Disord.,* 34 (Suppl.), S58–73, 2003.
66. Fairburn, C.G. and Brownell, K.D., *Eating Disorders and Obesity: A Comprehensive Handbook,* Guilford Press, New York, 2002.
67. Herman, C.P. and Polivy, J., A boundary model for the regulation of eating, in *Eating and its Disorders,* Stunkard, A.J. and Stellar, E., Eds., Raven Press, New York, 1984, pp. 141–156.
68. Wadden, T.A. and Butryn, M.L., Behavioral treatment of obesity, *Endocrinol. Metab. Clin. North Am.,* 32(4), 981–1003, 2003.
69. Kraemer, H.C., Wilson, G.T., Fairburn, C.G., and Agras, W.S., Mediator of moderators of treatment effects in randomized clinical trials, *Arch. Gen. Psychiatry,* 59, 877–883, 2002.

70. Lowe, M.R., Self-regulation of energy intake in the prevention and treatment of obesity: is it feasible? *Obes. Res.*, 11 (Suppl.), 44S–59S, 2003.
71. National Center for Health Statistics, *Health, United States, 2005 with Chartbook on Trends in the Health of Americans,* National Center for Health Statistics, Hyattsville, MD, 2005.

7 Orosensory Control of Feeding

Thomas R. Scott

CONTENTS

7.1 INTRODUCTION

The acquisition of nutrients is the most basic of biological requirements. Each creature must regularly assimilate an array of nutrients to serve the biochemical processes that define its existence. The single purpose of human appetite is to begin the alchemy of turning other organisms into humans.

The sexual motive is nearly as ancient as feeding, but more simply satisfied and less urgent. Indeed, successful reproduction is predicated on satisfactory nutrition, for insemination requires energy, and pregnancy only strains nutritional resources, which therefore must prove themselves adequate for conception to occur. Sex is an activity of the fed. Thirst is a newcomer among biological drives. It evolved only in the past few hundred million years as our ancestors emerged from the seas with the demand that they continue to bathe each cell in the very fluids they had forsaken.

The search for and acquisition of nutrients is a relentless task that has constituted a central pressure on the evolution of sensory, motor, and cognitive capacities of animals. In the lethal contest between predator and prey, three major types of sensory systems have evolved on each side: vision, sensitivity to vibration (touch, hearing, and lateral line systems), and chemical sensitivity.

The chemical senses are the most primitive of these three, having evolved specialized sensory organs as long as 500 million years ago in coelenterates.[1] They remain the dominant sensory systems across the animal kingdom as well as within the class Mammalia. We humans are unusual mammals in placing such reliance on vision and hearing. We come to this from our primate heritage, aloft in trees or raised up by our bipedal gait. The collection of sensory systems on our heads is lifted away from the odiferous earth and provided the long views that give value to vision. Yet chemical senses are central to mammalian evolution and so should have pervasive, if sometimes subtle, influences on human behavior. In accord with their age and status, smell and taste largely manage the two most fundamental biological functions: eating to preserve the individual and reproduction to preserve the species. The sense of taste has become more specialized to serve eating; the sense of smell, reproduction.

Animals sense chemicals that originate both within and beyond the body. Internal communication is accomplished largely through the release of chemicals from one site and their recognition at another, whether it is 200 Å away as in synaptic transmission, or perhaps a meter away as with leptin, insulin, cytokines, or glucose. In contrast, the capacity to detect those from outside the body is only poorly developed. Significant deviations from a pH of 7 can lead to sensations of acidity or causticity anywhere on the skin, and certain toxins (poison ivy, poison oak, etc.) may elicit a histamine response. The skin, however, is only a crude chemical detector. The exceptions to this are the points where most chemicals enter the body: the nose and mouth. Here, chemoreception is refined, complex, and subtle, for decisions must be made about which chemicals to admit. Smell and taste are the beginnings of a long chemosensory tube that extends from the face through the intestines, with receptors along its length that are sensitive to the products released by digestion. Consequently, the chemical senses should be responsive to feedback from the gut that is a continuation of their own function, an implication to be confirmed later in this chapter. This system represents a core of chemosensitivity that mediates between the vast array of chemicals around us, and the subset of them that serve our tightly regulated biochemical needs.

Chemoreceptors in the mouth are not fundamentally different from those in the rest of the body. The recognition of glucose by a taste receptor and by a β-cell in the pancreas both proceed by similar mechanisms, leading to a perception of sweetness in one case, to a release of insulin in the other. The passage of sodium ions through amiloride-sensitive channels produces a salty taste on the tongue, but sodium resorption in the kidney. The umami taste of monosodium glutamate and the recognition of glutamate throughout the central nervous system are probably managed by the same receptor, albeit tuned to different concentrations.

What distinguishes the chemical senses is not that they recognize these molecules, but that they do so before the irrevocable decision to swallow has been made. Taste is located at the interface between the uncontrolled external chemical world, and our highly regulated biochemical environment, and its primary role is to reduce the former to the latter. While preliminary assessments are provided by other senses

— notably touch, vision, and olfaction — and by central processes of familiarity and cultural norms, nonetheless, each chemical that enters the mouth goes before a gustatory judge whose only verdicts are swallow or not swallow.

As chemical gatekeeper, taste provides an assessment of the nutritional value or toxic consequences of a potential food. This input is sent to at least four locations: to the gut to help mediate gastrointestinal reflexes, to the hindbrain to control the somatic reflexes for ingestion or rejection, to the thalamus and insular cortex for a cognitive appreciation of the taste, and to the orbitofrontal cortex and ventral forebrain to be integrated with sight, smell, and texture to generate an hedonic response that provides among our most intense pleasure or revulsion. It is the hedonic value that determines whether a bite will be extended to a meal, a meal to a diet.

7.2 GUSTATORY ANATOMY

7.2.1 Receptors

Humans vary by a factor of 100 in the number of taste receptor cells they possess, but the mean is about 300,000.[2] They are gathered in groups of about 50 in goblet-shaped taste buds, of which the mean number in humans is about 6000. Approximately two thirds are located on the dorsal surface of the tongue, where they are housed in small swellings called papillae (Lat: nipple) (Figure 7.1). On the front of the tongue are about 200 fungiform (Lat: mushroom-shaped) papillae, each of which contains from 0 to 36 buds, with a mean of 3. Thus, a typical person has about 600 taste buds in fungiform papillae.

On each lateral margin of the tongue are 5 to 7 folds referred to as foliate (Lat: leaf-shaped) papillae. The groove between each pair of swellings may contain 100 buds, for a total of 1200. On the posterior tongue are 7 to 11 circumvallate (Lat: surrounded by a trench) papillae arranged in the form of a chevron. The moat that surrounds each papilla is lined with taste buds, a mean of 250 per papilla, or about 2200 altogether. Beyond these 4000 buds on the tongue surface are another 2000 embedded in the soft palate, pharynx, larynx, and epiglottis. Without papillae to fix their locations, they are broadly distributed.

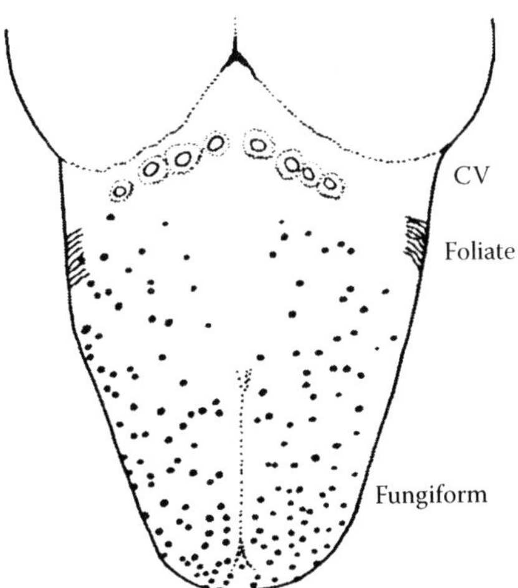

FIGURE 7.1 Sketch of the human tongue to illustrate the form and location of fungiform, foliate, and circumvallate (CV) papillae. (From Mistretta, C.M., *Ann. N.Y. Acad. Sci.*, 561, 277, 1989. With permission.)

Taste buds are of similar shape and composition wherever they occur in the mouth. Each is a collection of perhaps 50 taste cells, arranged like sections of an orange (Figure 7.2). The resulting globular structure is about 30 μm in diameter and 50 μm in length. At the base of the bud is a sturdy membrane surrounded

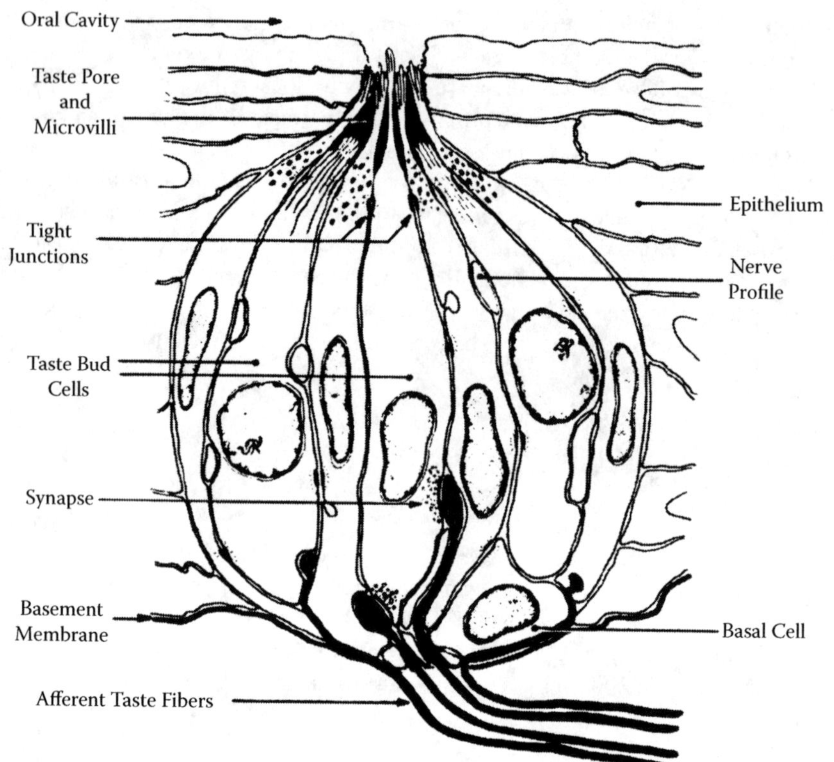

FIGURE 7.2 Sketch of a taste bud and its components. (From Mistretta, C.M., *Ann. N.Y. Acad. Sci.*, 561, 277, 1989. With permission.)

by flattened cells that join to create a shell in which the bud nestles. Thus, each is practically isolated, with no apparent electrical or diffusional interaction with its neighbors. At the top is a 6-μm-diameter pore through which the microvilli of its 50 receptor cells project to sample the environment.

Taste receptor cells are thought to be created continuously from basal cells at the periphery of the bud, and to migrate toward the center where they are dispatched after an average life span of 10 days.

7.2.2 Peripheral Nerves

The peripheral anatomy of the taste system offers such complexity that it was not clarified until the 1930s. Four cranial nerves drain the diverse gustatory receptive fields, and the information they carry is mixed with that from touch and motor fibers that travel in parallel with taste axons.

Taste fibers innervating the front of the tongue exit as part of cranial nerve V (trigeminal), but soon depart to join nerve VII (facial). They are joined by axons from the soft palate to form the sensory component of the predominantly motor nerve VII. At their central terminus, they enter the rostral division of the nucleus of the solitary tract (NTS).

Fibers serving the mid and posterior regions of the tongue join nerve IX (glossopharyngeal) and proceed to the NTS. Those that serve the esophagus and epiglottis become part of nerve X (vagus) and pass to the NTS.

7.2.3 Central Taste System

7.2.3.1 Nucleus of the Solitary Tract (NTS)

While the course of peripheral taste nerves remained controversial into the twentieth century, their destination did not (Figure 7.3). All three terminate in orderly fashion in the rostral division of the NTS in caudal medulla.[3–6] This crucial structure receives taste input in its rostral half, touch and temperature immediately lateral to taste, and visceral afferents more medially and caudally. Thus information concerning taste, which largely determines which chemicals enter the body, appropriately terminates in close contiguity with touch and temperature from the mouth (permitting an early integration of some components of flavor), and with fibers from the viscera through which the consequences of having swallowed a chemical may be reported.

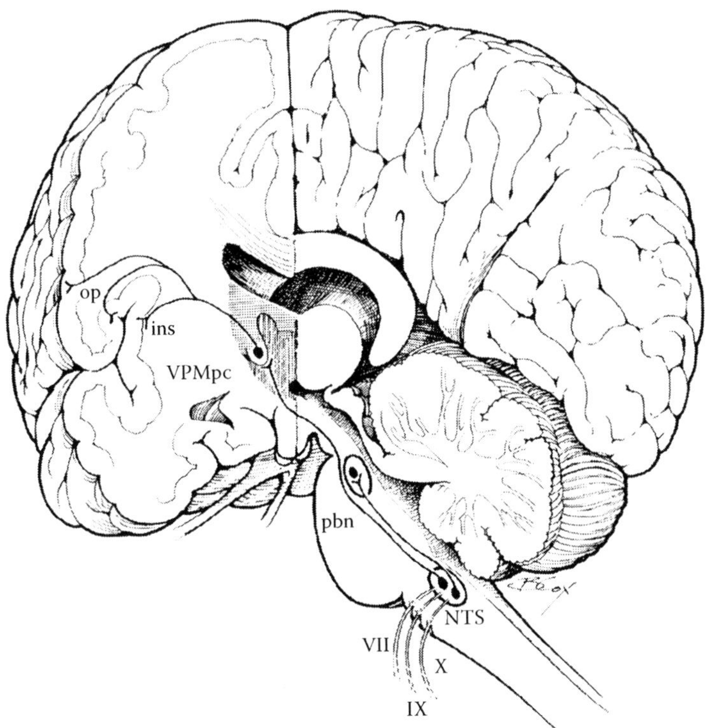

FIGURE 7.3 The human brain, showing the sensory pathways for taste through primary taste cortex (insula). NTS: nucleus of the solitary tract; pbn: parabrachial nucleus; op: operculum; ins: insula; VPMpc: parvicellular division of the ventroposteromedial nucleus of the thalamus. (From Pritchard, T.C., in *Taste and Smell in Health and Disease,* Getchell, T.V., Doty, R.L., Bartoshuk, L.M., and Snow, J.B. Jr., Eds., Raven Press, New York, 1991, p. 109. With permission.)

7.2.3.2 Thalamic Taste Area

Fibers from the NTS in primates project to a small region in the medial thalamus (Figure 7.3). About one-third of the cells here respond to taste stimulation,[7] while others are activated by touch and temperature in the mouth and by visceral stimulation of the vagus nerve. Thus, the intimate relationship, whereby taste is located between oral touch on the one side and visceral sensations on the other, is apparently maintained.

7.2.3.3 Primary Taste Cortex

Taste realizes its cortical representation along the sharp bend that extends from the anterior insula to the frontal operculum, known most commonly as insular cortex (Figure 7.3). The area has been explored extensively, revealing that only about 6% of its cells respond to taste stimuli.[8] Others are activated by jaw movements or touch in the mouth. Functional MRI studies have shown that humans shown expressions of disgust (literally, bad taste) experienced activation of the insula. Thus the same area that houses taste neurons also has cells that permit a visual appreciation of the social expression of a taste experience.[9] Insular cortex also receives visceral sensations and sends axons to regions that guide both oral and visceral reflexes associated with foods. It has the components to be labeled "ingestive cortex."

7.2.3.4 Beyond Primary Taste Cortex

In the macaque, neurons in insular cortex project forward to end in various subdivisions of the orbitofrontal cortex (OFC). These fibers are joined by those from vision, olfaction, and touch to form a sensory network from which an integrated appreciation of flavor can be extracted. The insula also projects to the central nucleus of the amygdala (CNA), which has robust reciprocal connections with OFC. The amygdala is an important site for processing taste information, as well as for the motivational aspects of eating.[10] Both OFC and CNA — receiving parallel input and themselves interconnected — project to the lateral hypothalamic area (LHA), which is also involved in the motivation to eat.

Finally, all forebrain taste areas send projections back to the NTS, establishing a circuit through which higher-order functions such as conditioning can affect the reflexive acceptance or rejection of foods.

7.3 GUSTATORY CONTROL OF EATING

7.3.1 The Organization of the Taste System

All sensory systems must build receptors that are sensitive to the physical environment they are charged to monitor. With taste, there are at least six receptor mechanisms. Four are committed to detecting the major components of our diet: carbohydrates (sweet), fats, proteins (umami), and sodium (salt); two others are vigilant to the primary threats to our biochemical welfare: acidity (sour) and toxins (bitter). Two of the mechanisms — for salt and sour — rely on the passage of small sodium and hydrogen ions through molecular membranes. The other four require specialized protein receptors.

This federation of receptor mechanisms stands in contrast to the strategies of vision, hearing, and olfaction, each of which employs a single receptor process, though with receptors tuned to different parts of the physical dimension they are assigned to detect (e.g., red versus blue). Taste is more akin to the skin senses, where touch, pressure, temperature, pain, and others are separate sensations. Failed attempts to integrate the basic taste sensations at the receptor level has even led to the suggestion that taste is not a single sense, but a series of half a dozen senses housed in a common location.

Yet there is a common organizing principle of taste. It eluded researchers because gustatory physiologists adopted the vision model to investigate their discipline, seeking to establish the relationship between the physical stimulus (wavelength) and the perceptual result (color). Taste is faced with a different requirement. Alone among the senses, it must evaluate whether a stimulus will become part of the body. Taste is charged not only with detecting a stimulus as other sensory systems are, but also with predicting the impact of that chemical on the animal's physiological welfare. The organizing principle of taste is not physical, but physiological.[11]

The effectiveness with which taste manages this obligation is demonstrated in a behavioral study in which naïve rats under 18-hour fluid deprivation were offered 15-second exposures to a wide sample of chemicals that appear in the natural environment.[12] In these brief tests, with neither experience nor postingestive feedback to guide them, rats rejected chemicals in direct proportion to toxicity. Rats inherit a taste system that permits accurate judgments about toxicity across a broad range of chemicals with diverse physical characteristics. While strychnine and cadmium possess entirely different molecular structures and poison the consumer by wholly different mechanisms, the taste system, as chemical guardian of the body, has the receptors to be vigilant to both. Moreover, the more assiduously a chemical was rejected by rats, the more likely it was to be described by humans as "bitter" or "nauseous"; chemicals avidly accepted by rats were labeled "food-like" or "pleasant." Thus the neural dimension of nutrition versus toxicity is directly related to acceptance versus rejection behavior in rats, and is perceptually coded in the hedonics of pleasant or unpleasant experiences by humans. With only a few exceptions, the better a chemical tastes, the more nutritious it is.

This basic assessment of whether a substance is nutritious or toxic is developed at birth, as demonstrated by the reactions of newborns to the delivery of sweet, salty, sour, or bitter tastes to tongues that had only moments before been cleared of amniotic fluid.[13] Sugars elicited licking and swallowing; quinine evoked gaping, rejection, and crying. Indeed, saccharin injected into the amniotic fluid 6 weeks before birth results in greater sucking and swallowing behavior in the fetus.

Anencephalic neonates, born with no forebrain, reacted identically to healthy babies, demonstrating that these acceptance–rejection reflexes are orchestrated in the hindbrain. The critical location would appear to be the NTS. This is the major hindbrain recipient of sensory information that originates within the body, including taste, respiration, blood pressure, blood pH, gastrointestinal activity, and pain.[14] Efferents from NTS regulate somatic reflexes both for acceptance and rejection, and autonomic reflexes associated with digestion.

To control somatic reflexes, clusters of cells in the ventral regions of gustatory NTS send projections to the retrofacial area, trigeminal motor nucleus, nucleus ambiguus, and hypoglossal nucleus. The contrary behavioral reactions of acceptance and rejection may be driven by anatomically distinct taste inputs.[15] The greater superficial petrosal and chorda tympani nerves are most sensitive to sweet and salty stimuli and could activate circuits that evoke acceptance responses. The glossopharyngeal nerve is responsive to sour and bitter qualities and could stimulate a separate population of NTS taste cells from which rejection reflexes were organized.

Autonomic reflexes are controlled by a second set of axons from ventral gustatory NTS, which travels caudally to viscerosensory NTS, to salivatory nuclei, and to the dorsal motor nucleus of the vagus to invoke parasympathetic processes associated with digestion.[16] These include salivation, gastric reflexes, and cephalic-phase releases of digestive enzymes and insulin. The dorsal motor nucleus of the vagus, whose output controls these processes, lies directly beneath the NTS and sends apical dendrites toward the taste area, though their contact with taste cells of the NTS has not yet been demonstrated. These cephalic-phase reflexes prepare the digestive system for the nutrients they are destined to receive when a sweet or other food-like taste is registered in NTS.

In the preceding section we found that the sense of taste is organized to perform a general differentiation of toxins from nutrients, and that this is accomplished at a brain stem level and is intact at, or before, birth in humans. Moreover, this analysis drives somatic reflexes of swallowing or rejection, parasympathetic reflexes that anticipate the digestive process and inform the hedonic reaction to the tasted chemical. While providing a broad and effective system for maintaining the biochemical welfare of the species, this organization would not allow for the idiosyncratic allergies or biochemical needs of the individual, or be sensitive to changes in those needs over time. The effects of experience — conditioned aversions or preferences — and of age, reproductive status, disease state, mineral needs, and level of satiety all affect behavioral reactions to foods. To serve these requirements, the taste code must be plastic.

7.3.2 Enduring Changes in Taste Based on Experience

An animal's experience has a pronounced and enduring effect on behavioral reactions to taste stimuli. The taste experiences of suckling rats establish preferences that persist to adulthood.[17,18] Preferences also develop through association of a taste with positive visceral reinforcement such as the delivery of a nutrient of which the animal has been deprived.[19–21] An efficient experimental paradigm has been developed to create conditioned preferences in rats.[22] Animals fitted with gastric cannulae are offered two taste solutions, equally preferred. Upon licking one, water is delivered into the stomach; with the other, a rich nutrient mix. After several days of trials, rats overwhelmingly select whichever taste solution was associated with the receipt of nutrients. Such learned preferences serve to bind members of a culture together through culinary identity. Each of the major cuisines of the world is characterized by unique flavors delivered with a nutritive carbohydrate load. Conditioned preferences for those tastes serve as the basis for the culinary rituals and social interactions identified with its culture.

The activity of single taste neurons in the NTS of rats reflects the neural changes that may underlie these conditioned preferences. Upon undergoing the experimental procedure described above, rats developed preferences for the taste solution associated with the gastric infusion of nutrients, as expected. Responses to these, as well as innately appetitive (glucose) and aversive (quinine) tastes were then monitored in the NTS. It was revealed that whichever taste had become preferred, its neural profile was less like those of aversive, and more like those of appetitive stimuli.[23] Thus, in rats, the taste system itself is altered at the brain stem level to reflect gustatory experiences, and this alteration may provide the basis for food preferences that develop throughout life.

Contrasted with the subtlety of conditioned preferences is the potent and instantaneous aversion resulting from a single pairing of a novel taste with nausea, the conditioned taste aversion (CTA). As opposed to gently guiding the animal toward tastes that have been associated with nutrients, the CTA is an intense alarm to protect the animal that survives its first encounter with a toxin from ever consuming that substance again.[24] It is so readily established, potent, and enduring that the CTA protocol has become a standard tool for studying taste behavior and physiology.

The mechanisms underlying the development of conditioned taste aversions have been studied mainly in rats. Taste-evoked activity in the NTS[25,26] and in the parabrachial nucleus (PBN)[27] rises to a taste that is paired with nausea. In the NTS, that increase is associated with a reorganization of inputs such that the incriminated taste no longer elicits swallowing reflexes and parasympathetic activity designed to ingest and assimilate the chemical, but rather rejection reflexes. In the PBN, the evoked activity shifts from a subnucleus associated with positive hedonics to one normally activated by aversive tastes.[28] Discrete subnuclei of the PBN are hypothesized to send separate projections to forebrain areas that analyze taste quality and hedonics. Thus, the shift in representation of the offending taste could serve as the basis for its reversed hedonic appeal, established in the brain stem but manifested in the forebrain.

7.3.3 Transient Changes in Taste Based on Physiological Needs

An animal's choice of foods is related to its physiological condition. The "body wisdom" demonstrated in cafeteria studies by Richter appears to be related to taste-directed changes in food preferences. Animals deprived of thiamine,[29] threonine,[30] or histidine[31] will experiment with different tasting foods until chancing upon one that supplies the missing nutrient.

Another need, reflected in a more constant and perhaps innate preference, is for sodium, whose concentration must be maintained at about 0.14 *M* to serve its functions of electrical conductance and the provision of osmotic force. Mammals seek out and consume salt, and when plentiful, do so in excess of need, as the American diet demonstrates.[32,33] This preference becomes exaggerated under conditions of sodium deficiency. Humans depleted by pathological states[34] or experimental manipulation[35] show a pronounced craving for salt. Similarly, rats subjected to uncontrolled urinary sodium loss following adrenalectomy,[36,37] to acute loss of plasma volume,[38] or to sodium dietary restriction[39] show sharp increases in sodium consumption. This compensatory response to the physiological need for salt results from a change in the hedonic value of tasted sodium. Concentrations that are rejected when the animal is sodium replete are avidly accepted when deprived. This change in taste-based behavior can also be traced to changes in the neural response to salt.

Activity generated by sodium in the peripheral taste nerves declines when a rat is in particular need of salt,[40,41] a result that should lead to the observed shift of the acceptance curve for sodium to higher concentrations. Recordings in the NTS reveal a more complex adaptation to the need for sodium. Responses to sodium in salt-deprived rats declined moderately, as expected from the peripheral nerve reports. But an analysis of the contributions of individual neurons revealed that salt-responsive neurons showed a precipitous reduction in evoked activity, and that this was partially offset by an increased response in neurons normally tuned to sweet tastes. Thus, the net effect was to transfer the burden of signaling sodium from salt toward sweet-oriented cells.[42] Thus, sodium might taste "sweet," or if sweetness is only a human construct, perhaps "good" to such a rat. This interpretation transcends a mere change in intensity perception and explains the eagerness with which deprived rats consume sodium, an avidity not created simply by decreasing the concentration of sodium, as the peripheral nerve work would imply. Whether based on changes in intensity or on a shift in perceived quality, however, it is clear that adaptive alterations in taste preferences are governed by modifications in the sensory code.

7.3.4 Momentary Changes in Taste Based on Level of Hunger

While the appreciation of amino acid or sodium deficiency occurs and may be restored over a period of days, the availability of glucose and other sources of energy is of almost hourly concern. There must be an accommodation of the decision to swallow or reject, and in the hedonic evaluation that drives that decision, as the dangers of malnutrition weigh against those of ingesting a toxin. Common experience reinforces the results of psychophysical studies: as hunger increases, foods become more palatable; with satiety, less so.[43–45] There is now a body of data from rats and primates that demonstrate the neural mechanisms underlying these changes.

The first effect of consuming a meal is gastric distension. Experimentally distending a rat's stomach with air causes the taste response to sucrose, recorded in the NTS, to decline, implying a less rewarding experience to the rat.[46] The next effect of a meal is to raise blood sugar levels. When these are increased experimentally through an intravenous infusion of glucose, taste responses to sugar in the NTS also decline.[47] Similar but smaller effects on taste activity are seen with modest infusions of insulin[48] or glucagon,[49] both of which result in the greater availability of glucose to the muscles. Thus, each procedure that delivers glucose to the body causes a transient reduction in sensitivity to sugars in the NTS. This implies a partial loss of the pleasure that sustains eating, making termination of a meal more likely.

If sensory activity in NTS, deep in the hindbrain, declines with satiety, the perceived intensity of a taste should also be reduced. This has indeed been shown to occur in rats.[50] Humans, however, respond differently. They report that the hedonic value of foods decreases with satiety, but intensity judgments are affected to a lesser extent, or not at all.[51,52] This prompted a series of studies in macaques, who had proven to be worthy surrogates for human gustation,[53] on the impact of satiety at various synaptic levels, from hindbrain to cortex.

The initial recordings were from the NTS to mimic those from the rat. A neuron was isolated, and its responses to sugar, salt, acid, and quinine were recorded. The monkey was then fed 50-ml aliquots of glucose, after each of which the responses to the same four taste stimuli in the NTS were reassessed.[54] As the monkey proceeded through this sequence, and as avid acceptance of the glucose eventually progressed to active rejection, the responsiveness of NTS neurons remained constant. In contradiction to the findings in rats, hindbrain taste neurons in primates were not influenced by the induction of satiety (Figure 7.4).

Recordings proceeded to primary taste cortex in the anterior insula with the same result.[55] Even as the macaque progressed from eager acceptance of glucose to total rejection, the responsiveness of taste cells in insular cortex to each of the four basic tastes remained constant. The insula has proven to house taste cells that give the most precise cognitive evaluation of stimulus quality.[56] These results would imply that this evaluation is unfettered with implications for liking or disliking these tastes.

From the insula, projections proceed forward to orbitofrontal cortex (OFC), where taste has at least two representations.[57] The first, with the higher concentration of taste cells and purer representation of taste, is toward the midline, in medial OFC.[58] Here, taking a macaque from hunger to satiety caused variable effects on the responsiveness of taste cells. Most showed a decline in sensitivity, but others were unmodified (as were those at earlier synaptic levels). Moreover, when a decline occurred, it was generic to all stimuli.[59] In addition, a subpopulation of neurons that had been silent began responding to taste stimuli as the monkey neared satiety, implying the existence of an active component to satiety.

The transitional state found in medial OFC — a partial reflection of hedonic decline, though not specific to the satiating stimulus — was refined in the caudolateral OFC to which medial OFC may project. Here, taste cells were tuned more narrowly than at earlier synapses and responded more specifically to changing hedonics.[60] Feeding a macaque to satiety on glucose was associated with a total loss of response to glucose in the caudolateral OFC, while the activity evoked by other stimuli was nearly unchanged (Figure 7.5). Just as humans report the loss of appeal of foods that they have consumed to satiety, they still derive pleasure from others, a phenomenon dubbed sensory-specific satiety.[61,62] Thus a filling entrée may still be complemented by an appealing dessert.

Cells in caudolateral OFC demonstrated other properties that relate to human food choices. A portion of the taste cells also responded to the sight, smells, and textures of foods, though not to those of nonfood objects.[63–65] They would be ideally informed to integrate sensory activity into an amalgam we know as flavor. Thus in caudolateral OFC of macaques are neurons equipped to evaluate the full sensory experience of eating and to reflect — perhaps direct — changes in the desirability of foods as a meal progresses.

Imaging studies using positron emission tomography and functional MRI have been conducted on human subjects to identify areas associated with taste, flavor, and reward. Neurons in the orbitofrontal cortex were generally activated by affectively charged stimuli[66,67] or sensitive to the subject's level of hunger.[68,69] Whether a function of the technical approach (single-neuron electrophysiology versus imaging) or a true species difference, the region associated with hunger and satiety in humans

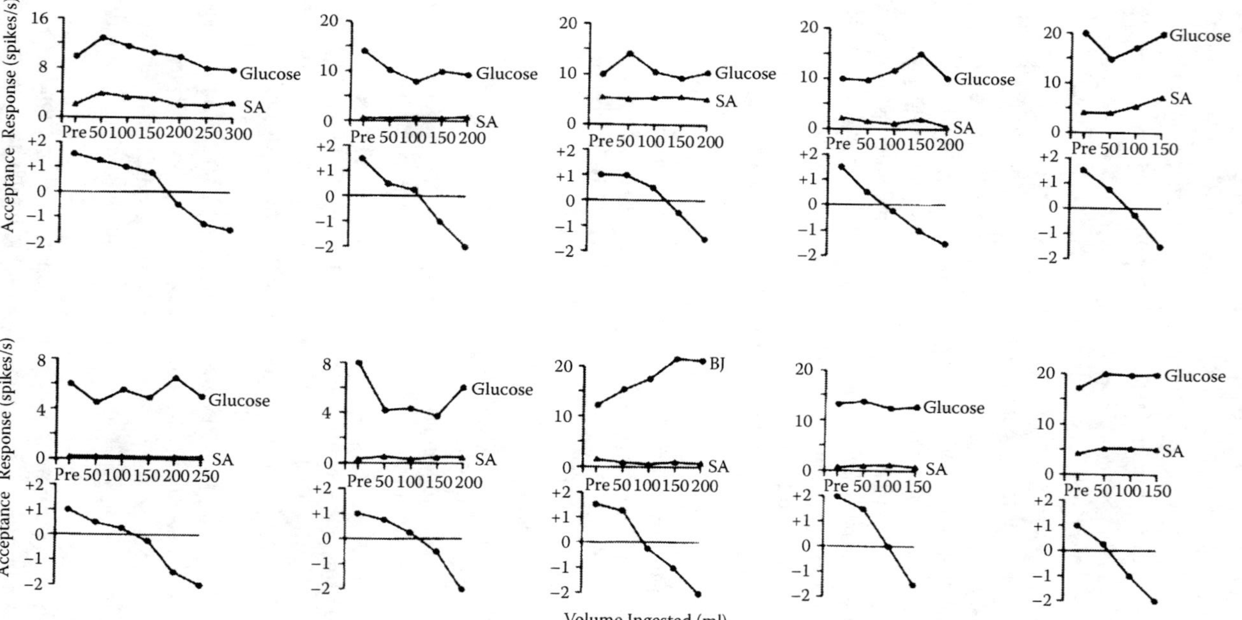

FIGURE 7.4 Ten independent trials of the effects of feeding monkeys to satiety on the neural response to the satiating solution in the nucleus of the solitary tract (NTS). SA: spontaneous activity. Under the neural response data for each trial, the willingness of the monkey to accept (+2) or reject (–2) the solution is shown as a function of the amount of solution delivered. The satiating solution was 20% glucose in each case except for one trial of black currant juice (BJ). Monkeys were fed 50 ml of the solution and tested neurally and behaviorally after each aliquot. Pre: the discharge rate of each neuron before the satiety trials began. (From Yaxley, S., Rolls, E.T., Sienkiewicz, Z.J., and Scott, T.R., *Brain Res.*, 347, 83, 1985. With permission.)

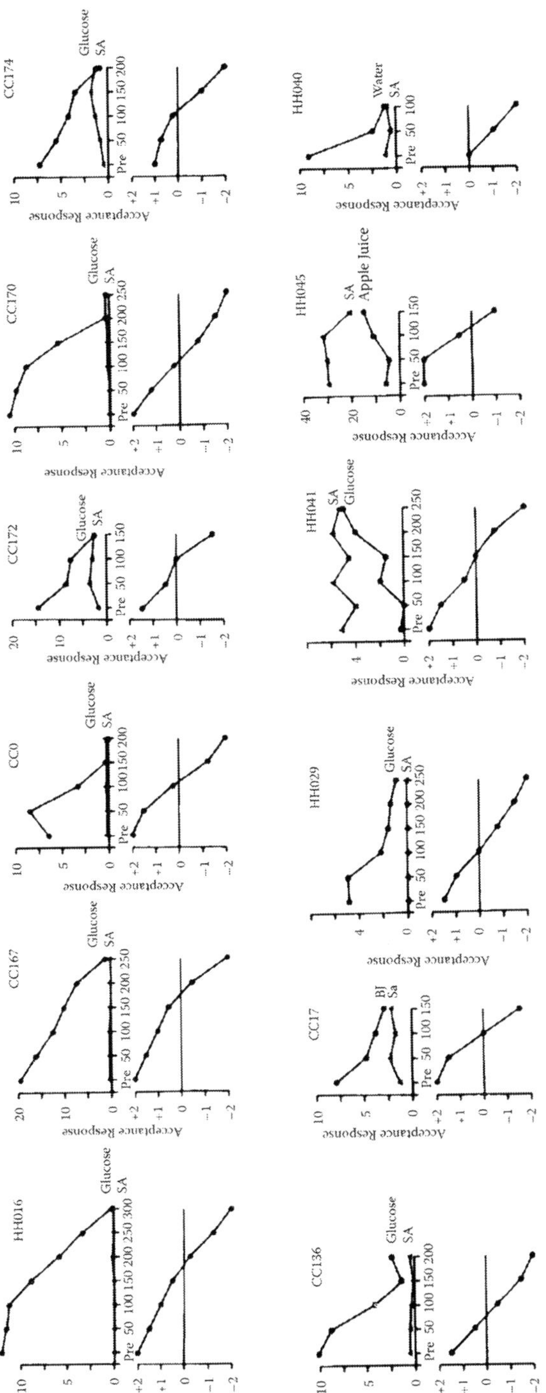

FIGURE 7.5 Twelve independent trials of the effects of feeding monkeys to satiety on the neural response to the satiating solution in the caudolateral orbitofrontal cortex (clOFC). The organization and abbreviations are as in Figure 7.4. (From Rolls, E.T., Sienkiewicz, Z.J., and Yaxley, S., *Eur. J. Neurosci.*, 1, 53, 1989. With permission.)

appears considerably larger than in macaque. Most of the caudal OFC is activated by hunger, and part of the anterior OFC by satiety.[70] It is likely that the broad distribution of activity associated with eating in human OFC reflects activation of reward systems, rather than flavor perception *per se*.[71,72]

Caudolateral OFC is part of a complex that also includes ventral forebrain regions, specifically the central nucleus of the amygdala[10] and the lateral hypothalamic area.[73,74] Recordings from each of these regions reveal activity much like that in caudolateral OFC, with reduced responsiveness to a taste on which a macaque is fed to satiety.[75,76]

7.4 CONCLUSIONS

A progression from recognition to analysis to integration takes place as we proceed up the nervous system. Recognition occurs at the receptors. Early analysis at the level of the nucleus of the solitary tract (NTS) permits the control of reflexes for acceptance or rejection, as well as of the parasympathetic reflexes that anticipate digestive processes. Cells in NTS and in the parabrachial nucleus (PBN) enable the associative processes involved in appetitive and aversive conditioning, and in the mediation of sodium appetite. In the rat, these hindbrain gustatory relays also reflect changes in physiological condition of the animal, from satiety to hunger over a period of hours, or the reverse over just minutes of eating.

In primates, represented in behavioral studies of humans and electrophysiological experiments in macaques, the reflexive responses to taste stimuli appear to be managed in the hindbrain, as in rats. Taste quality is most accurately represented in primary taste cortex in the insula. Beyond this level, integration is the major theme, both with other sensory systems and with central motivational states. In caudolateral orbitofrontal cortex, taste activity converges with that of the sight, smell, and texture of foods and is subject to modification according to the monkey's level of hunger. These properties are extended to subsequent processing stages in the amygdala and hypothalamus. Thus what begins as an analysis of chemical structure at the receptor becomes a component of the assessment of flavor and serves to drive the motivational systems that guide the selection and consumption of foods.

Throughout the history of scientific research on feeding, human and animal studies have approached the topic from different perspectives, asked different questions, and employed different techniques. Humans were addressed in psychophysical studies, animals in those that were behavioral and electrophysiological. This discrepancy is manifest in the content of the two chapters that address orosensory factors in feeding in this volume. There are three levels of ambiguity that intervene when investigators attempt to relate human and animal data on feeding:

1. *Species differences between human and the dominant animal model:* The rat. Differences in how humans and rats process orosensory information have been demonstrated both anatomically and functionally. Norgren and his colleagues[79,80] have reported that the PBN is a major obligatory synaptic relay for taste in rats, whereas gustatory fibers appear to bypass the PBN in primates. This difference gains significance in that the PBN in rats sends dual projections,

both to the thalamocortical axis and to a series of ventral forebrain sites, such that cognitive and hedonic components of a food may be processed in parallel. Lacking this relay in the PBN, taste in primates proceeds from the NTS to the thalamus and insular cortex before being relayed to orbitofrontal cortex and ventral forebrain, thus implying serial rather than parallel processing.

This presumed strategic difference has functional sequelae. Manipulations of hunger levels affected gustatory responsiveness in the hindbrains of rats[47–49] but not primates.[54] Rather, these inevitable impacts are reserved for later processing, after a cognitive analysis of taste quality has presumably been performed. This implies that primates may identify a taste and then independently determine its hedonic value, whereas in rats, these functions may be one. With the hindbrain accepting the responsibility of modifying its responsiveness to suit the animal's momentary needs, the rat may simply eat what tastes good and reject the rest.

2. *Neural level*: Cortex versus hindbrain. When a psychophysicist requests a verbal reply from a human subject, it is the cortex that is engaged. In contrast, most electrophysiology in rats has been performed in hindbrain relays: NTS and PBN. The rat's thalamic taste relay is small and difficult to access, and cortical taste responses have been compromised by the use of anesthetics (see below). Thus the majority of information from humans is cortically mediated and so vastly more processed than responses from the rodent's hindbrain.
3. *Anesthetic effects*: Taste, being phylogenetically old, lies deep in the nervous system, near the midline. It requires penetrating surgery to access taste nuclei and therefore general anesthesia. The resultant impact of suppressing activity at higher-order levels of the CNS is felt in hindbrain nuclei, whose responses are typically exaggerated by relief from the tonic inhibition placed on them by forebrain neurons. Therefore, anesthesia may both prevent recordings from rodent cortex and adulterate the quality of data obtained from hindbrain nuclei.

There have been signal advances from both the animal and human sides of this dichotomy that have served to reduce the ambiguities we face in interpreting gustatory data. Electrophysiological recordings may now be obtained from unanesthetized or lightly anesthetized rats, implanted with chronic recording chambers and actively licking tastants. But the major advance in mediating between human and animal studies is the development of an awake primate recording model. Species differences are minimized, as verified by reports demonstrating that taste processing in the macaque cortex is nearly identical to the taste experiences reported by humans in psychophysical studies.[56] The macaque cortex is readily accessible and may be investigated through hundreds of recording tracks over a period of months, providing an analogue to extended psychophysical tests with humans. Anesthetics are not required for the painless recording procedures, and the monkeys sit comfortably, tasting a variety of stimuli and offering behavioral reactions to them.

Just as studies of animals are becoming more expansive to approach those in humans, so experiments in humans now permit an investigation of activity elicited in the nervous system by taste stimuli, a domain formerly restricted to animal studies. As mentioned above, positron emission tomography and functional MRI experiments now provide insights into responses of the human nervous system to orosensory stimulation. The constraints with these techniques lie in the lack of precise localization of activated neurons and in the very newness of a field that is still seeking accepted standards against which further data may be compared. Nonetheless, imaging studies will eventually extend the study of human responses to orosensory stimulation from the psychophysical to the neural, to complete the bridge between human and animal studies.

REFERENCES

1. Garcia, J. and Hankins, W.G., The evolution of bitter and the acquisition of toxiphobia, in *Olfaction and Taste,* Vol. V, Denton, D.A. and Coughlan, J.P., Eds., Academic Press, Inc., New York, 1975, p. 39.
2. Miller, I.J., Jr., Variation in human fungiform taste bud densities among regions and subjects, *Anat. Rec.,* 216, 474, 1986.
3. Pfaffmann, C., Erickson, R., Frommer, G., and Halpern, B., Gustatory discharges in the rat medulla and thalamus, in *Sensory Communication,* Rosenblith, W.A., Ed., MIT Press, Cambridge, MA, 1961. p. 455.
4. Makous, W., Nord, S., Oakley, B., and Pfaffmann, C., The gustatory relay in the medulla, in *Olfaction and Taste,* Zotterman, Y., Ed., Pergamon Press, New York, 1963, p. 381.
5. Travers, J.B. and Smith, D.V., Gustatory sensitivities in neurons of the hamster nucleus tractus solitarius, *Sens. Proc.,* 3, 1, 1979.
6. Scott, T.R., Yaxley, S., Sienkiewicz, Z.J., and Rolls, E.T., Gustatory responses in the nucleus tractus solitarius of the alert cynomolgus monkey, *J. Neurophysiol.,* 55, 182, 1986.
7. Pritchard, T.C., Hamilton, R.B., and Norgren, R., Neural coding of gustatory information in the thalamus of *Macaca mulatta, J. Neurophysiol.,* 61, 1, 1989.
8. Scott, T.R., Yaxley, S., Sienkiewicz, Z.J., and Rolls, E.T., Gustatory responses in the frontal opercular cortex of the alert cynomolgus monkey, *J. Neurophysiol.,* 56, 876, 1986.
9. Phillips, M.L. et al., A specific neural substrate for perceiving facial expressions of disgust, *Nature,* 389, 495, 1997.
10. Scott, T.R. et al., Gustatory neural coding in the amygdala of the alert macaque monkey, *J. Neurophysiol.,* 69, 1810, 1993.
11. Scott, T.R. and Mark, G.P., The taste system encodes stimulus toxicity, *Brain Res.,* 414, 197, 1987.
12. Scott, T.R. and Giza, B.K., Issues of gustatory neural coding: where they stand today, *Physiol. Behav.,* 69, 65, 2000.
13. Steiner, J.E., The gustofacial response: observation on normal and anencephalic newborn infants, *Symp. Oral Sens. Percept.,* 254, 1973.
14. Smith, D.V. and Scott, T.R., Gustatory neural coding, in *Handbook of Olfaction and Gustation,* 2nd ed., Doty, R.L., Ed., Marcel Dekker, New York, 2003, p. 731.
15. Grill, H.J. and Norgren, R., The taste reactivity test. II. Mimetic responses to gustatory stimuli in chronic thalamic and chronic decerebrate rats, *Brain Res.,* 143, 281, 1978.
16. Travers, S.P., Orosensory processing in neural systems of the nucleus of the solitary tract, in *Mechanisms of Taste Transduction,* Simon, S.A. and Roper, S.D., Eds., CRC Press, Boca Raton, FL, 1993, p. 339.
17. Capretta, P.J. and Rawls, L.H., Establishment of a flavor preference in rats: importance of nursing and weaning experience, *J. Comp. Physiol. Psychol.,* 86, 670, 1974.
18. Galef, B.G., Jr., and Henderson, P.W., Mother's milk: a determinant of the feeding preferences of weaning rat pups, *J. Comp. Physiol. Psychol.,* 78, 213, 1972.

19. Booth, D.A., Stoloff, R., and Nicholls, J., Dietary flavor acceptance in infant rats established by association with effects of nutrient composition, *Physiol. Psychol.*, 2, 313, 1974.
20. Revusky, S.H., Smith, M.H., and Chalmers, D.V., Flavor preferences: effects of ingestion-contingent intravenous saline or glucose, *Physiol. Behav.*, 6, 341, 1971.
21. Rozin, P. and Rogers, W., Novel-diet preferences in vitamin-deficient rats and rats recovered from vitamin deficiency, *J. Comp. Physiol. Psychol.*, 63, 421, 1967.
22. Sclafani, A. and Nissenbaum, J.W., Robust conditioned flavor preference produced by intragastric starch infusions in rats, *Am. J. Physiol.*, 255, R672, 1988.
23. Giza, B.K. et al., Preference conditioning alters taste responses in the nucleus of the solitary tract of the rat, *Am. J. Physiol.*, 273, R1230, 1997.
24. Garcia, J., Kimmeldorf, D.J., and Koelling, R.A., Conditional aversion to saccharin resulting from exposure to gamma radiation, *Science,* 122, 157, 1955.
25. Chang, F.-C.T. and Scott, T.R., Conditioned taste aversions modify neural responses in the rat nucleus tractus solitarius, *J. Neurosci.*, 4, 1850, 1984.
26. McCaughey, S.A., Giza, B.K., Nolan, L.J., and Scott, T.R., Extinction of a conditioned taste aversion in rats. II. Neural effects in the nucleus of the solitary tract, *Physiol. Behav.*, 61, 373, 1997.
27. Shimura, T., Tanaka, H., and Yamamoto, T., Salient responsiveness of parabrachial neurons to the conditioned stimulus after the acquisition of taste aversion learning in rats, *Neurosci.*, 81, 239, 1997.
28. Yamamoto, T., Neural mechanisms of taste aversion learning, *Neurosci. Res.*, 16, 181, 1993.
29. Seward, J.P. and Greathouse, S.R., Appetitive and aversive conditioning in thiamine-deficient rats, *J. Comp. Physiol.*, 83, 157, 1973.
30. Halstead, W.C. and Gallagher, B.B., Autoregulation of amino acids intake in the albino rats, *J. Comp. Physiol. Psychol.*, 55, 107, 1962.
31. Sanahuja, J.C. and Harper, A.E., Effect of amino acid imbalance on food intake and preference, *Am. J. Physiol.*, 202, 165, 1962.
32. Denton, D.A., Hypertension: a malady of civilization? In *Systemic Effects of Hypertensive Agents,* Sambhi, M.P., Ed., Stratton Intercontinental Medical Books, New York, 1976, p. 577.
33. Richter, C.P., Increased salt appetite in adrenalectomized rats, *Am. J. Physiol.*, 115, 155, 1936.
34. Wilkins, L. and Richter, C.P., A great craving for salt by a child with corticoadrenal insufficiency, *J. Am. Med. Assoc.*, 114, 866, 1940.
35. McCance, R.A., Experimental sodium chloride deficiency in man, *Proc. R. Soc. Lond.*, 119, 245, 1936.
36. Clark, W.G. and Clausen, D.F., Dietary "self-selection" and appetites of untreated and treated adrenalectomized rats, *Am. J. Physiol.*, 139, 70, 1943.
37. Epstein, A.N. and Stellar, E., The control of salt preference in adrenalectomized rat, *J. Comp. Physiol. Psychol.*, 46, 167, 1955.
38. Stricker, E.M. and Jalowiec, J.E., Restoration of intravascular fluid volume following acute hypovolemia in rats, *Am. J. Physiol.*, 218, 191, 1970.
39. Fregley, M.J., Harper, J.M., and Radford, E.P., Jr., Regulation of sodium chloride intake by rats, *Am. J. Physiol.*, 209, 287, 1965.
40. Contreras, R., Changes in gustatory nerve discharges with sodium deficiency: a single unit analysis, *Brain Res.*, 121, 373, 1977.
41. Contreras, R. and Frank, M., Sodium deprivation alters neural responses to gustatory stimuli. *J. Gen. Physiol.*, 73, 569, 1979.
42. Jacobs, K.M., Mark, G.P., and Scott, T.R., Taste responses in the nucleus tractus solitarius of sodium-deprived rats, *J. Physiol.*, 406, 393, 1988.

43. Cabanac, M., Physiological role of pleasure, *Science,* 173, 1103, 1971.
44. Campbell, B.A., Absolute and relative sucrose preference thresholds in hungry and satiated rats, *J. Comp. Physiol. Psychol.,* 51, 795, 1958.
45. Rolls, B.J., Rolls, E.T., Rowe, E.A., and Sweeney, K., Sensory specific satiety in man, *Physiol. Behav.,* 27, 137, 1981.
46. Glenn, J.F. and Erickson, R.P., Gastric modulation of gustatory afferent activity, *Physiol. Behav.,* 16, 561, 1976.
47. Giza, B.K. and Scott, T.R., Blood glucose selectively affects taste-evoked activity in rat nucleus tractus solitarius, *Physiol. Behav.,* 31, 643, 1983.
48. Giza, B.K. and Scott, T.R., Intravenous insulin infusions in rats decrease gustatory-evoked responses to sugars, *Am. J. Physiol.,* 252, R994, 1987.
49. Giza, B.K., Deems, R.O., VanderWeele, D.A., and Scott, T.R., Pancreatic glucagon suppresses gustatory responsiveness to glucose, *Am. J. Physiol.,* 265, R1231, 1993.
50. Giza, B.K. and Scott, T.R., Blood glucose level affects perceived sweetness intensity in rats, *Physiol. Behav.,* 41, 459, 1987.
51. Sharma, K.N., Jacobs, H.L., and Gopal, V., Nutritional state/taste interactions in food intake: behavioral and physiological evidence for gastric/taste modulation, in *The Chemical Senses and Nutrition,* Kare, M.R. and Maller, O., Eds., Academic Press, New York, 1977, p. 167.
52. Thompson, D.A., Moskowitz, H.R., and Campbell, R.G., Effects of body weight and food intake on pleasantness for a sweet stimulus, *J. Appl. Physiol.,* 41, 77, 1976.
53. Smith-Swintosky, V.L., Plata-Salamán, C.R., and Scott, T.R., Gustatory neural coding in the monkey cortex: stimulus quality, *J. Neurophysiol.,* 66, 1156, 1991.
54. Yaxley, S., Rolls, E.T., Sienkiewicz, Z.J., and Scott, T.R., Satiety does not affect gustatory activity in the nucleus of the solitary tract of the alert monkey, *Brain Res.,* 347, 83, 1985.
55. Yaxley, S., Rolls, E.T., and Sienkiewicz, Z.J., The responsiveness of neurons in the insular gustatory cortex of the macaque monkey is independent of hunger, *Physiol. Behav.,* 42, 223, 1988.
56. Scott, T.R. and Plata-Salamán, C.R., Taste in the monkey cortex, *Physiol. Behav.,* 67, 489, 1999.
57. Carmichael, S.T. and Price, J.L., Sensory and premotor connections of the orbital and medial prefrontal cortex of macaque monkeys, *J. Comp. Neurol.,* 363, 642, 1996.
58. Pritchard, T.C. et al., Gustatory neural responses in the medial orbitofrontal cortex of the Old World monkey, *J. Neurosci.,* 25, 6047, 2005.
59. Pritchard, T.C., Schwartz, G.J., and Scott, T.R., Taste in the medial orbitofrontal cortex of the macaque, *Ann. N.Y. Acad. Sci.,* 2007, in press.
60. Rolls, E.T., Sienkiewicz, Z.J., and Yaxley, S., Hunger modulates the responses to gustatory stimuli of single neurons in the caudolateral orbitofrontal cortex of the macaque monkey, *Eur. J. Neurosci.,* 1, 53, 1989.
61. Rolls, E.T., Rolls, B.J., and Rowe, E.A., Sensory-specific and motivation-specific satiety for the sight and taste of food and water in man, *Physiol. Behav.,* 30, 185, 1983.
62. Rolls, B.J., Sensory-specific satiety, *Nutr. Rev.,* 44, 93, 1986.
63. Rolls, E.T., Critchley, H.D., and Browning, A.S., Responses to the sensory properties of fat of neurons in the primate orbitofrontal cortex, *J. Neurosci.,* 19, 1532, 1999.
64. Verhagen, J.V., Rolls, E.T., and Kadohisa, M., Neurons in primate orbitofrontal cortex respond to fat texture independently of viscosity, *J. Neurophysiol.,* 90, 1514, 2003.
65. Rolls, E.T., Critchley, H.D., Browing, A., and Hernadi, I., The neurophysiology of taste and olfaction in primates, and umami flavor, *Ann. N.Y. Acad. Sci.,* 855, 426, 1998.
66. De Araujo, I.E.T., Kringelbach, M.L., and Rolls, E.T., Human cortical responses to water in the mouth, and the effects of thirst, *J. Neurophysiol.,* 90, 1865, 2003.
67. Small, D.M., Gregory, M.D., and Mak, Y.E., Dissociation of neural representation of intensity and affective valuation in human gestation, *Neuron,* 39, 701, 2003.

68. Gautier, J.-F., Chen, K., and Salbe, A.D., Differential brain responses to satiation in obese and lean men, *Diabetes,* 49, 838, 2000.
69. Del Parigi, A., Gautier, J.-F., and Chen, K., Neuroimaging and obesity: mapping the brain responses to hunger and satiation in humans using positron emission tomography, *Ann. N.Y. Acad. Sci.,* 967, 389, 2002.
70. Tataranni, P.A., Gautier, J.-F., and Chen, K., Neuroanatomical correlates of hunger and satiation in humans using positron emission tomography, *Proc. Natl. Acad. Sci. USA,* 96, 4569, 1999.
71. O'Doherty, J.P., Deichmann, R., and Critchley, H.D., Neural responses during anticipation of a primary taste reward, *Neuron,* 33, 815, 2002.
72. Kringelbach, M.L. and Rolls, E.T., The functional neuroanatomy of the human orbitofrontal cortex: evidence from neuroimaging and neurophysiology, *Prog. Neurobiol.,* 72, 341, 2004.
73. Burton, M.J., Rolls, E.T., and Mora, F., Effects of hunger on the responses of neurons in the lateral hypothalamus to the sight and taste of food, *Expl. Neurol.,* 51, 668, 1976.
74. Norgren, R., Gustatory responses in the hypothalamus, *Brain Res.,* 21, 63, 1970.
75. Yan, J. and Scott, T.R., The effect of satiety on responses of gustatory neurons in the amygdala of alert cynomolgus macaques, *Brain Res.,* 740, 193, 1996.
76. Karadi, Z. et al., Responses of lateral hypothalamic glucose-sensitive and glucose-insensitive neurons to chemical stimuli in behaving rhesus monkeys, *J. Neurophysiol.,* 67, 389, 1992.
77. Mistretta, C.M., Anatomy and neurophysiology of the taste system in aged animals, *Ann. N.Y. Acad. Sci.,* 561, 277, 1989.
78. Pritchard, T.C., The primate gustatory system, in *Taste and Smell in Health and Disease,* Getchell, T.V., Doty, R.L., Bartoshuk, L.M., and Snow, J.B. Jr., Eds., Raven Press, New York, 1991, p. 109.
79. Norgren, R. and Leonard, C.M., Taste pathways in rat brainstem, *Science,* 173, 1136, 1971.
80. Norgren, R., Taste pathways to hypothalamus and amygdala, *J. Comp. Neurol.,* 166, 17, 1976.

8 The Role of Orosensory Factors in Eating Behavior as Observed in Humans

Didier Chapelot and Jeanine Louis-Sylvestre

CONTENTS

8.1 INTRODUCTION

The role of orosensory factors (OSF) in eating behavior is pivotal to the adaptation of an organism to its nutritional environment. They must provide reliable information on the most beneficial selection and amount of food to ingest. If a given food (a mix of macro and micronutrients) has proved to be appropriate, then OSF associated with this food will be considered as pleasant and the food will be sought, selected, and consumed when the need to eat recurs. Actually, as we will see, the conditioned processes underlying the adaptive function of eating behavior can sometimes lead to inconsistent results and have produced difficulties in the interpretation of data gathered in animals and in humans. This emphasizes that we have to be careful in inferring the effects of OSF on eating behavior and on energy homeostasis and adiposity level. Moreover, experimental tools are few, but vary among authors working in this field of research. In the present chapter, we will focus on the relation between OSF and the different events involved in eating behavior as observed in humans. Problems of terminology, methodology, and relevance of observation in free-living situations will be raised when necessary.

8.2 DEFINITIONS AND METHODOLOGICAL CONSIDERATIONS

8.2.1 OROSENSORY FACTORS

OSF are usually separated into distinct components, most frequently appearance, odor, taste temperature, and texture. Flavor is considered as the conjunction of gustatory (taste) and olfactory (odor) cues. Odors contribute greatly to flavor perception, this being clearly shown when olfaction is suppressed for various reasons (respiratory tract infection, etc.), resulting in hypo- or anosmia and yielding impaired perception of flavors.[1] The distinction between retronasal and orthonasal routes of olfaction are also important. They result in different activation patterns in the brain,[2] with odor intensity being modulated diversely in brain areas according to the alimentary or nonalimentary nature of the odor (e.g., chocolate versus lavender).[2,3]

8.2.2 Pleasure, Pleasantness, and Palatability

The two main variables that define OSF have quantitative and qualitative attributes. Quantitative attributes are often assessed via their intensity, while the qualitative attributes are assessed via the pleasure they provide. The term *pleasantness* is used to describe this affective sensation, and the term "palatability" is the generic word for the hedonic value of a food. Although there is an assumption of a shared understanding of pleasure, this phenomenon is highly complex and difficult to accurately define. For example, a number of unpleasant sensations become pleasant with repeated experiences, usually due to the formation of associations with social, cultural, health, and religious experiences.[4] This makes understanding the role of the relation between OSF in appetite and feeding across different cultures especially problematic.

Palatability is highly idiosyncratic and not fixed over the lifecycle. It changes according to the various pleasant or unpleasant experiences that one has with a certain food. Moreover, the hedonic value of a food can change according to the internal state of the individual, most notably, energy balance. This suggests that it might be necessary to distinguish the general palatability of a food from the oscillating hedonic impressions over the day. Chocolate may be regarded as a highly palatable food by an individual, yet rated a low hedonic value when sated. Thus, failure to control for internal state may yield erroneous conclusions about individual preferences. The concepts of "intrinsic palatability" (constant across metabolic states and relatively stable in time except where it may be durably altered) and "response palatability" (modified according to various factors including circadian or metabolic factors) were proposed long ago,[5] but have rarely been incorporated in experiments. This has practical implications, since it seems that individuals distinguish the terms palatable and pleasant. In one study, 28% of subjects who were asked to rate the palatability and pleasantness of a test meal, reported "palatability" remained constant whereas "pleasantness" was dramatically decreased.[6]

The term preference should be applied only when comparing two foods (or more precisely, their OSF). It is important to note that, if two foods have low palatability, a preference judgment cannot be interpreted as reflecting high palatability. Even in this situation, preference is still too generic, since it can confuse the positive image of a food in one's representation and actual pleasure derived from its consumption.

8.2.3 Measuring Palatability and Hedonic Value

Some authors state that palatability should be considered as the hedonic evaluation of OSF cues under standardized conditions.[6] Palatability and hedonic value are therefore usually assessed by voluntary reports when, or immediately after, seeing, smelling, or tasting a food. The ratings are quantified by scores at various intervals. These scales have either fixed points (FPS) or are continuous, visual analog scales (VAS). The latter are usually considered to be more reliable[7] and therefore have been used more frequently in recent studies. Given that subjects are asked to refer to their sensations at the moment of tasting, these scores should be considered as a hedonic value more than palatability *per se*. Indeed, to be consistent with the proposed distinction between palatability and hedonic value, palatability should be assessed either without any tasting procedure or at the moment when this food is usually consumed or most desired. Even under these conditions, tasting different samples in the same session or only one sample per session leads to different results.[8] In some studies, subjects rate lists of foods considered to have low and high palatability.[9] However, this risks confusing preference for palatability since subjects probably modulate their rating according to the other listed foods. When a food is not familiar to the individual, or when a familiar food's sensory properties are modified, palatability and hedonic values represent a more homogeneous dimension.

Two tasting procedures are commonly used in studies: "taste and swallow" and "taste and spit" (sometimes called "sip and spit" or MSF, for modified sham feeding). Both may induce potential biases due to the metabolic feedback in the first and displeasure associated with spitting food in the second. However, the spitting process does not seem to invalidate the taste and spit method, which is increasingly used to investigate the relationships between OSF and palatability, food intake, or cephalic responses.

8.2.4 Altering Palatability and Hedonic Value

Palatability may be manipulated by varying familiar OSF (generally flavor, but also color or texture). Preferably, these OSF are novel and prevent subjects from referring to past experiences. Different techniques have been used. Palatability can be reduced by an exogenous flavor, such as citric acid,[10] that is generally considered unpalatable. Other flavors such as cumin may increase or decrease palatability according to the experimental food.[11] Some flavors can yield decreased or increased palatability according to their concentration in food.[12] For instance, monosodium glutamate (MSG) increases the palatability of a main dish (for example, spinach mousse and beef) when added at concentrations ranging from 0.3 to 1.2%, with the highest palatability observed at 0.6%.[13] At various other concentrations, MSG increases the palatability of a soup[14,15] and chicken broth, independent of salt levels.[16] Various concentrations of salt have also been used to enhance the palatability in sandwiches,[17] the highest palatability being for 2%, lower for 4%, and the lowest for 0%. Sweetness has also been used by several authors as a sensory tool to modulate palatability,[18–21] although sweetness has the disadvantage of being widely familiar and, consequently, highly susceptible to learned associations.

8.2.5 Modulation of Palatability

8.2.5.1 Effect of Metabolic State on Palatability

The fact that palatability was not an invariant property of a food, but built on the postabsorptive consequences of this food is an important conceptual observation.[22] Preference can be considered as a behavioral efferent axis on a retroactive loop with OSF as an afferent axis and nutrient utilization as a referential variable. This is of course a simplistic model and must be projected on a time scale, as the implications of metabolic state may differ across circadian cycles. However, in eating behavior, one essential criterion is the ability of previously eaten food, signaled by OSF, to sustain satiety at least until the next eating opportunity. This satiety power is not only dependent on food composition (proportional and absolute content of the various nutrients and type of macronutrients, other nonnutritive associated elements), but also on individual metabolic processes (for example, hormonal, enzymatic, or cellular) that use these substrates over time. In animals, this is clearly and repeatedly demonstrated using diabetic rats, where the relative or complete impairment of the capacity to use glucose leads to a marked preference for OSF signaling fat.[23] In humans, few studies have provided evidence for this mechanism. However, it has been demonstrated in children that the increased palatability for OSF associated with a novel high-fat food is only observed when the food is consumed in a hungry state during conditioning.[24,25] Some studies demonstrate the importance of metabolic state in preference conditioning for novel OSF. First reported in the laboratory,[26] it has recently been shown in free-living adults that a learning procedure can increase palatability for a flavor[27,28] associated with an energy-containing food if subjects are hungry, but not when they are sated. This suggests that the basic processes that allowed humans to survive in various dietary environments during history are still operating today. However, the current widespread availability of modern food challenges this mechanism and seems to frequently override its accuracy.

8.2.5.2 Effect of Habits on Palatability

When individuals are accustomed to eating foods with a high content of salt, fat, or sugar, they will choose such foods to alleviate their hunger sensations. However, if constrained to eat foods with less salt, fat, or sugar for a period of time, then they do not show decreased preference for this diet, but may develop a preference for the new orosensory version with the most commonly experienced sensory property.[29–32] The importance of the presence or absence of OSF associated with fat for the progressive shift in liking of fat was shown in a study where low-fat foods were substituted for high-fat versions. Without the OSF usually associated with fat, a reduction in fat palatability was seen, whereas maintaining the OSF of fat with products imitating fat did not alter palatability.[30] This is one of the strongest demonstrations published of the detrimental role of maintaining fat OSF in the diet if a reduction of dietary fat intake is desired.

8.3 MECHANISMS OF ADAPTATION TO OROSENSORY FACTORS

8.3.1 Innate Preferences and Intrauterine Exposure

The pleasantness of sweet taste is usually considered innate since facial expressions following oral sweet exposure suggest acceptance within hours of birth, without any prior exposure to a food item.[33] Differential suckling movement patterns in newborns also document that they can discriminate between stimuli with graded sweetness and selected other tastes.[34] Different intensities of sweetness lead to the ingestion of different amounts of stimuli.[35] Recently, comparisons between newborn human infants and nonhuman primates have shown that they share common facial patterns.[36] The fact that sour and bitter induce facial expressions of distaste demonstrates the existence of discriminative affective reaction in early life and without postprandial feedback. The term innate is used to convey that this preference, which is a hedonic value, is not the consequence of a conditioning process. However, this inference is challenged by the demonstration that the gustatory system operates as early as the fourth month of gestation,[37] and the amnion contains selected flavors of food eaten by the mother.[38,39] Furthermore, prior exposure to amniotic taste compounds can alter hedonic responses at birth, suggestive of intrauterine learning. This was shown for carrot flavor mediated by carrot juice consumed 4 days a week during the last trimester of pregnancy, resulting in enhanced palatability of the carrot flavor as judged by facial responses, perception by mothers, and intake.[40] The association between amniotic flavor and fetal development may initiate positive feedback for low-intensity sweetness that contributes to acceptance of milk as food. Recent data obtained in rats show how amniotic fluid can acquire appetitive properties when paired with a flavor.[41] The fact that anencephalic and normal infants display similar responses to these taste cues argues the importance of the hindbrain and, in particular, the nucleus of the solitary tract, and the existence of a primitive unconditioned mechanism that conditioning may modify afterward.

8.3.2 Spontaneous Diet Selection

One notable experiment took place some 80 years ago, when Clara Davis allowed three weaned children to self-select their diet from ages 6 to 12 months. They were presented a wide variety of food items prepared to be eaten easily by a child and, in combination, covered all nutritive needs.[42] Results showed that the children developed preferences, but acquired a personal dietary selection that always contained a variety of different food items and experienced normal growth. No deleterious consequences were reported of this precocious free-food choice, indicating than an adaptive mechanism was operant, even in the absence of social or familial transmission. The observation of their behavior was greatly in favor of the pivotal role of OSF in this acquisition. Children tried almost all food items during the first weeks, sometimes spitting them out, but trying again, adopting the food or not, and finally, choosing the amount eaten. When conducted on 15 children, similar results were reported some years later.[43] As stated by Clara Davis, "… there was not the faintest sign of 'instinct' directed choice" and "Patterns of selective appetite, then, were shown to develop on the basis of sensory experience, that is, taste, smell, and doubtless the feeling of comfort and well-being that followed eating …," according to a trial-and-error method. Children learned how to cope with their macro- and micronutrient needs unconsciously and without imitations of peers or adults, basing their behavior on OSF associated with the various food items. It should be noted, however, that no food contained any poisonous substance, and therefore, this could not be extrapolated to humans living in natural conditions such as our ancestors.

8.3.3 Neophobia

On first exposure to the OSF of a novel food, the quantity eaten will range from none to a limited, "cautious" amount (Figure 8.1). This is called neophobia and is defined as "the hesitancy to eat novel food."[44] Although teleological, the usual explanation is that this phenomenon facilitates avoidance of poisonous substances.

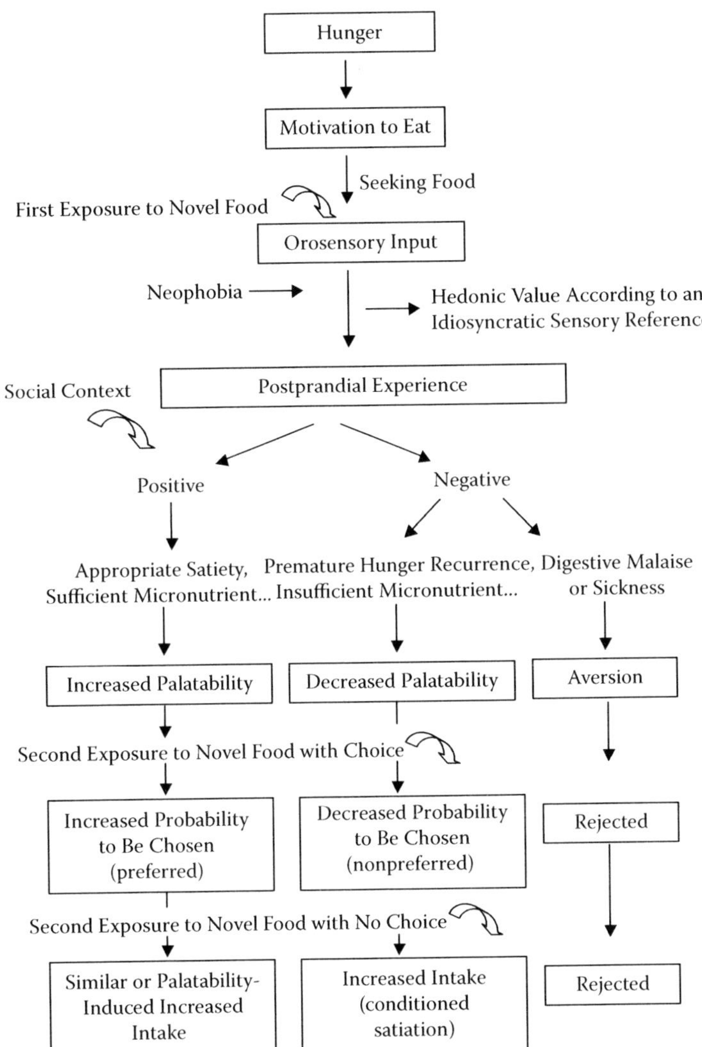

FIGURE 8.1 A theoretical model of the cascade leading to accept or reject a novel food item and determination of palatability for a given individual. Social context can counteract potential negative postingestive consequences if eating the food item provides some advantages in terms of social reward. Aversion is mainly caused by negative digestive consequences, post-absorptive effects altering primarily palatability. The consequences of postingestive events on palatability may vary according to the choice or no choice conditions when the food item is present again in the environment.

However, it should be noted that most poisonous substances can be lethal at lower doses than the amount eaten by the neophobic animal or human. Therefore, it may be appropriate to separate the neophobia leading to the rejection of a novel food from the neophobic response that leads to sampling only a small quantity of an item. The latter behavior is a cautious approach to avoid any digestive distress and allows any postabsorptive consequences of the food's intake to occur before determining the safe quantity to ingest. That this behavior is learned after experience rather than phylogenetically programmed, is suggested by the fact that food neophobia is weak before 2 years of age and fluctuates throughout childhood with increased levels between ages 2 and 9 years, followed by a progressive decrease.[45–48] Interestingly, a neophobic tendency, in regard to OSF associated with novel foods, will persist in a certain proportion of the population during childhood and adulthood and will have consequences for a variety of foods included in the diet.[49] With repeated exposures (familiarization), the acceptability of foods will be adjusted and variously incorporated in the diet. In children, it has been shown that the acceptance of foods increase with repeated exposures, requiring greater than 10 trials to stabilize.[50,51]

With age, true novel OSF become rare and most flavors or appearances can be related to familiar food items. Every individual develops an idiosyncratic referential sensory "panel" to which a novel complex OSF will be compared to determine a response on the first exposure. This may explain the common, wide interindividual variability of responses to novel foods, even with neophobic modulation by social factors, especially in children,[52–54] and reassuring visual cues are provided.

8.3.4 Food Aversion

Among the first postingestive consequences experienced after consumption of a food are the effects on the digestive tract. Any OSF associated with malaise such as nausea or vomiting, after food ingestion is likely to elicit a negative response upon subsequent reexposure. This occurs through a classical conditioning process[55] (OSF being the conditioned stimulus and illness the unconditioned stimulus) known as learned food aversion (LFA)[56] or, more specifically, conditioned taste aversion (CTA). In population-based studies,[57,58] it is usually reported that about one-third of individuals have experienced a LFA, with one-fourth showing a current aversion. This prevalence is more frequent in women than men. Sometimes, this conditioning is independent of the food, as in chemotherapy for cancer.[59] Here, the treatment, and not the food eaten prior to its administration, is the conditioned stimulus. The malaise associated with cancer treatment has often served as an experimental model to study LFA, although it is not fully analogous to the phenomenon in natural living conditions. Not only novel and less preferred foods, but also familiar and preferred items can be targets of LFA.[60] Moreover, the temporal pattern is much less rigid than in the classic Pavlovian model, since some foods consumed more than 24 hours prior to the malaise are targeted for chemotherapy-related LFA.[60,61] When not totally rejected, the pleasure component of a food is the primary target of LFA compared to intake.[62] Importantly, an aversion is not observed after postabsorptive deleterious effects, except if they have digestive consequences.

8.4 SOME PROBLEMS OF PERCEPTION OF OROSENSORY FACTORS

8.4.1 Genetic Variants in Perception of Orosensory Factors and Food Choices

After Fox discovered taste blindness to the bitter taste of phenylthiocarbamide (PTC), family studies showed that the ability to taste bitter thiourea compounds such as PTC and 6-n-propylthiouracil (PROP) is a Mendelian recessive trait. Approximately 70% of the Caucasian population is sensitive to these compounds (tasters) at low concentration, and 30% are not (nontasters). Polymorphisms in a single gene, TAS2R38 account for most of the variation among individuals. People who are heterozygous have lower sensitivities (tasters) compared with those who are homozygous for the taster form of the receptor (supertasters).[63] In some studies, the perceived saltiness of NaCl,[64] the burn of capsaicin,[65] and the intensity of ethyl alcohol[66] are perceived as stronger by tasters and supertasters. These groups also reportedly discriminate fat when nontasters cannot,[67,68] although this is not confirmed in all studies.[69]

These genetic variations could influence taste perception in humans,[70] and some individuals are specifically insensitive to MSG,[71] while some appear to be specifically insensitive to sucrose.[72]

Relations between taster status and preferences for foods have been examined in various studies.[73] In adults and children,[74] there is no robust relation between taster status and dietary selection, even in regard to intake of plant foods and beverages with bitter taste. Discrepant results were found for fat intake. The preference for fat and intake of fat-containing foods are guided more by gender and are product specific.

8.4.2 Perception of Fat

The paradox of fat has long been that people seemed to like its taste,[75] although fat was considered not to have taste *per se*. Rather, fat is commonly believed to be perceived only via texture and odor. When varied in milk, the differences between fat versions are primarily based on characteristics such as viscosity, since descriptive terms used by subjects are associated with this sensory dimension (e.g., thin, creamy, greasy). Moreover, removing olfactory cues with a nose clip does not impair the discrimination of subjects to detect fatness.[76] However, when viscosity of fat is changed, either by heat or different pressures,[77,78] discrimination is not altered, suggesting that viscosity is only one of the oral cues contributing to fat detection. Recently, it has been shown that perception of free fatty acids is multimodal, with independent contributions of olfactory, gustatory, and somatosensory components.[79] One important point when considering the orosensory properties of fat is their interaction with the overall flavor intensity, in particular aroma.[80] Viscosity may not be the principal factor, since it is shown not to exert a strong influence on aroma perception.[81] Finally, direct chemodetection of fat has been supported by the description of preference for nutritive oil over mineral oil in animals deprived of olfactory or texture cues[82] even after suppressing postingestive feedback.[83] A categorization of fat tasters and nonfat tasters has been proposed based on the ability to discriminate between oleic and linoleic acids.[84] However, this remains to be verified.

8.5 DIRECT EFFECT OF OROSENSORY FACTORS ON PRE- AND POSTABSORPTIVE EVENTS INVOLVED IN EATING BEHAVIOR

8.5.1 Roles and Mechanisms of Cephalic-Phase Reflexes

The accuracy of a biological system often requires feed-forward mechanisms that adjust system performance in anticipation of future inputs. Pavlov[85] demonstrated that the presence of food in the oral cavity stimulated neurally mediated reflexes named "psychic secretions" that enhance nutrient digestion, absorption, and metabolism. All functions concerned with nutrient loads and energy that disturb the internal milieu are activated by sensory stimulation. In humans, the rapid activation of physiological processes has been documented in multiple sites: salivary glands, gastrointestinal tract, pancreas (enzyme secretion and hormone release), thermogenic system, cardiovascular system, and renal system.[86] Cephalic-phase responses can be triggered by all OSF, but also by the mere thought of a palatable food.[87] They are neurally mediated physiologic reflexes to sensory stimulation. The vagus nerve is the "final common path" for many cephalic-phase responses, and its outflow is possibly modulated by the ascending visceral nervous afferents, by gut peptides, neuropeptides, and systemic signals. Signals reflecting metabolic status may also influence activity of forebrain sites and thereafter modulate the vagal outflow. Perhaps due to their small amplitude (as compared to the unconditioned responses) and to myriad of influences, cephalic-phase responses are occasionally difficult to document in human subjects. Nevertheless, they appear as a critical link between the sensory qualities of food and nutritional status. Three aspects of cephalic phases are of particular importance in eating behavior: salivary, insulin, and fat metabolism. However, other cephalic responses have been described in humans for hormones involved in eating behavior, such as glucagon[88] or ghrelin.[89]

8.5.2 Cephalic Phase of Salivary Response

Salivary function contributes to mechanical (formation of a food bolus facilitates swallowing), enzymatic (presence of enzymes such as alpha-amylase and lipase initiating digestion), and sensory (improved perception of gustatory stimuli) dimensions of eating behavior; the latter dimensions being interrelated.[90] It is a common experience that salivation is sensitive to OSF related to food, even to its thought,[91] and the activating signals have been explored experimentally.[92] Salivation has also been used to evaluate motivation to eat in ways other than subjective ratings or amount eaten, but this method is still questionable.[92] It was also proposed as an indicator of palatability,[93] but this raises interpretative problems, since unpleasant OSF can also produce a high salivary response. The cephalic-phase salivary response is, however, mainly a product of conditioning.[94] Some known physical and chemical characteristics of foods, such as pungency, are more predictive than palatability.[95] Although contradictory results are found, an increased salivary response is occasionally reported in restrained eaters[96–100] and in a hunger state.[101] This suggests that salivary flow is sensitive to metabolic state. However, simple repeated stimulation with the same OSF reduces salivation, whereas new OSF restore its flow,[102] raising the possibility of a link between intrameal motivation to eat according to the sensory-specific satiety mechanism (see Section 8.6.3).

8.5.3 Cephalic Phase of Insulin

Cephalic-phase insulin release (CPIR) has been well documented in normal humans.[103] It is vagally mediated,[104] but a noncholinergic contribution is also involved.[105] An increase in insulin secretion occurs within 2 minutes after oral sensory stimulation, peaks at 4 minutes, and returns to baseline 8 to 10 minutes after stimulation.[103] This increase is about 25% above baseline and, despite its small magnitude, reduces postprandial glucose levels. Thus, the oral sensory exposure dampens postprandial concentrations of glucose and insulin,[105,106] with implications for glucose tolerance and diabetes prevention. In some work, a greater frequency of CPIR occurred in response to highly palatable foods compared with less palatable foods,[107,108] but other studies with female subjects sham-fed with foods differing in palatability levels showed identical CPIR.[109] Sweetness was hypothesized to yield a specific CPIR, but this has not received convincing support.[110,111] Recent brain imaging has reported no early insulin response and no hypothalamic activity after sweet taste without glucose ingestion.[112]

8.5.4 Cephalic Phase of Fat Metabolism

The detection of fat via its OSF was clearly shown in a study where subjects ingested a capsule of 50 g of safflower oil followed by chewing and spitting full-fat, simulated-fat, or nonfat versions of cream cheese on crackers, crackers alone, or no oral stimulation.[113] The postprandial peak concentration of plasma triacylglycerol (TAG) and the duration of elevated levels (over the next 6 hours) were significantly higher when the oral cavity had been exposed to the full-fat version. In further research, unsaturated fats were reported to be the most effective stimuli to elicit this phenomenon.[114] Although butter was effective, saturated fat, carbohydrate (potatoes), and fat replacers were not.[115] It was also determined[116] that odor alone elicits a similar effect, but to a much lesser extent (only at the fourth hour). Fructose and glucose were also found to enhance this effect,[117] but this is not dependent on sweetness or palatability, since these factors were matched between conditions. Importantly, it was shown that this oral stimulation primarily triggered the release of fatty acids stored in the intestine and not from the absorption of fat immediately ingested.[118] The role of this cephalic phase response in satiety will have to be explored in coming years.

8.6 ROLE OF OROSENSORY FACTORS IN THE DIFFERENT PHASES OF EATING BEHAVIOR

The role of OSF in eating behavior was particularly well argued in a classic series of human studies conducted almost 40 years ago.[119] A pump delivered food either in the mouth or in the stomach while individuals were also allowed to drink a liquid meal. Energy balance was less accurate with gastric loading than when OSF were present. These studies demonstrated that without the temporal sequence of OSF followed by gastric stimulation, the response to the energy content of food was compromised. The importance of OSF in meal-induced subjective satiety was confirmed some years later.[120,121]

In recent years, a common view seems to have finally emerged for heuristically decomposing eating behavior into at least three different states, "hunger" (the physiological signal prompting the brain to initiate food seeking), "satiation" (the processes leading to the interruption of an eating occasion), and "satiety" (the nonhunger state between two meals), since they seem to be driven by different mechanisms.

8.6.1 Role of Orosensory Factors in Hunger

Among the proposed mechanisms for hunger, a triggering role of glucose has received a large amount of support due to the observation of a small and transient preprandial decline of blood glucose in animals[122] and humans,[123] even while following their usual meal pattern.[124] All eating occasions may not be the consequence of hunger. The simple availability of palatable foods, appropriate to the time of day can trigger intake even if individuals are sated.[124] As recently proposed,[125] palatability might be more specifically linked to the rewarding property of a food, a dimension exceeding the simple adequacy of its energy content to relieve hunger. There are two brain circuits that are distinct and possible to separate experimentally, even in human. However, via their roles on cephalic phase response, in particular CPIR, OSF may contribute to enhance glucopenia-induced hunger when food is seen, smelled, and tasted.

8.6.2 Role of Orosensory Factors in Satiation

8.6.2.1 Palatability and Conditioned Satiation

David Booth[126] demonstrated in humans that satiation is conditioned to the orosensory properties of foods, modifying the Pavlovian scheme in attributing to food cues the status of a conditioned stimulus. Having to supply immediate energy and a part of the energy for the passive period of the circadian cycle,[127–129] this behavior should be considered as partly homeostatic (motivated by need-state) and partly allostatic (anticipation of need-state).[130]

Relationships between palatability and satiation are more complex than usually described. It is often said that they are linked by an inverse correlation: greater palatability is correlated with lower satiation. However, the relationship is not so strong and has to be analyzed in view of the metabolic state of the consumer, the place of the energy-manipulated food in the meal, the sensory properties of the test food, and prior exposure effects.[131] Conditioned satiation based on the OSF of foods has been demonstrated experimentally under laboratory conditions, but its accuracy is reduced when subjects are in free-living conditions.[132,133] Effectiveness was clearly demonstrated with three palatable versions of bread (according to preferred concentration of salt) incorporated in sandwich-based lunch meals.[17] Interestingly, lunch intake was lower with the less palatable version on the first exposure, but with repeated exposures, intakes became similar between conditions, due to an increased acceptance of the less palatable version. Thus, the relationship between palatability and intake is flexible and needs to be considered with caution.

A recent study showed the complexity of interpreting the interaction between energy content and OSF in conditioned satiety.[21] When two versions of a meal similarly palatable, but differing in energy density (high [HED] and low [LED]) and OSF (blueberry versus cinnamon, pink versus neutral) were provided to subjects, they ate a similar amount on the first exposure. An increase in pleasantness for the HED version was observed on the next exposure. After two training days with a fixed 300-g amount, an increase in intake and in pleasantness was noted for the LED compared to the HED version.

8.6.2.2 Effect of Modulation of Palatability on Satiation

Many studies assess how various levels of palatability influence intake of a given food in a one-time exposure. With very different methods used to alter palatability (see Table 8.1), results generally show that, on an individual basis, higher palatability leads to increased intake. Some studies report an impaired response to changes in the energy content of foods when palatability increases. Thus, 30 minutes after disguised low- or high-energy preloads (carbohydrate or fat), intake at a test meal was modified accordingly only when bland, but not when palatable.[134] To better understand the complexity of the role of palatability in eating behavior, efforts should be made to (1) improve its definition and use subclassifications of some dimensions that do not overlap (a first one being the distinction between palatability and hedonic value), (2) propose a typology of change in relation to each experimental situation, and (3) match procedures across laboratories to provide consistent results.

Olfactory and visual factors have been overlooked when investigating the role of OSF in satiation. The odor and appearance (color) of a test food (e.g., custard) are more predictive of the amount eaten than the oral flavor and texture *per se* when the food is familiar, but the textural visual cue is the major determinant when it is not familiar.[135] However, all these dimensions become rapidly interrelated, since with repetition, odors paired with a taste compound acquire its sensory characteristic such as sweetness.[136] The hedonic value for the odor consistently follows this evolution with respect to pleasantness or unpleasantness.[137] Therefore, it may be important in the future to evaluate whether studies in laboratories (where olfactory factors are often reduced before meals to limit their effect on the main studied variable) are relevant to naturalistic situations, where food odors strongly influence the environment of individuals. The importance of previous experience and memories in the rating of odor[138] may provide new intervention approaches for dietary improvement.

8.6.3 Orosensory Factors and Sensory-Specific Satiety

8.6.3.1 Characteristics of Sensory-Specific Satiety

Rolls et al.[139] established a procedure in which various food samples with different sensory characteristics are tasted and the pleasantness perceived is rated on hedonic scales. After that, one of the foods is eaten either *ad libitum* or in a fixed, but

TABLE 8.1
Effect of Modifying Palatability on Food Intake

	Subjects	Method	Intake
Price & Grinker, 1974	20 (14F/6M)	5 different crackers leading to various P across individuals	Increased as a function of P
Bellisle & Le Magnen, 1981	10 (7F/3M)	5 different sandwiches leading to various P across individuals	Correlation between P and intake in 5 out of 10 subjects
Bellisle et al., 1984	10 (5F/5M)	P+: preferred sandwiches; P-: least preferred sandwiches	Increased in P+
Hill et al. 1984	12 F	P+: preferred sandwiches and biscuits meals	NR
Bobroff & Kissileff, 1986	16 (8F/8M)	Yogurt. P-: cumin	100 g more for each 2 point difference in P
Bellisle et al., 1989	36 (18F/18M)	Spinach mousse and jelly beef. P++: 0.6% and P+: 1.2% monosodium glutamate	Increased in P+ only
Spiegel et al., 1989	9 F	Sandwiches cut in SFU of 5 g. Different flavors leading to a P+ and a P– across individuals	Increased in P+
Monneuse et al., 1991	21 (10F/11M)	P+: various preference among 5 concentrations of aspartame in a yogurt	Increased in 10 / 21 subjects for the P+ (correlation ns for the group)
Perez et al., 1994	32 (17F/15M)	P+: various preferences among 5 concentrations (0, 5, 10, 20 and 40g/100 g) of sucrose in a yogurt	Low correlation between P and intake
Guy-Grand et al., 1994	7 F	Conventional, semiliquid and sandwich meals P+ or P– according to subject preferences	Increased in conventional P+, but not semiliquid or sandwiches
Yeomans, 1996	54 (27F/27M)	Pasta and tomato. P+: 0.27% oregano, P–: 0.54% oregano	Increased in P+, decreased in P–
Yeomans et al., 1997	16 M	Pasta and tomato. P+: 0.27% oregano	Increased in P+
De Graaf et al., 1999	35 (26F/9M)	Tomato soup. P–: 7.5mg/g, P–: 15mg/g citric acid	Decreased in P– (65%) and P– (40%)
Yeomans & Symes, 1999	50 M	Macaroni cheese flavored by mustard or cheese leading to P+ and P– across individuals	Increased in P+
Zandstra et al., 2000	35 (25F/10M)	Bread. Different NaCl concentrations (0, 2 and 4%) leading to 3 levels of P across individuals	Increased as a function of P
Yeomans et al., 2005	16 M	Porridge: High (H) and low (L) energy density (ED), P+ and P– by sweetness	Increased intake in the HED condition when P+ compared to P–

Note: M: males; F: females; P+: higher palatability; P–: lower palatability; NR: not recorded; SFU: solid food units substantial amount. As soon as 2 minutes after the end of consumption, it is observed that pleasantness (hedonic value) for the eaten food declines, whereas no change is reported for other food items tasted and not eaten. It is worth noting that pleasantness for texture[140–142] and odor[141,143] of the eaten food also decrease. Desire to eat is usually consistent and exhibits a significant decline. This decline is generalized to foods sharing some orosensory characteristics with the eaten food.[143] The perceived intensity of the taste of the eaten food is generally not, or only weakly decreased, arguing for a change in affective more than objective facets of taste.[144] This was interpreted as a demonstration that the decreased hedonic value of a food is the driving force of satiation. OSF are essential contributors to this mechanism via their progressive decreasing power to stimulate eating. This phenomenon was called sensory-specific satiety (SSS).[139] According to the terminology adopted in this chapter, satiety may seem inappropriate, and satiation, the term for the mechanisms interrupting eating, more appropriate. This hedonic decline persists for 20 to 60 minutes[140] and, in some studies, as long as 120 minutes,[145] perhaps contributing to satiety.

The sensory origin of this phenomenon was highly suggested by the fact that SSS was often at its maximum 2 minutes after the end of consumption (prior to postingestive feedback).[139] Chewing without swallowing food over a time interval comparable to a meal (tantamount to a sham feeding) also induces SSS and eliminates a causal role of postingestive nutritive factors.[146] However, SSS was smaller when food was chewed and spit out versus chewed and swallowed.[147] Smelling food for the duration it would have been in the mouth while eating also produced SSS.[146]

The magnitude of the SSS does not reach its peak at 2 minutes for all foods; in particular those with more complex or high-fat contents may not reach a maximum for up to 20 minutes.[142] This suggests that the hedonic decline may also have postingestive and postabsorptive determinants.

If a greater intake (of mass or energy) increases the magnitude of this hedonic decline,[148,149] it is usually reported that macronutrient composition and energy density of the food do not contribute significantly to SSS.[145,150] Some authors have reported that OSF associated with proteins accentuate SSS.[148,151,152] The confounding of macronutrient composition and OSF makes the distinction between them difficult. However, it has never been clearly shown that this hedonic drop was causal in the interruption of intake. No study has shown simultaneity between a change in pleasantness and the cessation of eating.

8.6.3.2 Variety and Intake

SSS could contribute to the way OSF enhance intake. The fact that OSF have the power to stimulate intake when they differ from the ones associated with the eaten food raises the possibility that the variety of OSF may promote overeating. This had been clearly shown in humans with energy intake increased by as much as 60% when the meal consisted of foods with varying OSF.[153] Variety in the fillings of sandwiches (3 versus 1) consistently induced an increase in intake of 14 to 18%.[154,155] This intake-enhancing effect of OSF variety has been repeatedly reported[153,155–162] and can be considered robust. This effect is so strong that the simple tasting of foods with OSF different from those consumed, can increase intake and slow the hedonic reduction of the eaten food.[163,164] Related to this phenomenon, is the concept of priming. Subjects briefly tasting a food of high palatability, consumed it in larger amount than without priming (tasting).[165] This mechanism warrants further study.

If OSF are augmented to increase food variety and therefore promote nutrient adequacy in populations at risk,[166] they may also contribute to overconsumption. In one study,[167] three nutritionally similar diets with low, medium, or high variety (5, 10, and 15 items per day, respectively) provided during 7 days showed that daily intake was positively associated with variety and induced significant weight gain (about 430 g). However, this effect seems to require a high level of variety, since it was not significant after 8 days of meals composed either of one or three food items.[168] Therefore, variety in the diet should not be promoted without caution. Recommendations to increase variety should focus on healthy foods.[169]

8.6.4 Role of Orosensory Factors in the Microstructure of the Meal

Meals may be deconstructed into several subcomponents to observe the effect of various environmental factors, such as OSF, on each of them. Components recorded vary across studies (for example, chewing time, chewing movement, chewing or eating rate, number of swallows, bite rate, bite size, bite number, bite duration, pause number, pause duration, intake during 2-minute bouts, meal duration and meal size). Studies conducted on this topic have consistently shown that palatability exerts a significant influence on the pattern of intake during a meal and, more specifically, at the beginning of the meal in enhancing eating rate.[11,12,157,158,170–173] This is usually considered a positive-feedback reward mechanism and is consistent with the role of OSF in enhancing motivation to eat.[174] However, alterations in the microstructure of the meal do not always induce consistent changes in energy intake. For example, palatability of a conventional meal increases intake, but not the microstructure of the meal, whereas the reverse is observed for semiliquid or sandwich meals.[175]

8.6.5 Role of Orosensory Factors in Satiety

There is a body of evidence that satiety is a state with strong postabsorptive determinants and in particular the immediate glucose availability for cells. Any change that precipitates or delays this glucose shortage consistently alters the duration of satiety.[176–178]

8.6.5.1 Methodological Considerations

A role of OSF in satiety would mean that OSF may interact with postabsorptive events to modify satiety produced by a food or a meal. However, satiety is comprised of three main dimensions that we will term: intensity, duration, and next-meal satiation. For assessing intensity, scales are completed by subjects at regular intervals during the postprandial period. Hunger, appetite, desire to eat, gastric fullness, and prospective consumption ratings are recorded on VAS. However, the interpretation of possible differences between scores in terms of actual eating behavior is quite speculative. As noted above, the simple availability of highly palatable food during a period with customarily low hunger state can induce intake.[124] It would be necessary to show that, for two different subjective satiety states, the power of palatable food to trigger intake (stimulate "wanting") varies, and different palatable versions of a food lead to different eating initiation thresholds. Such studies are still missing, although some authors introduce a scale assessing "appetite for a snack"[17] that may help to answer this question. In the latter study, the low-palatability version of a meal actually induced a higher mean appetite for a snack over the next 90 minutes than the two more palatable meals. However, it is important to note that mean energy intake at this meal was lower than usual, this being a confounding factor.

The second dimension of satiety is duration. An influence of OSF would be exemplified by earlier or later hunger and eating following varying orosensory stimulations. To date, this procedure has been sparsely used and mainly to determine the satiety power of various energy or macronutrient compositions of foods or meals[176–182] but not for OSF. The fine sensitivity of this variable and its physiological relevance should encourage the use of this procedure.

The third dimension incorporates both satiation and satiety, since the measured variable is the amount eaten (in mass and energy) at a test meal consumed at a fixed delay after the preload. Intake being the consequence of a satiation process, this variable is an assessment of how satiety (metabolic state) induced by the previous meal interacts with satiation. This design is used by most authors in this research area.

8.6.5.2 Effect of Palatability on Satiety

In a study where a number of preload attributes (energy and macronutrient content, weight, volume, texture, and taste) varied and subsequent satiety was tracked, OSF had some influence, but was lower than energy content.[183] However, in this study palatability was not assessed.

A palatability-induced decrease in satiety has been reported by Hill et al.[9] 120 minutes after the consumption of a preferred sandwich and biscuit meal compared to a less preferred version, but intake was not measured. Two studies[19,184] (using aspartame and sugar, respectively, to modify palatability) resulted in increased intake after the preferred version of a yogurt. Since the yogurts were consumed *ad lib* and therefore represented different preloads between conditions, it is not possible to infer any specific effect of palatability on satiety. This distinction between satiation and satiety was made by other researchers[10] using tomato soup with two concentrations of citric acid to reduce palatability. They did not find an effect of reduced palatability on subsequent subjective satiety or intake at the following meal (19 or 90 minutes later). But again, these results revealed that the reduced palatability of a food, such as a soup cannot be extrapolated to the putative intake-stimulating effect of highly palatable foods.

Even when palatability stimulates hunger, it generally does not influence gastric fullness to a similar magnitude,[12,21,134,173] although it has been reported.[20]

One possible explanation for these discrepant results may be the appropriateness of the test food. If liquid or semiliquid meals are used to equate consumption across conditions and subjects, their lack of ecological validity may introduce a confounding factor.

8.6.5.3 Effect of Sweet Taste on Satiety

The putative effect of sweet taste on satiety was extensively studied when artificial sweetener use expanded. Sweetening often enhances the palatability of a food, and therefore it is difficult to distinguish between sweet taste and palatability. For example, hunger was reduced 120 minutes after aspartame-sweetened and more palatable breakfasts were consumed compared to unsweetened and less palatable versions.[18] The difference occurred immediately after the most palatable version of the breakfast was consumed and lasted at least 5 hours.[20]

In most published studies, no decreased satiety (intensity and satiation at next meal(s)) is reported after a sweetened versus unsweetened preload (reviewed by Sorensen et al.[185]). When the daily energy balance is considered, the substitution of aspartame for sucrose-sweetened beverages seems to disassociate the energy content sugar.[186,187] A delayed enhanced intake effect has been reported in one study [188] but not in another.[189] This strategy to maintain sweet taste without the usual associated energy appears beneficial in populations most concerned by artificially sweetened beverages.[190] When sugar is used, the problem is discriminating sensory and postingestive factors due to the presence of carbohydrate in the digestive tract and the influence of chemoperception. A recent study has attempted to solve this using a sip and spit procedure[191] and incremental sucrose concentration (0, 2.5, 5, 10, and 20%). No alteration of taste sensitivity was noted. Group mean intake increased with sucrose concentration up to the 10% concentration. However, palatability followed the same pattern, so it is not possible to determine if sweet taste or palatability was responsible for this effect. Moreover, on an individual basis, responses varied widely, which questions a robust role for sweetness on intake. To separate palatability from sweetness intensity, future studies should focus on novel foods and select subjects who similarly like them with several intensities of sweetness. Although quite difficult to accomplish, this would shed important insight on the relation between sweetness and food intake. In addition, the development of conditioned satiation may strongly modulate short-term results. Biological correlates are greatly needed. In a study where blood glucose and spontaneous meal initiation were closely monitored, a lower suppression of hunger and a smaller change in postprandial glucose were found when sweet intensity was rated higher.[179]

8.6.5.4 Effect of Oral Fat Sensation on Satiety

There is increasing evidence that the orosensory stimulation by fat influences not only utilization of fat[113] but also satiety.[192] In the latter study, chewing and spitting a high-fat lunch induced a modification in blood glucose and insulin consistent with a cephalic-phase response and also increased subjective satiety as rated on a VAS during the following 90 minutes, compared to a water stimulus condition.

A distinction of individuals into two fat-intake subtypes of the population was proposed: usual high-fat eaters (HFE) (about 47% of daily energy) did not distinguish high-fat test foods from their low-fat versions and ate a relatively constant amount of food, whereas usual low-fat eaters (LFE, about 20% of daily energy) did detect the difference in fat versions and adapted energy intake to the change in energy content and density of foods.[193] Although based on a small sample of subjects (eight in each phenotype) and the inability to determine whether the phenotype precedes or follows consumption of the high-fat diet, this is an interesting proposal.

Further study is also needed on whether different OSF-induced TAG elevations in blood have consequences in terms of satiety. Adding butter to a lunch increased duration of satiety and delayed the onset of the next meal.[178] The effect was linked to increased disposal of fatty acids for oxidation and a sparing effect on glucose. An increased presence of TAG due to oral stimulation by fatty OSF could, in theory, mimic this effect and contribute to enhanced satiety. However, adding fat to a meal usually leads to a reduction in insulin secretion. Alternatively, some authors[147,192,194] have reported significant increases in insulin induced by OSF (via chew and spit methods) although others have not.[114,195] If insulin secretion is actually stimulated by fat OSF, this may favor fat storage, reduce satiety, and progressively lead to weight gain. This is an important area of research for the near future.

8.7 CONCLUSIONS

One of the most debated dimensions of OSF is palatability. Some authors have denied any involvement of palatability in the metabolic control of food intake,[130] attributing this role to nonhomeostatic intake. This may be questioned, since it is clearly established that modulation of palatability according to postingestive effects is a pivotal step in the adaptive properties of eating behavior.[196] A global perspective of its involvement in the integrative mechanism of the central nervous system is proposed in Figure 8.2. It must be remembered that, prior to obtaining palatability judgments, the development of a retroactive loop, based on the adequacy of the food signaled by OSF to the body needs, is necessary. The reward process requires some reinforcement, and the satisfaction of body needs, to this day, provides the strongest experimental support. If palatability leads to the consumption of a food only for its reward effect, resulting in positive energy balance, this should not preclude a homeostatic role for palatability. It is important to remember that, in the Bertino et al. study,[197] the palatability of a regularly tasted soup increased as the time of the next meal approached and hunger increased. This change was inhibited by an opioid antagonist. Furthermore, when hunger was triggered by 2-deoxy-*d*-glucose in humans, antagonizing opioids reduced food intake.[198] This provides some support for a contribution of palatability to the physiological control of eating behavior.

Thus, based on the various data presented in this chapter, palatability seems to have several different consequences for eating behavior:

- Helps the selection of foods of those items more adapted to body needs.
- Stimulates intake at the beginning of the eating occasion in order to increase the amount consumed of a food item.
- Enhances the feeling of satisfaction of eating.
- Improves the accuracy of the association between the energy content of a food item and its OSF.

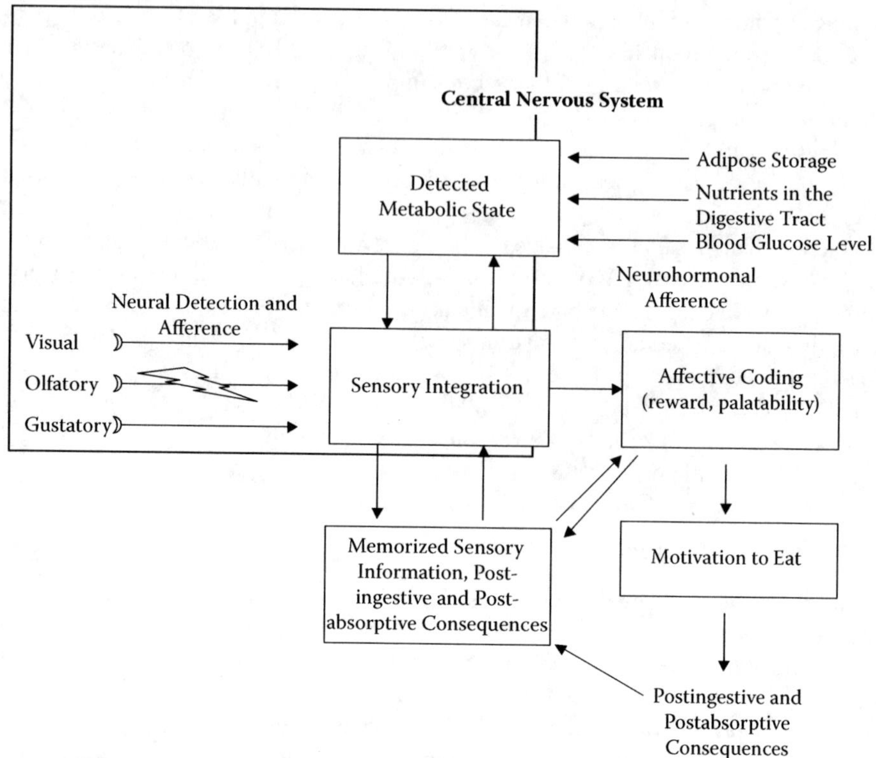

FIGURE 8.2 Integration of orosensory and metabolic cues in the central nervous system in relation to food intake. A codification in reward and palatability will complete this integration and modulate motivation to eat. Memorization is a pivotal step for this mechanism to be operant.

- Elevates the threshold of satiety under which a food item can trigger intake.
- Maintains intake of a food item even when the metabolic state may tend to reduce its consumption.

These various functions may seem redundant, but complete understanding of their mechanisms may benefit from this subdivision.

REFERENCES

1. Bonfils, P., Avan, P., Faulcon, P., and Malinvaud, D., Distorted odorant perception: analysis of a series of 56 patients with parosmia, *Arch. Otolaryngol. Head Neck Surg.*, 131, 107–112, 2005.
2. Small, D.M., Gerber, J.C., Mak, Y.E., and Hummel, T., Differential neural responses evoked by orthonasal versus retronasal odorant perception in humans, *Neuron,* 47, 593–605, 2005.
3. Heilmann, S. and Hummel, T., A new method for comparing orthonasal and retronasal olfaction, *Behav. Neurosci.,* 118, 412–419, 2004.

4. Rozin, P. and Vollmecke, T.A., Food likes and dislikes, *Annu. Rev. Nutr.*, 6, 433–456, 1986.
5. Kissileff, H., in *The Chemical Senses and Nutrition,* Kare, M.R. and Brand, J.B., Eds., Academic Press, New York, 1986, pp. 293–317.
6. Yeomans, M.R. and Symes, T., Individual differences in the use of pleasantness and palatability ratings, *Appetite,* 32, 383–394, 1999.
7. Bond, L. and Lader, M., The use of analogue scales in rating subjective feelings, *Br. J. Med. Psychol.*, 47, 211–218, 1974.
8. McBride, R., Hedonic rating of food: single or side-by-side sample presentation? *J. Food Technol.*, 21, 355–363, 1986.
9. Hill, A.J., Magson, L.D., and Blundell, J.E., Hunger and palatability: tracking ratings of subjective experience before, during and after the consumption of preferred and less preferred food, *Appetite,* 5, 361–371, 1984.
10. De Graaf, C., De Jong, L.S., and Lambers, A.C., Palatability affects satiation but not satiety, *Physiol. Behav.*, 66, 681–688, 1999.
11. Bobroff, E.M. and Kissileff, H.R., Effects of changes in palatability on food intake and the cumulative food intake curve in man, *Appetite,* 7, 85–96, 1986.
12. Yeomans, M.R., Palatability and the micro-structure of feeding in humans: the appetizer effect, *Appetite,* 27, 119–133, 1996.
13. Bellisle, F., Tournier, A., and Louis-Sylvestre, J., Monosodium glutamate and the acquisition of food preferences in a European context, *Food Qual. Prefer.*, 1, 103–108, 1989.
14. Rogers, P.J. and Blundell, J.E., Umami and appetite: effects of monosodium glutamate on hunger and food intake in human subjects, *Physiol. Behav.*, 48, 801–804, 1990.
15. Prescott, J., Effects of added glutamate on liking for novel food flavors, *Appetite,* 42, 143–150, 2004.
16. Okiyama, A. and Beauchamp, G.K., Taste dimensions of monosodium glutamate (MSG) in a food system: role of glutamate in young American subjects, *Physiol. Behav.*, 65, 177–181, 1998.
17. Zandstra, E.H., De Graaf, C., Mela, D.J., and Van Staveren, W.A., Short- and long-term effects of changes in pleasantness on food intake, *Appetite,* 34, 253–260, 2000.
18. Mattes, R., Effects of aspartame and sucrose on hunger and energy intake in humans, *Physiol. Behav.*, 47, 1037–1044, 1990.
19. Monneuse, M.O., Bellisle, F., and Louis-Sylverstre, J., Responses to an intense sweetener in humans: immediate preference and delayed effects on intake, *Physiol. Behav.*, 49, 325–330, 1991.
20. Warwick, Z.S., Hall, W.G., Pappas, T.N., and Schiffman, S.S., Taste and smell sensations enhance the satiating effect of both a high-carbohydrate and a high-fat meal in humans, *Physiol. Behav.*, 53, 553–563, 1993.
21. Yeomans, M.R., Weinberg, L., and James, S., Effects of palatability and learned satiety on energy density influences on breakfast intake in humans, *Physiol. Behav.*, 86, 487–499, 2005.
22. Le Magnen, J., in *Eating Habits,* Boakes, R.A., Popplewell, D.A., and Burton, J.M., Eds., Wiley, Chichester, pp. 131–154, 1987.
23. Tordoff, M.G., Tepper, B.J., and Friedman, M.I., Food flavor preferences produced by drinking glucose and oil in normal and diabetic rats: evidence for conditioning based on fuel oxidation, *Physiol. Behav.*, 41, 481–487, 1987.
24. Birch, L.L., Effects of experience on the modification of food acceptance patterns, *Ann. N.Y. Acad. Sci.*, 561, 209–216, 1989.
25. Kern, D.L., McPhee, L., Fisher, J., Johnson, S., and Birch, L.L., The postingestive consequences of fat condition preferences for flavors associated with high dietary fat, *Physiol. Behav.*, 54, 71–76, 1993.

26. Booth, D.A., *Psychology of Nutrition*, Taylor and Francis, London, 1994.
27. Mobini, S., Chambers, L.C., and Yeomans, M.R., Effects of hunger state on flavour pleasantness conditioning at home: flavour–nutrient learning verus flavour–flavour learning, *Appetite,* 48, 20–28, 2007.
28. Appleton, K.M., Gentry, R.C., and Shepherd, R., Evidence of a role for conditioning in the development of liking for flavours in humans in everyday life, *Physiol. Behav.,* 87, 478–486, 2006.
29. Bertino, M., Beauchamp, G.K., and Engelman, K., Long-term reduction in dietary sodium alters the taste of salt, *Am. J. Clin. Nutr.,* 36, 1134–1144, 1982.
30. Mattes, R.D., Fat preference and adherence to a reduced-fat diet, *Am. J. Clin. Nutr.,* 57, 373–81, 1993.
31. Conner, M., Tolerated sensory changes, *Appetite,* 17, 155, 1991.
32. Specter, S.E. et al., Reducing ice cream energy density does not condition decreased acceptance or engender compensation following repeated exposure, *Eur. J. Clin. Nutr.,* 52, 703–710, 1998.
33. Steiner, J.E., The gustofacial response: observation on normal and anencephalic newborn infants, *Symp. Oral. Sens. Percept.,* 254–278, 1973.
34. Lipsitt, L. and Behl, G., in *Taste, Experience and Feeding,* Capaldi, E. and Powley, T., Eds., American Psychological Association, Washington DC, pp. 75–93, 1990.
35. Desor, J., Maller, O., and Turner, R., Taste in acceptance of sugars by human infants, *J. Comp. Physiol. Psychol.,* 84, 496–501, 1973.
36. Steiner, J.E., Glaser, D., Hawilo, M.E., and Berridge, K.C., Comparative expression of hedonic impact: affective reactions to taste by human infants and other primates, *Neurosci. Biobehav. Rev.,* 25, 53–74, 2001.
37. Mistretta, C.M., in *Smell and Taste in Health and Disease,* Getchell, T.V., Bartoshuk, L.M., Doty, R.L., and Snow, J.B., Eds., Raven Press., New York, pp. 35–64, 1991.
38. Hauser, G.J., Chitayat, D., Berns, L., Braver, D., and Muhlbauer, B., Peculiar odours in newborns and maternal prenatal ingestion of spicy food, *Eur. J. Pediatr.,* 144, 403, 1985.
39. Mennella, J.A., Johnson, A., and Beauchamp, G.K., Garlic ingestion by pregnant women alters the odor of amniotic fluid, *Chem. Senses,* 20, 207–209, 1995.
40. Mennella, J.A., Jagnow, C.P., and Beauchamp, G.K., Prenatal and postnatal flavor learning by human infants, *Pediatrics,* 107, E88, 2001.
41. Arias, C. and Chotro, M.G., Amniotic fluid can act as an appetitive unconditioned stimulus in preweanling rats, *Dev. Psychobiol.,* 49, 139–149, 2007.
42. Davis, C., Self-selection of diet by newly weaned infants. An experimental study, *Am. J. Dis. Child.,* 36, 651–679, 1928.
43. Davis, C., Results of the self-selection of diets by young children, *Can. Med. Assoc. J.,* 257–261, 1939.
44. Barnett, S., *The rat. A study in behaviour,* Aldine Publishing Company, Chicago, 1963.
45. Koivisto, U.K. and Sjoden, P.O., Food and general neophobia in Swedish families: parent-child comparisons and relationships with serving specific foods, *Appetite,* 26, 107–118, 1996.
46. Cooke, L., Wardle, J., and Gibson, E.L., Relationship between parental report of food neophobia and everyday food consumption in 2–6-year-old children, *Appetite,* 41, 205–206, 2003.
47. Hursti Uk, K. and Sjoden, P., Food and general neophobia and their relationship with self-reported food choice: familial resemblance in Swedish families with children of ages 7 to 17 years, *Appetite,* 29, 89–103, 1997.
48. Loewen, R. and Pliner, P., Effects of prior exposure to palatable and unpalatable novel foods on children's willingness to taste other novel foods, *Appetite,* 32, 351–366, 1999.

49. Nicklaus, S., Boggio, V., Chabanet, C., and Issanchou, S., A prospective study of food variety seeking in childhood, adolescence and early adult life, *Appetite,* 44, 289–297, 2005.
50. Birch, L.L. and Marlin, D.W., I don't like it; I never tried it: effects of exposure on two-year-old children's food preferences, *Appetite,* 3, 353–360, 1982.
51. Sullivan, S.A. and Birch, L.L., Infant dietary experience and acceptance of solid foods, *Pediatrics,* 93, 271–277, 1994.
52. Hendy, H.M. and Raudenbush, B., Effectiveness of teacher modeling to encourage food acceptance in preschool children, *Appetite,* 34, 61–76, 2000.
53. Hendy, H.M., Effectiveness of trained peer models to encourage food acceptance in preschool children, *Appetite,* 39, 217–225, 2002.
54. Harper, L. and Sanders, K., The effect of adults' eating on young children's acceptance of unfamiliar foods, *J. Exp. Child Psychol.,* 20, 206–214, 1975.
55. Garcia, J., Lasiter, P.S., Bermudez-Rattoni, F., and Deems, D.A., A general theory of aversion learning, *Ann. N.Y. Acad. Sci.,* 443, 8–21, 1985.
56. Logue, A.W., Conditioned food aversion learning in humans, *Ann. N.Y. Acad. Sci.,* 443, 316–329, 1985.
57. Mattes, R.D., Curran, W.J., Jr., Powlis, W., and Whittington, R., A descriptive study of learned food aversions in radiotherapy patients, *Physiol. Behav.,* 50, 1103–1109, 1991.
58. Nordin, S., Broman, D.A., Garvill, J., and Nyroos, M., Gender differences in factors affecting rejection of food in healthy young Swedish adults, *Appetite,* 43, 295–301, 2004.
59. Bernstein, I.L. and Webster, M.M., Learned taste aversions in humans, *Physiol. Behav.,* 25, 363–366, 1980.
60. Andrykowski, M.A. and Otis, M.L., Development of learned food aversions in humans: investigation in a "natural laboratory" of cancer chemotherapy, *Appetite,* 14, 145–158, 1990.
61. Mattes, R.D., Arnold, C., and Boraas, M., Learned food aversions among cancer chemotherapy patients. Incidence, nature, and clinical implications, *Cancer,* 60, 2576–2580, 1987.
62. Schwartz, M.D., Jacobsen, P.B., and Bovbjerg, D.H., Role of nausea in the development of aversions to a beverage paired with chemotherapy treatment in cancer patients, *Physiol. Behav.,* 59, 659–663, 1996.
63. Reed, D.R., Bartoshuk, L.M., Duffy, V., Marino, S., and Price, R.A., Propylthiouracil tasting: determination of underlying threshold distributions using maximum likelihood, *Chem. Senses,* 20, 529–533, 1995.
64. Bartoshuk, L.M., Duffy, V.B., Lucchina, L.A., Prutkin, J., and Fast, K., PROP (6-n-propylthiouracil) supertasters and the saltiness of NaCl, *Ann. N.Y. Acad. Sci.,* 855, 793–796, 1998.
65. Karrer, T. and Bartoshuk, L., Capsaicin desensitization and recovery on the human tongue, *Physiol. Behav.,* 49, 757–764, 1991.
66. Bartoshuk, L.M., Genetic and pathological taste variation: what can we learn from animal models and human disease? *Ciba Found. Symp.,* 179, 251–262; discussion 262–267, 1993.
67. Tepper, B.J. and Nurse, R.J., Fat perception is related to PROP taster status, *Physiol. Behav.,* 61, 949–954, 1997.
68. Nasser, J.A., Kissileff, H.R., Boozer, C.N., Chou, C.J., and Pi-Sunyer, F.X., PROP taster status and oral fatty acid perception, *Eat. Behav.,* 2, 237–245, 2001.
69. Yackinous, C. and Guinard, J.X., Relation between PROP taster status and fat perception, touch, and olfaction, *Physiol. Behav.,* 72, 427–437, 2001.
70. Reed, D.R., Tanaka, T., and McDaniel, A.H., Diverse tastes: genetics of sweet and bitter perception, *Physiol. Behav.,* 88, 215–226, 2006.
71. Lugaz, O., Pillias, A.M., and Faurion, A., A new specific ageusia: some humans cannot taste l-glutamate, *Chem. Senses,* 27, 105–115, 2002.

72. Henkin, R.I. and Shallenberger, R.S., Aglycogeusia: the inability to recognize sweetness and its possible molecular basis, *Nature,* 227, 965–966, 1970.
73. Bartoshuk, L.M., Psychophysical advances aid the study of genetic variation in taste, *Appetite,* 34, 105, 2000.
74. Keller, K.L., Steinmann, L., Nurse, R.J., and Tepper, B.J., Genetic taste sensitivity to 6-n-propylthiouracil influences food preference and reported intake in preschool children, *Appetite,* 38, 3–12, 2002.
75. Drewnowski, A. and Greenwood, M.R., Cream and sugar: human preferences for high-fat foods, *Physiol. Behav.,* 30, 629–633, 1983.
76. Mela, D.J., Sensory assessment of fat content in fluid dairy products, *Appetite,* 10, 37–44, 1988.
77. Mela, D.J., Langley, K.R., and Martin, A., Sensory assessment of fat content: effect of emulsion and subject characteristics, *Appetite,* 22, 67–81, 1994.
78. Mela, D.J., Langley, K.R., and Martin, A., No effect of oral or sample temperature on sensory assessment of fat content, *Physiol. Behav.,* 56, 655–658, 1994.
79. Chale-Rush, A., Burgess, J.R., and Mattes, R.D., Multiple routes of chemosensitivity to free fatty acids in humans, *Am. J. Physiol. Gastrointest. Liver Physiol.,* 292, G1206–1212, 2007.
80. Bayarri, S., Taylor, A.J., and Hort, J., The role of fat in flavor perception: effect of partition and viscosity in model emulsions, *J. Agric. Food Chem.,* 54, 8862–8868, 2006.
81. Lethuaut, L., Weel, K.G., Boelrijk, A.E., and Brossard, C.D., Flavor perception and aroma release from model dairy desserts, *J. Agric. Food Chem.,* 52, 3478–3485, 2004.
82. Takeda, M., Imaizumi, M., and Fushiki, T., Preference for vegetable oils in the two-bottle choice test in mice, *Life Sci.,* 67, 197–204, 2000.
83. Takeda, M., Sawano, S., Imaizumi, M., and Fushiki, T., Preference for corn oil in olfactory-blocked mice in the conditioned place preference test and the two-bottle choice test, *Life Sci.,* 69, 847–854, 2001.
84. Kamphuis, M.M., Saris, W.H., and Westerterp-Plantenga, M.S., The effect of addition of linoleic acid on food intake regulation in linoleic acid tasters and linoleic acid non-tasters, *Br. J. Nutr.,* 90, 199–206, 2003.
85. Pavlov, I., *The Work of the Digestive Glands,* Charles Griffin, London, 1902.
86. Mattes, R.D., Physiologic responses to sensory stimulation by food: nutritional implications, *J. Am. Diet. Assoc.,* 97, 406–413, 1997.
87. Goldfine, I.D., Abraira, C., Gruenewald, D., and Goldstein, M.S., Plasma insulin levels during imaginary food ingestion under hypnosis, *Proc. Soc. Exp. Biol. Med.,* 133, 274–276, 1970.
88. Secchi, A. et al., Cephalic-phase insulin and glucagon release in normal subjects and in patients receiving pancreas transplantation, *Metabolism,* 44, 1153–1158, 1995.
89. Arosio, M. et al., Effects of modified sham feeding on ghrelin levels in healthy human subjects, *J. Clin. Endocrinol. Metab.,* 89, 5101–5104, 2004.
90. de Wijk, R.A., Prinz, J.F., Engelen, L., and Weenen, H., The role of alpha-amylase in the perception of oral texture and flavour in custards, *Physiol. Behav.,* 83, 81–91, 2004.
91. Wooley, S.C. and Wooley, O.W., Salivation to the sight and thought of food: a new measure of appetite, *Psychosom. Med.,* 35, 136–142, 1973.
92. Mattes, R.D., Nutritional implications of the cephalic-phase salivary response, *Appetite,* 34, 177–183, 2000.
93. Wooley, S. and Wooley, O., Relationship of salivation in humans to deprivation, inhibition and the encephalization of hunger, *Appetite,* 2, 331–350, 1981.
94. Navazesh, M. and Christensen, C.M., A comparison of whole mouth resting and stimulated salivary measurement procedures, *J. Dent. Res.,* 61, 1158–1162, 1982.

95. Christensen, C.M. and Navazesh, M., Anticipatory salivary flow to the sight of different foods, *Appetite,* 5, 307–315, 1984.
96. Tepper, B.J., Dietary restraint and responsiveness to sensory-based food cues as measured by cephalic phase salivation and sensory specific satiety, *Physiol. Behav.,* 52, 305–311, 1992.
97. Klajner, F., Herman, C.P., Polivy, J., and Chhabra, R., Human obesity, dieting, and anticipatory salivation to food, *Physiol. Behav.,* 27, 195–198, 1981.
98. Legoff, D.B. and Spigelman, M.N., Salivary response to olfactory food stimuli as a function of dietary restraint and body weight, *Appetite,* 8, 29–35, 1987.
99. Sahakian, B.J., Lean, M.E., Robbins, T.W., and James, W.P., Salivation and insulin secretion in response to food in non-obese men and women, *Appetite,* 2, 209–216, 1981.
100. Brunstrom, J.M., Yates, H.M., and Witcomb, G.L., Dietary restraint and heightened reactivity to food, *Physiol. Behav.,* 81, 85–90, 2004.
101. Wooley, O.W., Wooley, S.C., and Dunham, R.B., Deprivation, expectation and threat: effects on salivation in the obese and nonobese, *Physiol. Behav.,* 17, 187–193, 1976.
102. Epstein, L.H., Paluch, R., and Coleman, K.J., Differences in salivation to repeated food cues in obese and nonobese women, *Psychosom. Med.,* 58, 160–164, 1996.
103. Teff, K., Nutritional implications of the cephalic-phase reflexes: endocrine responses, *Appetite,* 34, 206–213, 2000.
104. Teff, K.L. and Townsend, R.R., Early phase insulin infusion and muscarinic blockade in obese and lean subjects, *Am. J. Physiol.,* 277, R198–208, 1999.
105. Ahren, B. and Holst, J.J., The cephalic insulin response to meal ingestion in humans is dependent on both cholinergic and noncholinergic mechanisms and is important for postprandial glycemia, *Diabetes,* 50, 1030–1038, 2001.
106. Teff, K.L. and Engelman, K., Oral sensory stimulation improves glucose tolerance in humans: effects on insulin, C-peptide, and glucagon, *Am. J. Physiol.,* 270, R1371–1379, 1996.
107. Bellisle, F., Louis-Sylvestre, J., Demozay, F., Blazy, D., and Le Magnen, J., Reflex insulin response associated to food intake in human subjects, *Physiol. Behav.,* 31, 515–521, 1983.
108. Bellisle, F., Louis-Sylvestre, J., Demozay, F., Blazy, D., and Le Magnen, J., Cephalic phase of insulin secretion and food stimulation in humans: a new perspective, *Am. J. Physiol.,* 249, E639–645, 1985.
109. Teff, K.L. and Engelman, K., Palatability and dietary restraint: effect on cephalic phase insulin release in women, *Physiol. Behav.,* 60, 567–573, 1996.
110. Abdallah, L., Chabert, M., and Louis-Sylvestre, J., Cephalic phase responses to sweet taste, *Am. J. Clin. Nutr.,* 65, 737–743, 1997.
111. Teff, K.L., Devine, J., and Engelman, K., Sweet taste: effect on cephalic phase insulin release in men, *Physiol. Behav.,* 57, 1089–1095, 1995.
112. Smeets, P.A., de Graaf, C., Stafleu, A., van Osch, M.J., and van der Grond, J., Functional magnetic resonance imaging of human hypothalamic responses to sweet taste and calories, *Am. J. Clin. Nutr.,* 82, 1011–1016, 2005.
113. Mattes, R.D., Oral fat exposure alters postprandial lipid metabolism in humans, *Am. J. Clin. Nutr.,* 63, 911–917, 1996.
114. Tittelbach, T.J. and Mattes, R.D., Oral stimulation influences postprandial triacylglycerol concentrations in humans: nutrient specificity, *J. Am. Coll. Nutr.,* 20, 485–493, 2001.
115. Mattes, R.D., Oral exposure to butter, but not fat replacers elevates postprandial triacylglycerol concentration in humans, *J. Nutr.,* 131, 1491–1496, 2001.
116. Mattes, R.D., The taste of fat elevates postprandial triacylglycerol, *Physiol. Behav.,* 74, 343–348, 2001.
117. Singleton, M.J., Heiser, C., Jamesen, K., and Mattes, R.D., Sweetener augmentation of serum triacylglycerol during a fat challenge test in humans, *J. Am. Coll. Nutr.,* 18, 179–185, 1999.

118. Mattes, R.D., Oral fat exposure increases the first phase triacylglycerol concentration due to release of stored lipid in humans, *J. Nutr.,* 132, 3656–3662, 2002.
119. Jordan, H.A., Voluntary intragastric feeding: oral and gastric contributions to food intake and hunger in man, *J. Comp. Physiol. Psychol.,* 68, 498–506, 1969.
120. Cecil, J.E., Francis, J., and Read, N.W., Relative contributions of intestinal, gastric, oro-sensory influences and information to changes in appetite induced by the same liquid meal, *Appetite,* 31, 377–390, 1998.
121. Cecil, J.E., Castiglione, K., French, S., Francis, J., and Read, N.W., Effects of intragastric infusions of fat and carbohydrate on appetite ratings and food intake from a test meal, *Appetite,* 30, 65–77, 1998.
122. Louis-Sylvestre, J. and Le Magnen, J., Fall in blood glucose level precedes meal onset in free-feeding rats, *Neurosci. Biobehav. Rev.,* 4 (Suppl. 1), 13–15, 1980.
123. Campfield, L.A., Smith, F.J., Rosenbaum, M., and Hirsch, J., Human eating: evidence for a physiological basis using a modified paradigm, *Neurosci. Biobehav. Rev.,* 20, 133–137, 1996.
124. Chapelot, D., Marmonier, C., Aubert, R., Gausseres, N., and Louis-Sylvestre, J., A role for glucose and insulin preprandial profiles to differentiate meals and snacks, *Physiol. Behav.,* 80, 721–731, 2004.
125. Lowe, M.R. and Levine, A.S., Eating motives and the controversy over dieting: eating less than needed versus less than wanted, *Obes. Res.,* 13, 797–806, 2005.
126. Booth, D.A., Lee, M., and McAleavey, C., Acquired sensory control of satiation in man, *Br. J. Psychol.,* 67, 137–147, 1976.
127. Le Magnen, J. and Devos, M., Metabolic correlates of the meal onset in the free food intake of rats, *Physiol. Behav.,* 5, 805–814, 1970.
128. Le Magnen, J., Devos, M., Gaudilliere, J.P., Louis-Sylvestre, J., and Tallon, S., Role of a lipostatic mechanism in regulation by feeding of energy balance in rats, *J. Comp. Physiol. Psychol.,* 84, 1–23, 1973.
129. Le Magnen, J. and Devos, M., Meal to meal energy balance in rats, *Physiol. Behav.,* 32, 39–44, 1984.
130. Yeomans, M.R., Blundell, J.E., and Leshem, M., Palatability: response to nutritional need or need-free stimulation of appetite? *Br. J. Nutr.,* 92 (Suppl. 1), S3–14, 2004.
131. Booth, D.A., Mather, P., and Fuller, J., Starch content of ordinary foods associatively conditions human appetite and satiation, indexed by intake and eating pleasantness of starch-paired flavours, *Appetite,* 3, 163–184, 1982.
132. Louis-Sylvestre, J. et al., Learned caloric adjustment of human intake, *Appetite,* 12, 95–103, 1989.
133. Zandstra, E.H., Stubenitsky, K., De Graaf, C., and Mela, D.J., Effects of learned flavour cues on short-term regulation of food intake in a realistic setting, *Physiol. Behav.,* 75, 83–90, 2002.
134. Yeomans, M.R., Lee, M.D., Gray, R.W., and French, S.J., Effects of test-meal palatability on compensatory eating following disguised fat and carbohydrate preloads, *Int. J. Obes. Relat. Metab. Disord.,* 25, 1215–1224, 2001.
135. de Wijk, R.A., Polet, I.A., Engelen, L., van Doorn, R.M., and Prinz, J.F., Amount of ingested custard dessert as affected by its color, odor, and texture, *Physiol. Behav.,* 82, 397–403, 2004.
136. Stevenson, R.J., The acquisition of odour qualities, *Q. J. Exp. Psychol. A,* 54, 561–77, 2001.
137. Yeomans, M.R., Mobini, S., Elliman, T.D., Walker, H.C., and Stevenson, R.J., Hedonic and sensory characteristics of odors conditioned by pairing with tastants in humans, *J. Exp. Psychol. Anim. Behav. Process.,* 32, 215–228, 2006.
138. Stevenson, R.J. and Boakes, R.A., A mnemonic theory of odor perception, *Psychol. Rev.,* 110, 340–364, 2003.

139. Rolls, B.J., Rolls, E.T., Rowe, E.A., and Sweeney, K., Sensory specific satiety in man, *Physiol. Behav.,* 27, 137–142, 1981.
140. Hetherington, M., Rolls, B.J., and Burley, V.J., The time course of sensory-specific satiety, *Appetite,* 12, 57–68, 1989.
141. Rolls, B.J. and McDermott, T.M., Effects of age on sensory-specific satiety, *Am. J. Clin. Nutr.,* 54, 988–996, 1991.
142. Guinard, J.X. and Brun, P., Sensory-specific satiety: comparison of taste and texture effects, *Appetite,* 31, 141–157, 1998.
143. Rolls, B.J., Hetherington, M., and Burley, V.J., Sensory stimulation and energy density in the development of satiety, *Physiol. Behav.,* 44, 727–733, 1988.
144. Rolls, B.J., Sensory-specific satiety, *Nutr. Rev.,* 44, 93–101, 1986.
145. Rolls, B.J., Hetherington, M., and Burley, V.J., The specificity of satiety: the influence of foods of different macronutrient content on the development of satiety, *Physiol. Behav.,* 43, 145–153, 1988.
146. Rolls, E.T. and Rolls, J.H., Olfactory sensory-specific satiety in humans, *Physiol. Behav.,* 61, 461–473, 1997.
147. Smeets, A.J. and Westerterp-Plantenga, M.S., Oral exposure and sensory-specific satiety, *Physiol. Behav.,* 89, 281–286, 2006.
148. Johnson, J. and Vickers, Z., Effects of flavor and macronutrient composition of food servings on liking, hunger and subsequent intake, *Appetite,* 21, 25–39, 1993.
149. de Graaf, C., Schreurs, A., and Blauw, Y.H., Short-term effects of different amounts of sweet and nonsweet carbohydrates on satiety and energy intake, *Physiol. Behav.,* 54, 833–843, 1993.
150. Bell, E.A., Roe, L.S., and Rolls, B.J., Sensory-specific satiety is affected more by volume than by energy content of a liquid food, *Physiol. Behav.,* 78, 593–600, 2003.
151. Johnson, J. and Vickers, Z., Factors influencing sensory-specific satiety, *Appetite,* 19, 15–31, 1992.
152. Vandewater, K. and Vickers, Z., Higher-protein foods produce greater sensory-specific satiety, *Physiol. Behav.,* 59, 579–583, 1996.
153. Rolls, B.J., Van Duijvenvoorde, P.M., and Rolls, E.T., Pleasantness changes and food intake in a varied four-course meal, *Appetite,* 5, 337–348, 1984.
154. Norton, G.N., Anderson, A.S., and Hetherington, M.M., Volume and variety: relative effects on food intake, *Physiol. Behav.,* 87, 714–722, 2006.
155. Spiegel, T.A. and Stellar, E., Effects of variety on food intake of underweight, normal-weight and overweight women, *Appetite,* 15, 47–61, 1990.
156. Pliner, P., Polivy, J., Herman, C.P., and Zakalusny, I., Short-term intake of overweight individuals and normal weight dieters and non-dieters with and without choice among a variety of foods, *Appetite,* 1, 203–213, 1980.
157. Bellisle, F. and Le Magnen, J., The structure of meals in humans: eating and drinking patterns in lean and obese subjects, *Physiol. Behav.,* 27, 649–658, 1981.
158. Bellisle, F. and Le Magnen, J., The analysis of human feeding patterns: the edogram, *Appetite,* 1, 141–150, 1980.
159. Beatty, W.W., Dietary variety stimulates appetite in females but not in males, *Bull. Psychon. Soc.,* 19, 212–214, 1982.
160. Wisniewski, L., Epstein, L.H., and Caggiula, A.R., Effect of food change on consumption, hedonics, and salivation, *Physiol. Behav.,* 52, 21–26, 1992.
161. Rolls, B.J. et al., Variety in a meal enhances food intake in man, *Physiol. Behav.,* 26, 215–221, 1981.
162. Rolls, B.J., Rowe, E.A., and Rolls, E.T., How sensory properties of foods affect human feeding behavior, *Physiol. Behav.,* 29, 409–417, 1982.
163. Hetherington, M.M., Foster, R., Newman, T., Anderson, A.S., and Norton, G., Understanding variety: tasting different foods delays satiation, *Physiol. Behav.,* 87, 263–271, 2006.

164. Romer, M. et al., Does modification of olfacto-gustatory stimulation diminish sensory-specific satiety in humans? *Physiol. Behav.,* 87, 469–477, 2006.
165. Cornell, C.E., Rodin, J., and Weingarten, H., Stimulus-induced eating when satiated, *Physiol. Behav.,* 45, 695–704, 1989.
166. Torheim, L.E. et al., Validation of food variety as an indicator of diet quality assessed with a food frequency questionnaire for Western Mali, *Eur. J. Clin. Nutr.,* 57, 1283–1291, 2003.
167. Stubbs, R.J., Johnstone, A.M., Mazlan, N., Mbaiwa, S.E., and Ferris, S., Effect of altering the variety of sensorially distinct foods, of the same macronutrient content, on food intake and body weight in men, *Eur. J. Clin. Nutr.,* 55, 19–28, 2001.
168. Alfenas, R.C. and Mattes, R.D., Influence of glycemic index/load on glycemic response, appetite, and food intake in healthy humans, *Diabetes Care,* 28, 2123–2129, 2005.
169. McCrory, M.A. et al., Dietary variety within food groups: association with energy intake and body fatness in men and women, *Am. J. Clin. Nutr.,* 69, 440–447, 1999.
170. Kissileff, H.R., Thornton, J., and Becker, E., A quadratic equation adequately describes the cumulative food intake curve in man, *Appetite,* 3, 255–272, 1982.
171. Bellisle, F., Lucas, F., Amrani, R., and Le Magnen, J., Deprivation, palatability and the micro-structure of meals in human subjects, *Appetite,* 5, 85–94, 1984.
172. Spiegel, T.A., Shrager, E.E., and Stellar, E., Responses of lean and obese subjects to preloads, deprivation, and palatability, *Appetite,* 13, 45–69, 1989.
173. Yeomans, M.R., Gray, R.W., Mitchell, C.J., and True, S., Independent effects of palatability and within-meal pauses on intake and appetite ratings in human volunteers, *Appetite,* 29, 61–76, 1997.
174. Blundell, J.E. and Rogers, P.J., in *Chemical Senses: Vol 4. Appetite, and Nutrition,* Friedman, M.I., Tordoff, M.G., and Kare, M.R., Eds., Marcel Dekker, New York, pp. 127–148, 1991.
175. Guy-Grand, B., Lehnert, V., Doassans, M., and Bellisle, F., Type of test-meal affects palatability and eating style in humans, *Appetite,* 22, 125–134, 1994.
176. Marmonier, C., Chapelot, D., Fantino, M., and Louis-Sylvestre, J., Snacks consumed in a nonhungry state have poor satiating efficiency: influence of snack composition on substrate utilization and hunger, *Am. J. Clin. Nutr.,* 76, 518–728, 2002.
177. Marmonier, C., Chapelot, D., and Louis-Sylvestre, J., Metabolic and behavioral consequences of a snack consumed in a satiety state, *Am. J. Clin. Nutr.,* 70, 854–866, 1999.
178. Himaya, A., Fantino, M., Antoine, J.M., Brondel, L., and Louis-Sylvestre, J., Satiety power of dietary fat: a new appraisal, *Am. J. Clin. Nutr.,* 65, 1410–1418, 1997.
179. Melanson, K.J., Westerterp-Plantenga, M.S., Campfield, L.A., and Saris, W.H., Blood glucose and meal patterns in time-blinded males, after aspartame, carbohydrate, and fat consumption, in relation to sweetness perception, *Br. J. Nutr.,* 82, 437–446, 1999.
180. Melanson, K.J., Westerterp-Plantenga, M.S., Campfield, L.A., and Saris, W.H., Appetite and blood glucose profiles in humans after glycogen-depleting exercise, *J. Appl. Physiol.* 87, 947–954, 1999.
181. Marmonier, C., Chapelot, D., and Louis-Sylvestre, J., Effects of macronutrient content and energy density of snacks consumed in a satiety state on the onset of the next meal, *Appetite,* 34, 161–168, 2000.
182. Callahan, H.S. et al., Postprandial suppression of plasma ghrelin level is proportional to ingested caloric load but does not predict intermeal interval in humans, *J. Clin. Endocrinol. Metab.,* 89, 1319–1324, 2004.
183. Kirkmeyer, S.V. and Mattes, R.D., Effects of food attributes on hunger and food intake, *Int. J. Obes. Relat. Metab. Disord.,* 24, 1167–1175, 2000.
184. Perez, C., Dalix, A.M., Guy-Grand, B., and Bellisle, F., Human responses to five concentrations of sucrose in a dairy product: immediate and delayed palatability effects, *Appetite,* 23, 165–178, 1994.

185. Sorensen, L.B., Moller, P., Flint, A., Martens, M., and Raben, A., Effect of sensory perception of foods on appetite and food intake: a review of studies on humans, *Int. J. Obes. Relat. Metab. Disord.*, 27, 1152–1166, 2003.
186. Van Wymelbeke, V., Beridot-Therond, M.E., de La Gueronniere, V., and Fantino, M., Influence of repeated consumption of beverages containing sucrose or intense sweeteners on food intake, *Eur. J. Clin. Nutr.*, 58, 154–161, 2004.
187. Beridot-Therond, M.E., Arts, I., Fantino, M., and De La Gueronniere, V., Short-term effects of the flavour of drinks on ingestive behaviours in man, *Appetite,* 31, 67–81, 1998.
188. Lavin, J.H., French, S.J., and Read, N.W., The effect of sucrose- and aspartame-sweetened drinks on energy intake, hunger and food choice of female, moderately restrained eaters, *Int. J. Obes. Relat. Metab. Disord.*, 21, 37–42, 1997.
189. Holt, S.H., Sandona, N., and Brand-Miller, J.C., The effects of sugar-free vs sugar-rich beverages on feelings of fullness and subsequent food intake, *Int. J. Food Sci. Nutr.*, 51, 59–71, 2000.
190. Raben, A., Vasilaras, T.H., Moller, A.C., and Astrup, A., Sucrose compared with artificial sweeteners: different effects on ad libitum food intake and body weight after 10 wk of supplementation in overweight subjects, *Am. J. Clin. Nutr.*, 76, 721–729, 2002.
191. Klein, D.A., Schebendach, J.S., Devlin, M.J., Smith, G.P., and Walsh, B.T., Intake, sweetness and liking during modified sham feeding of sucrose solutions, *Physiol. Behav.*, 87, 602–606, 2006.
192. Smeets, A.J. and Westerterp-Plantenga, M.S., Satiety and substrate mobilization after oral fat stimulation, *Br. J. Nutr.*, 95, 795–801, 2006.
193. Cooling, J. and Blundell, J., Are high-fat and low-fat consumers distinct phenotypes? Differences in the subjective and behavioural response to energy and nutrient challenges, *Eur. J. Clin. Nutr.*, 52, 193–201, 1998.
194. Robertson, M.D., Jackson, K.G., Williams, C.M., Fielding, B.A., and Frayn, K.N., Prolonged effects of modified sham feeding on energy substrate mobilization, *Am. J. Clin. Nutr.*, 73, 111–117, 2001.
195. Tittelbach, T.J. and Mattes, R.D., Effect of orosensory stimulation on postprandial thermogenesis in humans, *Physiol. Behav.*, 75, 71–81, 2002.
196. Le Magnen, J., *Neurobiology of Feeding and Nutrition,* Academic Press, San Diego, 1992.
197. Bertino, M., Beauchamp, G.K., and Engelman, K., Naltrexone, an opioid blocker, alters taste perception and nutrient intake in humans, *Am. J. Physiol.*, 261, R59–63, 1991.
198. Thompson, D.A., Welle, S.L., Lilavivat, U., Penicaud, L., and Campbell, R.G., Opiate receptor blockade in man reduces 2-deoxy-d-glucose-induced food intake but not hunger, thirst, and hypothermia, *Life Sci.*, 31, 847–852, 1982.

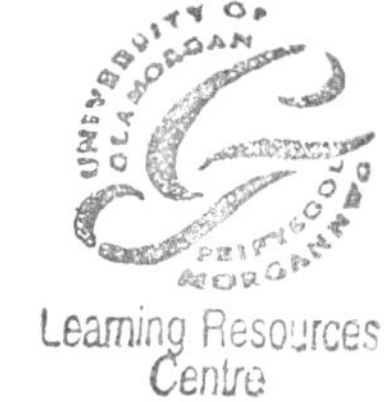

9 Gastrointestinal Factors in Appetite and Food Intake — Animal Research

Thomas A. Lutz and Nori Geary

CONTENTS

9.1 INTRODUCTION

9.1.1 Scope

Animal research in recent years has produced many advances in understanding of the operation of gastrointestinal (GI) controls of eating and their interactions with other mechanisms. The most progress has been made in hormonal controls in laboratory mouse and rat models. This chapter briefly reviews this literature. We emphasize the normal physiological operation of the controls because we believe this information is the most relevant aspect of animal models for the development of selective, therapeutically useful controls of disordered human eating.[1] Further information on this very active research area is available in several recent detailed reviews of GI controls of eating.[2–7]

In animals, one is limited to the study of behavior, although subjective processes, such as food hedonics, can be modeled with appropriate behavioral tests. The elemental movements of eating — licking, chewing, swallowing, and so forth — are functionally organized by the brain into the molar functional unit of eating, the meal. Thus, it seems to make neurological and psychological sense to analyze eating in terms of the controls of meal initiation (usually called hunger), maintenance of eating during the meal (one aspect of food reward), meal termination (satiation), and inhibition of eating following meals (postprandial satiety). The best investigated of these is the control of satiation.

Information related to many GI functions is relayed to the brain and affects eating. The principal means of communication between gut and brain are hormonal (gastrointestinal and pancreatic peptides whose release is affected by eating) and

TABLE 9.1
Gut Peptides Potentially Involved in the Physiological Control of Eating

Peptide	Site(s) of Production	Site(s) of Critical Receptors	Reference
Amylin	Pancreatic B-cell	Area postrema (AP)	[8]
Apolipoprotein A IV	Villus epithelia	?	[9]
Bombesin-like peptides (GRP; neuromedin B)	Stomach	Vagal and spinal visceral afferents	[10]
Cholecystokinin (CCK)	Proximal small intestine	Vagal afferents in pyloric area; pyloric smooth muscle; liver	[6]
Enterostatin	Exocrine pancreas	?	[11]
Ghrelin	Stomach	Arcuate nucleus (ARC); AP; vagal afferents	[12]
GLP-1	Ileum	Brain stem; hypothalamus	[13]
Glucagon	Pancreatic A-cell	Liver	[14]
Insulin	Pancreatic B-cell	ARC	[4]
(gastric) Leptin	Stomach	ARC; vagal afferents; brain stem	[4,15]
PYY 3-36	Ileum	Hypothalamus	[16]

neural (vagal and spinal visceral afferent neural signals originating in the gut). Table 9.1 lists gut peptides that presently appear to have signal functions controlling eating, and Table 9.2 lists potential neural controls arising from the stimulation of gut receptors. Because it is beyond our scope to review each of these in detail, we focus on a few examples that illustrate the key issues involved in establishing GI signals as normal physiological controls of eating. Further, we include the pancreatic hormone amylin, which acts as a satiating hormone similar to gut-derived signals and which interacts with them. We also discuss the operation of these GI signals in animal models of overeating and obesity. Finally, we close with a discussion of some perspectives relevant to the translation of animal physiology into human therapeutics.

TABLE 9.2
Gut Neural Receptors Potentially Involved in the Physiological Control of Eating

Receptor Site and Characteristics	Reference
Gastric mechanoreceptors	[17]
Hepatic chemoreceptors[a]	[18,19]
Hepatic thermoreceptors	[20]
Intestinal chemoreceptors[a]	[21,22]
Intestinal mechanoreceptors	[21]
Intestinal osmoreceptors	[7]

[a] Here, chemoreceptors are broadly defined to include specific nutrients (glucose) or their digestive and metabolic products or consequences (lactate, changes in hepatocyte membrane potential, or changes in pH).

9.1.2 Physiological Relevance of Gut Hormones in Eating

Hormones have been under consideration as physiological controls of eating for many years. Criteria for evaluating their physiological status have evolved together

TABLE 9.3
Criteria for the Physiological Action of Hormonal Controls of Eating[5]

1. Secretion	Eating changes the secretion of the hormone.
2. Receptor	Receptors are present at the primary site of action.
3. Physiological dose	The eating effect is reproduced by mimicking the secretion pattern of the endogenous hormone by administration of the hormone. This may perhaps only occur in synergy with other endogenous stimuli.
4. Removal, replacement	Removal of the hormone or the critical receptors prevents the eating effect. Appropriate hormone replacement or receptor rescue reproduces the effect.
5. Antagonism	The eating effect of the endogenous hormone is prevented by selectively antagonizing the hormone signaling. Selective antagonisms also prevent the eating effect of physiological doses of the exogenous hormone.

with progress in endocrinology in general. Table 9.3 provides a recent version of such criteria, which we use in evaluating the effects of the several hormones that we consider here.

9.1.3 Integrative Context

The GI tract is the source of numerous physiological signals controlling eating. GI signals, together with signals originating in the oropharynx, form a primordial mechanism controlling eating, present even in animals lacking a central nervous system. These primordial controls continue to operate in mammals, although they are modulated by numerous other, more recently evolved mechanisms related, for example, to the homeostatic control of metabolism and energy balance. In addition, phylogeny has strongly tended toward increasing plasticity in behavior and physiology, and eating is no exception. The evidence for this is obvious in human eating, which is so strongly individuated by culture and individual experience that the operation of the underlying physiology is often difficult to discern. Nevertheless, GI and other primordial controls of eating do operate in humans and form the basis on which other physiological controls, as well as the influences of learning and cognition, are overlaid.

9.2 GASTRIC SIGNALS

9.2.1 Gastric Volume

The upper gastrointestinal tract is richly innervated with mechanoreceptors that are stimulated by various aspects of gut loading during and after meals and that signal the brain via both vagal and splanchnic visceral afferents. The effects of gastric volume on eating in rats have been elegantly analyzed using gastric cannulas in combination with chronic pyloric cuffs that can be inflated during meals to limit food stimuli to the oropharynyx and stomach.[17] The key findings are as follows:

1. When gastric cannulas are used to prevent ingested liquid food from accumulating in the stomach, meal size is dramatically increased.
2. When ingested food is prevented from entering the intestines by inflating pyloric cuffs, meal size is about normal.
3. When fluid loads are infused into the stomach of rats with closed pyloric cuffs, eating is inhibited in proportion to the volume infused.
4. The effect of gastric fill on eating is identical whether nutrient or nonnutrient loads are used.

These data indicate that gastric volume is an adequate stimulus for mechanoreceptors that can contribute to the control of eating. The normal contribution of this signal to eating, however, appears to be small. First, intragastric infusions inhibit eating in rats with closed pyloric cuffs only when the total gastric fill (ingesta plus infusion) is markedly larger than the control meal size. Second, the dose–response relation between infusion volume and amount less eaten is relatively flat, such that the behavior does not nearly compensate for the infusion. And third, because normal gastric emptying is prevented in the cuff-closed condition, the gastric volume at meal end is markedly larger than the gastric volume at the end of a similarly sized meal in the cuff-open (normal) condition. Indeed, gastric emptying usually proceeds at a surprisingly brisk pace during the meal, especially when liquids are eaten. In both rats and rhesus monkeys, the intrameal rate of gastric emptying of liquid diet is about five times the postmeal rate.[17]

Because of its key role in the distribution of ingesta in the gastrointestinal tract, gastric emptying is a highly regulated and adaptable function with numerous hormonal and neural controls. The fact that some of these controls affect eating independent of their influence on gastric emptying (for example, cholecystokinin [CCK]) complicates analysis of the effects of gastric emptying *per se* on eating. The influence of gastric emptying on eating is further complicated by the obvious fact that gastric emptying both decreases the intensity of gastric signals and increases the intensity of intestinal and postabsorptive signals. Importantly, the fact that at meal end there are significant amounts of ingesta both in the stomach and at postgastric sites suggests the possibility that gastric and postgastric signals interact in the normal control of eating. Evidence for such interactions is considered in the following sections.

9.2.2 Food Viscosity

The speed of gastric emptying varies with the physical properties of a diet. Solid food empties more slowly from the stomach than low-viscosity, liquid food of similar energy content. Davidson and Swithers recently tested the effect of the viscosity of premeals on subsequent food intake in rats.[23] Their key findings were:

1. Rats ate more during a 1-hour test meal after a low-viscosity premeal than after a high-viscosity premeal.
2. This phenomenon was due to the physical viscosity of the premeal rather than the nature of the thickening agent used.

3. Rats chronically offered a low-viscosity food in addition to chow gained more body weight than rats that were offered a similarly palatable high-viscosity supplement or rats offered chow alone.

These findings in rats suggest that high-energy, low-viscosity foods, such as many soft drinks, may contribute to excessive body weight gain in humans.

9.2.3 Ghrelin

Ghrelin, a hormone discovered in 1999, is the endogenous ligand for the growth hormone secretagogue receptor (GHS-R). Ghrelin is expressed mainly in the stomach, but also in the brain and other tissues. Gastric ghrelin has attracted great interest because (1) it is the only gut peptide whose secretion is stimulated during fasting and inhibited by eating, and (2) it is the only gut peptide whose administration stimulates eating, as now shown in rats and humans.[24,25] Furthermore, chronic peripheral or central ghrelin administration stimulates food intake, decreases energy expenditure, and induces weight gain.

9.2.3.1 Physiological Relevance

According to the criteria of Table 9.3, the physiological status of ghrelin as a hunger signal is not fully established.

1. In several species including humans and rats, plasma ghrelin levels rise shortly before meals are initiated and fall rapidly when food is consumed. However, in humans there is also a nocturnal rise and fall in plasma ghrelin that is not associated with meals, so ghrelin alone is insufficient to account for meal initiation.
2. The preponderance of evidence[26] indicates that the eating-stimulatory effect of ghrelin is mediated by the GHS-Rs in the brain, especially those in the hypothalamic arcuate nucleus (ARC) and the brain stem. Since neurons in these areas also secrete ghrelin, the relative contributions of hormonal and neuronal ghrelin to its eating effect remain unclear.
3. It is unknown whether mimicking physiological ghrelin levels, especially the physiological preprandial rise in circulating ghrelin, is sufficient to trigger eating.
4. Removal of ghrelin secreting cells would require gastrectomy, clearly an intervention with numerous other effects. The ghrelin knockout mouse, however, exhibits the expected leaner phenotype under some conditions.[27] Thus, the criterion for removal and replacement is only partially fulfilled.
5. GHS receptor antagonists have been shown to reduce feeding in mice, but the potency and specificity of ghrelin antagonists are still not ideal.[28] Blocking endogenous ghrelin action by specific ghrelin spiegelmers may offer an interesting alternative.[29]

Because plasma ghrelin levels fall rapidly during meals, it is conceivable that the reduction in ghrelin signaling contributes to satiation. Indeed, recent data in humans suggest that the mealtime inhibition of ghrelin secretion is mediated by the increase in secretion of the satiation signal CCK.[30] Consistent with the hypothesis that reductions in plasma ghrelin secretion signal satiation, (1) ghrelin administration often increases meal size in rats and affects the timing of meals, and (2) ghrelin may interact with satiation signals in the control of eating.[3,31]

9.2.3.2 Ghrelin as an Inverse Adiposity Signal

Ghrelin may contribute to the control of body weight as well as to the initiation of individual meals. Indeed, initial reports suggest that ghrelin meets the three principal criteria proposed for an adiposity signal.[8,14] That is:

1. Endogenous fasting ghrelin levels are inversely correlated with body weight in humans and rats (although diet composition also appears to be a major determinant of ghrelin levels independent of body weight).[25]
2. Chronic ghrelin administration increases adiposity and body weight in mice and rats (although the relative contributions of eating and energy expenditure remain unclear).[32]
3. Chronic administration of specific ghrelin spiegelmers has recently been shown to reduce weight gain in mice offered a high-fat diet.[29]

Hence, we consider the hypothesis that ghrelin is an adiposity signal controlling eating to be plausible and in need of further verification.

9.2.3.3 Ghrelin and Obesity

In addition to the chronic spiegelmer results mentioned above, rats and mice that were actively immunized with an anti-ghrelin vaccine did not eat in response to peripheral ghrelin, although they did eat in response to central ghrelin, and gained slightly less body weight than control animals (T.A. Lutz, unpublished). Hence, it is possible that antagonism of endogenous ghrelin signaling is sufficient to control body weight in rats. Whether this is also true in animal models of obesity is not yet known.

9.3 INTESTINAL SIGNALS

9.3.1 Intestinal Chemoreception

Nutrient and osmotic stimuli acting in the small intestine appear to play physiological roles in satiation (see Ritter[7] for a critical review). Nutrients involved include long-chain fatty acids, most carbohydrates, and proteins. Both neural (especially vagal afferents) and endocrine (see following sections) signals relay this information to the brain. Nonnutritive osmotic stimuli have been shown to affect food intake within the physiological range of intrameal intraluminal osmotic pressure (700 mosmol/l in swine and rats).[7]

The most extensive information related to nutrient-related intestinal satiation or satiety exists for lipids.[7] The reduction in eating induced by intraduodenal lipids depends largely on preabsorptive sensing of fatty acids and monoglyceride. Inhibition of pancreatic lipase, for example by orlistat (Hoffman LaRoche, Basel, Switzerland) attenuates the reduction of food intake induced by intestinal triglyceride infusion. Furthermore, long-chain fatty acids seem to be preferentially involved, because intestinal infusions of glycerol or fatty acids with chain length of 12 C or less elicited less satiation. Thus, the full eating-inhibitory potential of fatty acids apparently is realized when fatty acids are absorbed via the chylomicron pathway rather than directly into the hepatic portal vein. The major mediators of intestinal lipid-induced satiation or satiety appear to be signals released during absorption, such as the peptides CCK, glucagon-like peptide-1 (GLP-1), peptide YY (PYY), and apolipoprotein A-IV (Apo A-IV), or oleoylethanolamide (OEA) (see sections that follow).

Among carbohydrates, glucose seems to be the major intestinal signal. Blockade of carbohydrate digestion (by acarbose, for example) reduced the effect of intraduodenal infusions of maltotriose on food intake.[7] The afferent signal induced by carbohydrates seems unrelated to glucose uptake into the enterocytes, because blockade of the sodium-linked glucose transporter with phlorizin did not affect carbohydrate-induced intestinal satiation. Some specific amino acids, especially l-phenylalanine and l-tryptophan, also seem to be important intestinal signals. The transduction mechanisms involved are unknown.

Finally, vagal afferents are clearly the major gut–brain pathway mediating intestinal nutrient-related signals. After subdiaphragmatic vagal deafferentation, the most selective and complete method for lesions of gut vagal afferents, rats no longer ate less in response to intraduodenal infusions of lipid, carbohydrate, or fat.

9.3.2 Cholecystokinin (CCK)

CCK is synthesized by I cells in the proximal small intestinal mucosa. Their apical surfaces are exposed to intraluminal stimuli, and CCK is secreted through the basolateral membrane. Gibbs and colleagues were the first to show that intraperitoneal injections of CCK selectively inhibit eating.[33] CCK seems to be a pure satiation signal because administration of CCK at meal onset decreases meal size in animals and humans with little effect on the following intermeal interval[5,6] and, except at high doses, without causing aversive or toxic effects. CCK remains the most investigated gut peptide that controls eating (see work by the groups of G.P. Smith and J.G. Gibbs, T. Moran and P. McHugh, R. Ritter, R. Reidelberger, C. Beglinger).

9.3.2.1 Physiological Relevance

Here, we briefly summarize the evidence that, in both rats and humans, CCK meets the criteria of Table 9.3 for a physiological satiation signal.

1. In contrast to humans, plasma CCK concentration has rarely been demonstrated to increase during a meal in rats.[5] Together with other data, in particular that intraperitoneal administration of CCK is relatively more potent than intravenous CCK to inhibit eating, this suggests that CCK acts mainly as a paracrine rather than as an endocrine signal in rats. The paracrine action also suggests that CCK secreted from enteric neurons may be important in CCK satiation. Eisen et al. suggested that CCK may, in part, have

an endocrine mode of action in rats, with a target site in the liver, and that the form of the CCK peptide may be a factor influencing the site of action.[34] In any case, however, measurements of neither the molecular form nor the concentrations of prandial CCK in the extracellular fluid of the proximal gut or in the hepatic portal vein have been reported.

2. In rats, the results of close-arterial infusions, pylorectomies, and selective vagotomies suggest that the satiating action of CCK is mediated by CCK_A receptors in vagal afferents and in the pyloric circular muscle. CCK_A receptors in the liver may also be involved. The role of CCK_A receptors in several brain areas, including the nucleus of the solitary tract (NTS) remains uncertain.
3. As mentioned earlier, in rats the data required to establish a physiological paracrine mode of action are not available. In contrast, in humans CCK apparently acts via an endocrine mode, and physiological doses of CCK are sufficient to inhibit eating.
4. To study removal and replacement is difficult because CCK-producing cells are distributed widely. Surgical removal of CCK would require removal of much of the small intestine. Findings in rats with a spontaneously mutated CCK_A receptor at least in part support the criterion (reviewed by Geary[5] and Moran[6]). In these rats, meal size, total daily food intake, and body weight are all increased. However, CCK_A receptor knockout mice have an unchanged adult body weight and daily food intake. Unfortunately, meal patterns have not been determined. Whether this species difference is due to different receptor distributions is unknown at present.[6]
5. The criterion of antagonism has been well established in rats, because CCK receptor antagonists increase meal size and block the satiating effect induced by intraduodenal infusions of fat, which at least in part is mediated by CCK. This evidence also indicates a peripheral site of action of endogenous CCK, because it includes tests both with antibodies, which do not cross the blood–brain barrier, and with local infusions of receptor antagonists into the gut circulation.

9.3.2.2 Mechanisms of CCK's Satiation Effect

Peripheral CCK_A receptors signal the brain via all four subdiaphragmatic vagal branches.[35] The involvement of CCK_A and CCK_B receptors in the dorsal vagal complex or in the area postrema (AP) have also been suggested. These receptors, however, may be activated by neural, locally released CCK. The same is true for the CCK_A receptors in the dorsomedial hypothalamus. This situation may be part of a more general phenomenon in which the same molecules are released from peripheral nerves or glands as well as from neurons in the brain. Thus in the case of CCK, central receptors, perhaps in the AP, may mediate the decreases in food intake and conditioned taste aversions that can be elicited by larger doses of CCK (intraperitoneal injection of >8 μg/kg CCK-8), even in vagotomized rats.

For CCK, as well as for most other eating-control signals, little is known about information processing in the brain or about the extensive convergence of the many signals that are activated simultaneously. Neural signals from the gut, including the vagally mediated CCK signal, project to the NTS. In the case of CCK, central processing seems to involve catecholaminergic and GLP-1-ergic neurons in the NTS, NTS neurons that express the melanocortin-4 receptor (MC4R) that apparently originate in the hypothalamus,[36] and at least in females, NTS neurons expressing estrogen receptor-α (ERα).[37] Further, CCK satiation also depends on brain serotonin. Importantly, most of this work has involved tests of exogenous CCK, and it is not clear whether the neural processing of exogenous CCK is identical to that of endogenous CCK. For example, it seems likely that smaller doses of CCK or endogenous CCK, which signal via the vagus, and larger doses of CCK, which signal at least in part independent of the vagus, do not activate identical neural networks.

9.3.2.3 CCK and Obesity

Numerous studies suggest that CCK is acutely effective in a wide variety of models of obesity, including rats with lesions of the ventromedial hypothalamus (which included the ARC), *ob/ob* mice, Zucker *fa/fa* rats, and rats with dietary-induced obesity. However, in Koletsky fa^k/fa^k rats, CCK decreased meal size less than in lean control rats[39] (but see Wildman et al.[38]). The deficit in CCK satiation was rescued by leptin receptor expression via adenoviral gene therapy into the ARC. Therefore, leptin may control meal size through an obligatory interaction with CCK, consistent with Smith's theory of the direct and indirect control of meal size.[40]

The effects of repeated CCK administration on eating and body weight suggest that CCK effectively reduces meal size, total food intake, and body weight when meal frequency is controlled, but not in freely feeding rats. West et al. showed that, when CCK was infused intraperitoneally before each spontaneous meal for six days in rats, meal size was reduced throughout the study with no sign of tolerance.[41] However, meal frequency rapidly increased to return total daily food intake to control level. Body weight gain was reduced for only one day. Similar results have been reported in free-feeding rats when CCK was continuously infused for several days and when CCK_A receptor agonists were tested chronically. In contrast, when CCK was intraperitoneally injected before each of three scheduled daily meals for three weeks, CCK consistently reduced meal size and led to significant weight loss.[42]

9.3.3 Intestinal Glucagon-Like Peptide-1 (GLP-1)

Glucagon-like peptide-1 (GLP-1) is a product of the preproglucagon gene that is produced mainly in intestinal L-cells and also in a specific group of neurons in the NTS in the brain stem.[43] Exendin-4 is a GLP-1 analogue which has an extended half-life over GLP-1 because, especially in rodents, the active form of GLP-1 (GLP-1[7-36amide]) is rapidly degraded through action of dipeptidyl-peptidase IV.

9.3.3.1 Effects of GLP-1 on Food Intake

In rodents and humans, food intake results in an immediate release of GLP-1 into the blood. Central and peripheral GLP-1 each produce dose-dependent reductions in food intake in rats and mice.[44] The reduction in food intake results mainly from a decrease in meal size, but meal number is also reduced, at least at higher doses. Chronic delivery of exendin-4 reduces body weight gain in mice by specifically reducing body fat mass.[45] Interestingly, however, mice lacking the GLP-1 receptor have unaltered body weight compared to controls. Hence, the GLP-1 receptor is probably not a single critical component in the control of food intake.

9.3.3.2 Physiological Relevance

Four of the five criteria (Table 9.3) qualifying an anorectic substance to be of physiological relevance have been investigated in rats.[43]

1. Eating increases GLP-1 secretion: the amount of GLP-1 secreted during a meal in rats, however, has not yet been carefully characterized.
2. GLP-1 receptors are present in GLP-1's presumed site(s) of action (the gastrointestinal tract and certain brain nuclei, including the brain stem).
3. To our knowledge, this criterion has not been investigated in rats.
4. The criterion of removal and replacement is difficult to investigate because it would require ablation of the GLP-1 producing cells. Obviously, this has been done neither in humans nor in experimental animals. The effect of removal of receptors has been tested in GLP-1 receptor knockout mice. These mice are insensitive to exogenous GLP-1, but their body weight was unchanged compared to controls. Whether this represents opposing effects on spontaneous meal size and meal frequency, as discussed in the case of CCK, is not known. Surprisingly, however, the fasting-induced feeding response in the knockout mice was also similar to that in wild-type controls. Hence, at least under these conditions, endogenous GLP-1 does not seem to play a necessary role in the regulation of eating.
5. The final criterion of receptor antagonism has been investigated using the GLP-1 receptor antagonist exendin 9-39. *Ad libitum*–fed rats that were treated with exendin-9-39 centrally ate more than control animals.[44] Hence, blockade of endogenous central GLP-1 signaling seems to lead to increased food intake. Whether antagonism of peripheral GLP-1 signaling has a similar effect is not known.

In summary, GLP-1 does not yet fully meet all criteria that are required for a hormone to be a physiological regulator of eating, but the available data are encouraging. It is important to note in this context, however, that the relationship of the aversive effects of GLP-1 and its agonist exendin-4 that occur under certain conditions (see below) and the hypothesized satiation effect needs to be clarified.

9.3.3.3 Site of GLP-1 Action

Central or peripheral delivery of GLP-1 or exendin-4 activate neurons, as characterized by c-Fos immunocytochemistry, in specific brain areas in the brain stem (e.g., AP, NTS) and hypothalamus (e.g., ARC, paraventricular nucleus).[44] The central c-Fos pattern induced by peripheral exendin-4 and amylin (see below) is similar, and amylin and GLP-1 coactivate AP neurons.[8] However, the anorectic effect of exendin-4, unlike amylin, is not blocked in AP-lesioned rats, while vagal blockade by vagotomy or capsaicin-pretreatment abolished exendin-4's but not amylin's effect. Consistent with a peripheral component in GLP-1's anorectic effect, central administration of the GLP-1 antagonist exendin-9-39 was unable to block the anorectic effect of exendin-4. Surprisingly, however, peripheral coadministration of exendin-9-39 also did not block exendin-4's effect. Only simultaneous central and peripheral application of the antagonist blocked exendin-4's effect on feeding in rats (T.A. Lutz, unpublished). The potential interaction of central and peripheral GLP-1 receptors remains to be clarified.

9.3.3.4 Role of Brain GLP-1

The peripheral and the central GLP-1 system in the NTS do not seem to interact directly because an anorectic dose of peripheral exendin-4 did not activate GLP-1ergic NTS neurons. In contrast, high doses of peripheral CCK (100 μg/kg), which clearly produced nonspecific, aversive effects, did activate these neurons.[46] Thus, whether central GLP-1 mediates the physiological satiating effect of GLP-1, CCK, or other anorectic satiating hormones is questionable.

Central GLP-1 may mediate the anorectic effect of leptin, because the feeding-inhibitory effect of central leptin was attenuated by central administration of exendin-9-39. Further, restricted feeding decreased preproglucagon mRNA in the NTS compared to controls, and this effect was prevented by central leptin. The hypothalamic content of immunoreactive GLP-1 paralleled preproglucagon mRNA expression in the NTS. Leptin may therefore stimulate GLP-1ergic neurons in the NTS; the physiological importance of these findings, however, requires further work.

9.3.3.5 GLP-1 and Conditioned Taste Aversions

It seems likely that central GLP-1 is involved in mediating the anorectic effects of some aversive stimuli.[46] Rinaman has shown, for example, that peripheral administration of sickness-producing agents (for example, LiCl, lipopolysaccharide, high doses of CCK) all produce a strong c-Fos response in GLP-1ergic neurons of the NTS, whereas other feeding-related stimuli, such as gastric distension, did not. Furthermore, both central GLP-1 administration and peripheral exendin-4 administration (T.A. Lutz, unpublished) produced strong conditioned taste aversions in rats in two-bottle reference tests.

Situational effects and species differences appear to be important in GLP-1's aversive effects. For example, Mack et al. reported that a dose of 10 μg/kg exendin-4 (five times higher than the doses we found aversive in a conditioned taste aversion test) failed to affect another measure of aversion, kaolin intake.[45] As to species differences, central GLP-1, similar to rats, produced conditioned taste aversion in wild-type mice, but not in GLP-1 receptor knockout mice. This points to a GLP-1 receptor-mediated effect. However, LiCl produced taste aversion in both groups of mice, indicating that the GLP-1 receptor may not be involved in this aversive behavior under these conditions in mice. Furthermore, the GLP-1 antagonist exendin-9-39 reduced the aversive effect of GLP-1, but not that of LiCl in mice. Both effects clearly differ from rats.[47]

9.3.4 Peptide YY (PYY)

Peptide YY is synthesized and released mainly by intestinal L-cells, the same cells that synthesize GLP-1. Some data indicate that the two peptides are not always cosecreted, although the mechanisms for the dissociation are unclear. Two main forms of PYY appear in the circulation, full-length PYY1-36 (which we call PYY here) and its more active cleavage product, PYY3-36. Interestingly, the same enzyme, dipeptidyl peptidase-IV (DPP IV), that inactivates circulating GLP-1[7-36amide] catalyzes the formation of PYY3-36, so that the active GLP-1 has a much shorter plasma half-life than PYY3-36. L-cells release PYY, like GLP-1, in response to food intake, especially lipids. Beglinger and his colleagues have recently shown that, in humans, secretion of PYY3-36 after intraduodenal lipid infusions depends on CCK release — that is, if a CCK_A receptor antagonist was administered, PYY3-36 did not appear in the plasma following the lipid infusions.[30]

PYY has affinity to all subtypes of Y receptors, whereas PYY3-36 predominantly activates Y2 receptors. Centrally administered PYY has long been known to increase food intake, presumably via activation of Y1 or Y5 receptors. Batterham and colleagues recently provided the first evidence that peripheral PYY3-36 also decreases eating in rats.[48] This effect is apparently mediated by Y2 receptors, because it was attenuated by Y2 receptor antagonist and absent in Y2 receptor knockout mice.[48] Many investigators have reported that they were unable to reproduce the eating-inhibitory effect of peripheral PYY in rats.[16,49] This is likely due to differences in adaptation to test conditions, circadian timing, or other procedural differences.[3]

The site where PYY3-36 acts to inhibit eating is not clear. Evidence in favor of both a central site of action in the ARC as well as a peripheral, vagally mediated action has been presented. In the original publication by Batterham and colleagues, it was reported that PYY3-36 specifically increased the firing rate of POMC neurons located in the ARC in an *in vitro* slice preparation in mice.[48] Further, a Y2 receptor agonist increased the release of the splicing product of the POMC gene, alpha-melanocyte stimulating hormone (alpha-MSH), from rat hypothalamic explants containing the ARC. Hypothalamic alpha-MSH decreases feeding by acting on paraventricular neurons. Hence, the increase in firing rate in POMC neurons may coincide with the release of alpha-MSH. At the same time, neuropeptide Y (NPY) expression and the release of NPY from hypothalamic explants was decreased. The latter effects correspond to our own findings that full-length PYY inhibited ghrelin-activated neurons in rat brain slices of the medial ARC.[50] These neurons presumably express NPY and mediate the orexigenic effect of ghrelin. In apparent contrast to these indications that PYY may have a direct action in the ARC, Abbott et al. showed that the anorectic effect of peripheral PYY3-36 was blocked in vagotomized rats and in rats with lesions of the "brain stem-hypothalamic pat[h]way."[51]

Peripheral PYY3-36 induced expression of c-Fos protein in the brain stem, specifically in the AP and NTS,[16] and in the ARC.[51] Vagotomy prevented PYY3-36-induced expression of c-Fos protein in the ARC. Whether NTS c-Fos expression also depends on the vagus has, to our knowledge, not been investigated. Interestingly, however, and unlike GLP-1, PYY3-36's effect on feeding was not blocked by capsaicin, so that it seems unlikely that vagal afferents are directly involved in the anorectic action.[52] Clearly, more research is needed to define the primary site of action (periphery? brain stem? ARC?) of peripheral PYY and PYY3-36.

In contrast to the original report,[48] high doses of PYY3-36 have been reported to induce conditioned taste aversion in rodents and to cause nausea in humans.[16] However, low-dose intravenous infusions of PYY3-36 reduced feeding without aversive effects in rats.[16]

9.3.5 Interaction of GLP-1 and PYY3-36

Because food intake triggers the release of numerous hormones from the gastrointestinal tract that individually have been implicated in the control of food intake, understanding their functional and mechanistic interactions is of both physiological and pharmacological interest. One of the more interesting interactions is exemplified by the feeding effects of simultaneous administration of PYY3-36 and GLP-1. Combined subthreshold doses of GLP-1 and PYY3-36 (10 and 1 nmol/kg, respectively) significantly reduced feeding in rats.[53] (See also Talsania et al.[52]) In addition, suprathreshold doses of GLP-1 and PYY3-36 (100 nmol/kg each), which individually each decreased food intake significantly, led to a significantly stronger effect when combined. These findings are consistent with immunohistochemical studies showing that the combination of GLP-1 and PYY3-36, but neither peptide alone, increased c-Fos expression in the ARC.[53]

9.3.6 Apolipoprotein A-IV

Apolipoprotein A-IV (Apo A-IV) is produced in enterocytes during the digestion of lipids containing long chain ($C > 12$) fatty acids and is released into the lymph, thus reaching the bloodstream much slower than the gut hormones considered before. Fujimoto and colleagues were the first to show that Apo A-IV reduces food intake in rats.[7,9] Apo A-IV may contribute to the reduction in food intake that is seen after intestinal fat infusion in rats. Infusion of chylous lymph that was collected from animals after intestinal application of fat, but not after intraintestinal saline, reduced feeding in rats, and this effect was not observed if Apo A-IV was removed from lymph by immunoprecipitation. Interestingly, Apo A-IV is also synthesized in the ARC. Additionally, centrally administered Apo A-IV inhibited eating, and administration of Apo A-IV antibodies into the third cerebral ventricle stimulated eating and reduced Apo A-IV expression in the hypothalamus. Despite these promising data, the role of Apo A-IV in the physiological control of food intake is far from being resolved.

9.3.7 Oleoylethanolamide (OEA)

Recently, the eating-inhibitory effect of the endogenous lipid oleoylethanolamide (OEA), which is synthesized in enterocytes in response to food intake, has drawn increased attention.[54,55] OEA is synthesized in duodenal and jejunal mucosal cells during and after meals, but not in fasted rats. Peripheral, but not central, administration of OEA decreases food intake. OEA apparently acts by binding to the transcription factor peroxisome proliferator-activated receptor-alpha (PPAR-alpha), which then activates a neural pathway. Whether this occurs directly or indirectly and whether vagal afferents, spinal visceral afferents, or both are involved is not yet clear. Interestingly, long-lasting forms of OEA selectively decrease meal frequency, suggesting that this molecule is involved in signaling postprandial satiety.

9.4 PANCREATIC SIGNALS

The pancreatic hormones insulin, amylin, glucagon, and somatostatin are all released in response to food intake and appear to act as satiating hormones (amylin, glucagon, possibly somatostatin and insulin) and adiposity signals (insulin, possibly amylin). In this section, we briefly discuss amylin in the control of food intake because amylin interacts with CCK to control meal size and because recent advances have made it a likely candidate for the first hormonal treatment of obesity.

9.4.1 Amylin

Amylin (or islet amyloid polypeptide) is synthesized by the pancreatic B-cells and cosecreted with insulin. It is considered an important complement to insulin in the control of glucose metabolism.[56] Amylin also controls the supply of metabolites by controlling eating.[4,8,14] Like ghrelin, amylin appears to have a dual role, such that prandial amylin secretion contributes to meal-ending satiation and basal plasma amylin levels may act as an adiposity signal.

9.4.1.1 Physiological Relevance

Amylin has been shown to meet most of the criteria summarized in Table 9.3 for a physiological satiation signal in rats.

1. Food intake results in a marked increase in plasma amylin concentration that begins within 5 minutes and whose magnitude is correlated with amount eaten.
2. All the components of the amylin receptor complex —calcitonin receptor core (CT-R) together with several receptor-activity modifying proteins (RAMPs) that confer amylin affinity and selectivity — are expressed in the AP, where amylin appears to act to inhibit eating.[57,58]
3. Amylin infusions that yielded plasma amylin levels close to those measured postprandially were sufficient to inhibit eating.[59]
4. There is currently no method for acute removal of amylin without damaging B-cell function. The amylin knockout mouse shows the expected phenotype of overeating and increased adiposity,[8] but the effect of physiological doses of amylin on eating in these mice has not yet been tested.
5. Finally, peripheral or central delivery of amylin antagonists increases eating. For example, administration of the amylin receptor antagonist AC 187 into the AP blocked the anorectic effect of intraperitoneally injected amylin and, when administered alone, stimulated eating by increasing meal size.[60,61]

9.4.1.2 Amylin as an Adiposity Signal

Amylin also appears to meet all the criteria proposed for an adiposity signal[8,14] in rats.

1. Basal plasma amylin level is (positively) correlated with body adiposity.
2. Chronic continuous amylin infusion reduces food intake and body weight.
3. Chronic peripheral or central infusion of amylin antagonists increased body adiposity.

In addition, the amylin knockout mouse is heavier than wild-type controls.

9.4.1.3 Mechanism of Amylin Action

Amylin acts in the AP to inhibit eating.

1. Eating was inhibited or stimulated, respectively, by injection of amylin or the amylin receptor antagonist AC187 directly into the AP.[60]
2. After AP/NTS lesions, peripheral amylin no longer inhibited eating.[58] Lesions of peripheral neural afferents, in contrast, had no effect.[8,62]
3. Both peripheral amylin and postdeprivation refeeding increased neuronal activation in the AP, as gauged by expression of c-Fos protein, and both responses were effectively blocked by AC187.[63]
4. Direct application of amylin onto AP neurons in slice preparations led to dose-dependent increases in electric activity.
5. c-Fos responses rostral to the AP that were elicited by peripheral administration of amylin were eliminated after AP lesions.

Dopamine (presumably acting in the AP/NTS region), histamine (ventromedial hypothalamus), orexin, and melanin concentrating hormone (lateral hypothalamic area) neuronal systems have been implicated in amylin signaling.[8]

9.4.1.4 Amylin and Obesity

Amylin or its agonist salmon calcitonin (sCT) effectively reduced eating in the *ob/ob* mouse, the obese Zucker *fa/fa* rat, and the melanocortin-4 receptor knockout mouse.[62,64,65] Amylin antagonism with peripheral AC187 also increased eating in Zucker rats.[65] Recent reports of anti-obesity actions in humans (for example, acute administration of the amylin analogue pramlintide decreased the size of test meals by about 20% in nondiabetic obese individuals[66,67]) strongly encourage further research in this direction.

9.5 PERSPECTIVES

9.5.1 The Translation of Animal Physiology into Human Therapeutics

9.5.1.1 Animal Models

Although the value of animal models for human eating is a matter of ongoing discussion, the clear consensus among researchers is that progress in the physiology of eating absolutely requires animal models.[68–71] Many questions can be addressed only with methodologies that are difficult or impossible in human subjects. Furthermore, it is a validated strategy; physiology is replete with examples of successful translation of analyses of physiological mechanisms in animals to those in humans.

Accepting that animal models are useful in general leaves open the question as to which particular animal model(s) is best suited. On first glance, it would seem logical to use phylogenetic relationships as a criterion, but in fact, this is probably not so. Our closest primate relatives, great apes and old-world primates, are not appropriate research animals for many reasons. In addition, most of these species have quite different nutritional adaptations; in particular, only a few are omnivores. Several omnivores have been used in eating research, including dogs, swine, rats, and mice. Among these species, both classical structural taxonomy and more recent molecular phylogenetics place the order of rodents closer to primates than are either carnivores or even-toed ungulates (the order including swine).[72] This general relationship, however, is not necessarily true for any specific ancestral gene or phenotype.[73,74] The rat, for example, does not have a gall bladder, whereas carnivores and swine do.

Many of these points are illustrated by the case of CCK. As described above, the pharmacological satiating effect of CCK, discovered in rats in 1973,[33] was quickly translated into normal-weight and obese human subjects.[75] A similar progression occurred for the satiating effect of endogenous CCK. In this case, a specific behavioral assay — the satiating action of intestinal nutrient infusions — that was developed in rats proved illuminating in monkeys and humans as well.[76,77] This procedure also revealed a species difference: although intestinal infusions of lipids increased CCK secretion in all three species, intestinal infusions of l-phenylalanine produced CCK release in rats, but not in monkeys.[78] Work with animals lacking CCK_A receptors suggests a similarly important species difference in two even more closely related species. That is, as mentioned above, rats with null deletions of the CCK_A receptor gene are obese, whereas mice with similar mutations are not, apparently because of a difference in the distribution of the CCK_A receptor in the brain.[6,79]

Finally, CCK physiology also illustrates the potential of back translation, from humans to animals. That is, rats, rather than humans, will presumably be the species of choice to determine the mechanisms underlying the necessary role of CCK release for the stimulation of PYY3-36 secretion and inhibition of ghrelin secretion by intraduodenal lipid recently discovered in humans.[30]

9.5.1.2 Physiology, Pharmacology, and Selectivity

As the foregoing sections make clear, numerous manipulations inhibit eating in animals or humans under some conditions. Such demonstrations provide no real evidence that the function modeled, such as gastric distension or gut hormone secretion during or after eating, physiologically controls eating. Rather, such demonstrations merely encourage a program of research to investigate the issue.

Consider three alternatives. (1) The manipulation may mimic a normal or physiological endogenous mechanism of appetite. (2) The manipulation may stimulate a normal appetitive behavior, but in a way or at a time that does not occur physiologically (i.e., it has a selective but pharmacological effect). For example, an exogenous hormone may produce satiation even if the endogenous hormone is not secreted, or is not secreted in sufficient amounts, during meals. (3) The manipulation may affect appetite, but do so by eliciting a response that is not part of the normal physiological control of eating, such as illness, aversion, etc. This is a nonselective effect on appetite. Such effects can and do occur even in the case of exogenous administration of physiological signals, if they are given in too high a dose (for example, CCK) or in the wrong context.

Distinguishing among these alternatives can be very difficult, especially in animal research. Many theoretical and practical criteria have been proposed and continue to evolve as new methodologies emerge. It is important to note that, even if a peptide does not appear to be a likely physiological control of eating, this does not preclude it from being a potential pharmaceutical target for appetite control, as long as eating and body weight can be influenced without triggering major side effects.

9.5.2 Potentials and Problems of Gut–Brain Axis Signals in the Treatment of Obesity

9.5.2.1 Redundancy and Synergy

The controls of eating are multifactorial and redundant. This may mean that manipulations of individual signals will be ineffective because of functionally antagonistic, adaptive responses of others. On the other hand, this also creates the potential for therapies based on simultaneous manipulation of several signals. "Cocktail" therapies may provide a means to counteract side effects or antagonistic adaptive responses. For example, simultaneous use of a ghrelin-based therapy may perhaps prevent increases in meal frequency that might otherwise neutralize the decreases in meal size produced by a CCK- or amylin-based therapy.

Therefore, we consider the study of interactions of the many signals that control ingestive behavior an especially important area in the context of their therapeutic potential. Similar to other areas of pharmacological therapeutics, it seems plausible that combination therapies for obesity may have the same advantages of increased potency and decreased side effects. CCK, the best investigated signal in this regard, has been reported to functionally interact with several other peripheral signals (listed in Table 9.4). Functional synergy between CCK and gastric loads has been reported in rats, primates, and humans. As to the mechanisms underlying these synergies, CCK and gastrointestinal mechanostimulation synergistically increased the electrophysiological activity of vagal afferent neurons. The interaction may depend on activation of 5HT3 receptors in the periphery and n-methyl-d-aspartate (NMDA) receptors in the dorsal vagal complex. At the hormonal level, the amylin-induced neural signaling may be a necessary part of CCK signaling, because CCK satiation was reduced by amylin antagonist pretreatment in rats and in amylin knockout mice, in which it was rescued by subthreshold doses of amylin. The reverse appears not to be true, because CCK antagonists had no effect on amylin satiation.[8]

TABLE 9.4
Functional Interactions between CCK and Other Peripheral Signals Controlling Eating

Signal	Nature of Interaction	Reference
Amylin	Synergy	[8,80]
Estradiol	Synergy	[37]
Gastric load	Synergy	[6]
GLP-1	None	[13,81]
Pancreatic glucagon	Antagonism	[82]
(Central) Insulin	Synergy	[4]
Leptin	Synergy	[4]

Note: Here, synergy is defined as a further decrease in eating when CCK and the other signal are applied simultaneously in comparison CCK alone. Antagonism is a smaller decrease in eating when CCK and the other signal are applied simultaneously.

9.5.2.2 Side Effects

Gut–brain axis signals may offer several advantages to the currently available therapies in the treatment of obesity in relation to side effects. Many details of the physiology of several gut–brain controls have been established, so that the types and severity of side effects might be more predictable. Peripheral side effects may be more tractable to treatment, and peripheral signals can be manipulated peripherally, which is in general more accessible, selective, predictable, and perhaps more safe than manipulation of central neurotransmitter systems. Further, many of the hormonal gut–brain signals are fully coupled hormonal controls.[5] This means that ideal timing of agonistic or antagonistic therapies can be predicted. As indicated above, perhaps a ghrelin antagonist should, for example, be applied several hours before meals, whereas a CCK or amylin agonist should be applied immediately before eating.

Gut–brain axis manipulation often causes gastrointestinal dysfunction and nausea as side effects. However, this is dose dependent, and CCK and amylin, for example, at least acutely reduce eating in the absence of such effects. Whether the same is true of other gut–brain axis hormones such as GLP-1, its analogues, or PYY3-36 is less clear. Although they potently reduce food intake, this effect is often accompanied by presumably gastrointestinal side effects leading to conditioned taste aversions in animals or nausea in humans.

9.5.2.3 Route of Administration

A disadvantage of brain–gut axis signals is that the peptide or peptidergic agonists or antagonists cannot be administered orally. This, of course, would not apply to nonpeptide analogs. Furthermore, the increasing recognition of the medical severity of obesity together with the advantages of gut–brain peptide therapies may soon be felt to justify injections as a route of administration.

9.5.3 Relative Strengths of Animal and Human Studies

This chapter reviewed the control of eating in animals by gut–brain axis signals, focusing especially on hormonal gut–brain signals. One may reasonably ask if animal research has particular strengths in this area. We believe that it does.

As is the case with all other areas of behavioral neuroscience, one can perform many types of experiments in animals that cannot be done in humans. This includes long-term control of behavioral and physiological functions, for example, adaptation to particular diets, that help isolate phenomena of interest. Similarly, one can perform injurious or potentially injurious procedures in animals, including, for example, surgical, pharmacological and genetic lesions, and to name an example germane to behavioral endocrinology, cannulations of vasculature and endocrine organs, and so forth. These procedures permit less well-controlled physiological studies in humans to be carefully validated in animals. As well, they permit extension and reduction of behavioral data to physiological and neurophysiological functions.

This pertains particularly to gastrointestinal controls of eating. Gut–brain axis signals, and especially hormonal signals, are easily accessible to experimental investigation in both animals and humans. This permits the use of essentially identical experimental designs, so that studies performed in animals can be done in parallel in humans. This allows a degree of direct validation of animal results in human subjects that is rarely possible in physiological research. Excellent examples of this can be found in the study of the satiating effects of CCK and other gut peptides (for example, studies on synergistic actions between preloads and CCK in rats, monkeys, and humans; intestinal satiation with intraduodenal infusions of fat combined with CCK antagonism in rats and humans).

Finally, it is important to note that, in both animals and humans, one can study not only pharmacological hormone action but also normal endogenous hormone release simply by taking a blood sample. Thus, if one can sample a hormone between its site of release and the relevant receptors, then the ability to monitor and manipulate physiological signaling is limited only by the temporal resolution of infusions and measures. Nonetheless, this is not a trivial issue, as many hormones related to eating are released into the hepatic portal vein, which is less accessible than the systemic circulation, and moreover, most have pulsatile patterns of release. Pulsatile release, of course, is a general phenomenon in endocrinology and not limited to gut–brain signals. Nevertheless, even considering these complications, the accessibility of hormonal signaling molecules remains incomparably greater than that of central neural signals. We have detailed information as to the relevant prandial patterns of release of several endocrine controls of eating; with few exceptions, such as recent reports of dopamine release in the nucleus accumbens measured during sucrose or fat meals,[83,84] almost no comparable information is available for any brain neurotransmitter.

REFERENCES

1. Diamond, J.M., How to be physiological, *Nature,* 376, 117, 1995.

2. Stanley, S. et al., Hormonal regulation of food intake, *Physiol. Rev.,* 85, 1131, 2005.
3. Cummings, D.E. and Overduin, J., Gastrointestinal regulation of food intake, *J. Clin. Invest.,* 117, 13, 2007.
4. Woods, S.C., Signals that influence food intake and body weight, *Physiol. Behav.,* 86, 709, 2005.
5. Geary, N., Endocrine controls of eating: CCK, leptin, and ghrelin, *Physiol. Behav.,* 81, 719, 2004.
6. Moran, T.H., Gut peptide signaling in the controls of food intake, *Obesity,* 14 (Suppl. 5), 250S, 2006.
7. Ritter, R.C., Gastrointestinal mechanisms of satiation for food, *Physiol. Behav.,* 81, 249, 2004.
8. Lutz, T.A., Pancreatic amylin as a centrally acting satiating hormone, *Curr. Drug Targets,* 6, 181, 2005.
9. Qin, X. and Tso, P., The role of apolipoprotein AIV on the control of food intake, *Curr. Drug Targets,* 6, 145, 2005.
10. Yamada, K., Wada, E., and Wada, K., Bombesin-like peptides: studies on food intake and social behaviour with receptor knock-out mice, *Annals Med.,* 32, 519, 2000.
11. Berger, K. et al., Enterostatin and its target mechanisms during regulation of fat intake, *Physiol. Behav.,* 83, 623, 2004.
12. Cummings, D.E., Foster-Schubert, K.E., and Overduin, J., Ghrelin and energy balance: focus on current controversies, *Curr. Drug Targets,* 6, 153, 2005.
13. Gutzwiller, J.P. et al., Glucagon-like peptide 1 (GLP-1) and eating, *Physiol. Behav.,* 82, 17, 2004.
14. Woods, S.C. et al., Pancreatic signals controlling food intake — insulin, glucagon and amylin, *Philosoph. Transact. Royal Soc. B Biol. Sci.,* 361, 1219, 2006.
15. Berthoud, H.R., A new role for leptin as a direct satiety signal from the stomach, *Am. J. Physiol.,* 288, R796, 2005.
16. Murphy, K.G. and Bloom, S.R., Gut hormones and the regulation of energy homeostasis, *Nature,* 444, 854, 2006.
17. Kaplan, J.M. and Moran, T.H., Gastrointestinal signaling in the control of food intake, in *Handbook of Behavioral Neurobiology, Vol. 14, Neurobiology of Food and Fluid Intake,* 2nd ed., Stricker, E. and Woods, S.C., Eds., Kluwer Academic, Plenum Publishers, New York, 2004, p. 275.
18. Langhans, W., Role of the liver in the control of glucose-lipid utilization and body weight, *Curr. Opin. Clin. Nutr. Metab. Care,* 6, 449, 2003.
19. Scharrer, E., Control of food intake by fatty acid oxidation and ketogenesis, *Nutrition,* 15, 704, 1999.
20. De Vries, J. et al., Patterns of body temperature during feeding in rats under varying ambient temperatures, *Physiol. Behav.,* 53, 229, 1993.
21. Schwartz, G.J., The role of gastrointestinal vagal afferents in the control of food intake: current prospects, *Nutrition,* 16, 866, 2000.
22. Savastano, D.M., Carelle, M., and Covasa, M., Serotonin-type 3 receptors mediate intestinal polycose- and glucose-induced suppression of intake, *Am. J. Physiol.,* 288, R1499, 2005.
23. Davidson, T.L. and Swithers, S.E., Food viscosity influences caloric intake compensation and body weight in rats, *Obes. Res.,* 13, 537, 2005.
24. Kojima, M. and Kangawa, K., Ghrelin: structure and function, *Physiol. Rev.,* 85, 495, 2005.
25. Williams, D.L. and Cummings, D.E., Regulation of ghrelin in physiologic and pathophysiologic states, *J. Nutr.,* 135, 1320, 2005.
26. Arnold, M. et al., Gut vagal afferents are not necessary for the eating-stimulatory effect of intraperitoneally injected ghrelin in the rat, *J. Neurosci.,* 26, 11052, 2006.

27. Wortley, K.E. et al., Absence of ghrelin protects against early-onset obesity, *J. Clin. Invest.,* 115, 3393, 2005.
28. Asakawa, A. et al., Antagonism of ghrelin receptor reduces food intake and body weight gain in mice, *Gut,* 52, 947, 2003.
29. Helmling, S. et al., Inhibition of ghrelin action *in vitro* and *in vivo* by an RNA-spiegelmer, *Proc. Natl. Acad. Sci. USA,* 7, 101, 13174, 2004.
30. Degen, L. et al., Effect of CCK-1 receptor blockade on ghrelin and PYY secretion in man, *Am. J. Physiol.,* 292, R1391, 2007.
31. Kobelt, P. et al., CCK inhibits the orexigenic effect of peripheral ghrelin, *Am. J. Physiol.,* 288, R751, 2005.
32. Tschöp, M., Smiley, D.L., and Heimann, M.L., Ghrelin induces adiposity in rodents, *Nature,* 407, 908, 2000.
33. Gibbs, J., Young, R.C., and Smith, G.P., Cholecystokinin decreases food intake in rats, *J. Comp. Physiol. Psychol.,* 84, 488, 1973.
34. Eisen, S. et al., Inhibitory effects on intake of cholecystokinin-8 and cholecystokinin-33 in rats with hepatic proper or common hepatic branch vagal innervation, *Am. J. Physiol.,* 289, R456, 2005.
35. Berthoud, H.R. et al., Neuroanatomy of extrinsic afferents supplying the gastrointestinal tract, *Neurogastroenterol. Motil.,* 16 (Suppl. 1), 28, 2004.
36. Zheng, H. et al., Brain stem melanocortinergic modulation of meal size and identification of hypothalamic POMC projections, *Am. J. Physiol.,* 289, R247, 2005.
37. Asarian, L. and Geary, N., Modulation of appetite by gonadal steroid hormones, *Philos. Trans. Royal Soc. B Biol. Sci.,* 361, 1251, 2006.
38. Wildman, H.F. et al., Effects of leptin and cholecystokinin in rats with a null mutation of the leptin receptor Lepr(fak), *Am. J. Physiol.,* 278, R1518, 2000.
39. Morton, G.J. et al., Leptin action in the forebrain regulates the hindbrain response to satiety signals, *J. Clin. Invest.,* 115, 703, 2005.
40. Smith, G.P., The direct and indirect controls of meal size, *Neurosci. Biobehav. Rev.,* 20, 41, 1996.
41. West, D.B., Fey, D., and Woods, S.C., Cholecystokinin persistently suppresses meal size but not food intake in free-feeding rats, *Am. J. Physiol.,* 246, R776, 1984.
42. Smith, G.P. and Gibbs, J., The satiety effect of cholecystokinin. Recent progress and current problems, *Ann. N.Y. Acad. Sci.,* 448, 417, 1985.
43. Drucker, D.J., Biologic actions and therapeutic potential of the proglucagon-derived peptides, *Nat. Clin. Pract. Endocrinol. Metab.,* 1, 22, 2005.
44. Turton, M.D. et al., A role for glucagon-like peptide-1 in the central regulation of feeding, *Nature,* 379, 69, 1996.
45. Mack, C.M. et al., Antiobesity action of peripheral exenatide (exendin-4) in rodents: effects on food intake, body weight, metabolic status and side-effect measures, *Int. J. Obes.,* 30, 1332, 2006.
46. Rinaman, L., Interoceptive stress activates glucagon-like peptide-1 neurons that project to the hypothalamus, *Am. J. Physiol.,* 277, R582, 1999.
47. Lachey, J.J. et al., The role of central glucagon-like peptide-1 in mediating the effects of visceral illness: differential effects in rats and mice, *Endocrinology,* 146, 458, 2005.
48. Batterham, R.L. et al., Gut hormone PYY3-36 physiologically inhibits food intake, *Nature,* 418, 650, 2002.
49. Boggiano, M.M. et al., PYY3-36 as an anti-obesity drug target, *Obes. Rev.,* 6, 307, 2005.
50. Riediger, T. et al., Peptide YY directly inhibits ghrelin-activated neurons of the arcuate nucleus and reverses fasting-induced c-Fos expression, *Neuroendocrinology,* 79, 317, 2004.
51. Abbott, C.R. et al., The inhibitory effects of peripheral administration of peptide YY_{3-36} and glucagon-like peptide-1 on food intake are attenuated by ablation of the vagal-brainstem-hypothalamic pathway, *Brain Res.,* 1044, 127, 2005.

52. Talsania, T. et al., Peripheral exendin-4 and peptide $YY^{3\text{-}36}$ synergistically reduce food intake through different mechanisms in mice, *Endocrinology,* 146, 3748, 2005.
53. Neary, N.M. et al., Peptide $YY_{3\text{-}36}$ and glucagon-like peptide$1_{7\text{-}36}$ inhibit food intake additively, *Endocrinology,* 146, 5120, 2005.
54. Fu, J. et al., Food intake regulates oleoylethanolamide formation and degradation in the proximal small intestine, *J. Biol. Chem.,* 282, 1518, 2007.
55. Yang, Y. et al., Mechanism of oleoylethanolamide on fatty acid uptake in small intestine after food intake and body weight reduction, *Am. J. Physiol.,* 292, R235, 2007.
56. Weyer, C. et al., Amylin replacement with pramlintide as an adjunct to insulin therapy in type 1 and type 2 diabetes mellitus: a physiologic approach toward improved metabolic control, *Curr. Pharmaceut. Design,* 7, 1353, 2001.
57. Sexton, P.M. et al., *In vitro* autoradiographic localization of amylin binding sites in rat brain, *Neurosci.,* 62, 553, 1994.
58. Lutz, T. A. et al., Lesion of the area postrema/nucleus of the solitary tract (AP/NTS) attenuates the anorectic effects of amylin and calcitonin gene-related peptide (CGRP) in rats, *Peptides,* 19, 309, 1998.
59. Arnelo, U. et al., Sufficiency of postprandial plasma levels of islet amyloid polypeptide for suppression of feeding in rats, *Am. J. Physiol.,* 275, R1537, 1998.
60. Mollet, A. et al., Infusion of the amylin antagonist AC 187 into the area postrema increases food intake in rats, *Physiol. Behav.,* 81, 149, 2004.
61. Reidelberger, R.D. et al., Amylin receptor blockade stimulates food intake in rats, *Am. J. Physiol.,* 287, R568, 2004.
62. Morley, J.E. et al., Modulation of food intake by peripherally administered amylin, *Am. J. Physiol.,* 267, R178, 1994.
63. Riediger, T. et al., The anorectic hormone amylin contributes to feeding-related changes of neuronal activity in key structures of the gut-brain axis, *Am. J. Physiol.,* 286, R114, 2004.
64. Eiden, S. et al., Salmon calcitonin — a potent inhibitor of food intake in states of impaired leptin signaling in laboratory rodents, *J. Physiol.,* 541, 1041, 2002.
65. Grabler, V. and Lutz, T.A., Chronic infusion of the amylin antagonist AC 187 increases feeding in Zucker fa/fa rats but not in lean controls, *Physiol. Behav.,* 81, 481, 2004.
66. Hollander, P. et al., Effect of pramlintide on weight in overweight and obese insulin-treated type 2 diabetes patients, *Obesity Res.,* 12, 661, 2004.
67. Chapman, I. et al., Effect of pramlintide on satiety and food intake in obese subjects, *Diabetologia,* 48, 838, 2005.
68. Corwin, R.L. and Buda-Levin, A., Behavioral models of binge-type eating, *Physiol. Behav.,* 82, 123, 2004.
69. Geary, N., A new animal model of binge eating, *Int. J. Eat. Disord.,* 34, 183, 2003.
70. Smith, G.P., Animal models of human eating disorders, *Ann. N.Y. Acad. Sci.,* 575, 63, 1989.
71. Thibault, L., Woods, S.C., and Westerterp-Plantenga, M.S., The utility of animal models of human energy homeostasis, *Br. J. Nutr.,* 92 (Suppl. 1), S41, 2004.
72. Murphy, W.J. et al., Resolution of the early placental mammal radiation using Bayesian phylogenetics, *Science,* 294, 2348, 2001.
73. Li, W.H. et al., Molecular phylogeny of rodentia, lagomorpha, primates, artiodactyla, and carnivora and molecular clocks, *Proc. Natl. Acad. Sci. USA,* 87, 6703, 1990.
74. Hoyle, C.H., Neuropeptide families and their receptors: evolutionary perspectives, *Brain Res.,* 848, 1, 1999.
75. Pi-Sunyer, X., Kissileff, H.R., Thornton, J., and Smith, G.P., C-terminal octapeptide of cholecystokinin decreases food intake in obese men, *Physiol. Behav.,* 29, 627, 1982.
76. Liebling, D.S., Eisner, J.D., Gibbs, J., and Smith, G.P., Intestinal satiety in rats, *J. Comp. Physiol. Psychol.,* 89, 955, 1975.

77. Beglinger, C. and Degen, L., Fat in the intestine as a regulator of appetite- role of CCK, *Physiol. Behav.,* 83, 617, 2004.
78. Gibbs, J. and Smith, G.P., Cholecystokinin and satiety in rats and rhesus monkeys, *Am. J. Clin. Nutr.,* 30, 758, 1977.
79. Bi, S. and Moran, T.H., Actions of CCK in the controls of food intake and body weight: lessons from the CCK-A receptor deficient OLETF rat, *Neuropeptides,* 36, 171, 2002.
80. Bhavsar, S., Watkins, J., and Young, A., Synergy between amylin and cholecystokinin for inhibition of food intake in mice, *Physiol. Behav.,* 64, 557, 1998.
81. Gutzwiller, J.P. et al., Interaction between GLP-1 and CCK-33 in inhibiting food intake and appetite in men, *Am. J. Physiol.,* 287, 562, 2004.
82. Geary, N. et al., Individual, but not simultaneous, glucagon and cholecystokinin infusions inhibit feeding in men, *Am. J. Physiol.,* 262, R975, 1992.
83. Hajnal, A., Smith, G.P., and Norgren, R., Oral sucrose stimulation increases accumbens dopamine in the rat, *Am. J. Physiol.,* 286, R31, 2004.
84. Liang, N.-C., Hajnal, A., and Norgren, R., Sham feeding corn oil increases accumbens dopamine in the rat, *Am. J. Physiol.,* 291, R1236, 2006.

10 The Role of the Gastrointestinal Tract in Satiation, Satiety, and Food Intake: Evidence from Research in Humans

Harry P.F. Peters and David J. Mela

CONTENTS

10.1 INTRODUCTION

The gastrointestinal (GI) tract is the site of origin of a wide range of signals that ultimately act to influence and contribute toward regulation of hunger, food intake, and satiety.[1] Stimulation of the GI tract leads to activation of vagal afferents or release of gut peptides,[2] and the effects of these are integrated with signals originating from other parts of the body, such as adipocytes, and combine with sensory and cognitive influences to influence eating behavior.

The response of the GI tract to the entry of nutrients is traditionally divided into cephalic, gastric, and intestinal phases, reflecting anatomical and physiological mediators and events. Although these phases are not truly separable, they can be roughly aligned with chronologically and behaviorally corresponding aspects of satiation, satiety, and food intake.

In this chapter, we focus on how events within the GI tract can affect satiation, satiety, and food intake. We use "satiation" to refer to processes that act to reduce or terminate eating within a meal and the (acute) feeling state associated with this, generally occurring within 20 to 60 minutes of initiating ingestion. "Satiety" refers to processes that act to inhibit eating postprandially and reduce intake at later meals, and the associated feeling state (hunger suppression), typically observed up to 4 to 6 hours. We also use "appetite" as a more generic term for the motivational state or drive to seek food and eat. "Food intake" can include a variety of measures of actual ingestive behavior, including rate, volume, choice, and energy content.

Our emphasis is on evidence derived from experimentation with humans, without going into too much depth on underlying biochemical or neural mechanisms, or characteristics of specific hormones. The applicability of this evidence under normal physiological circumstances is considered, using some specific examples with different macronutrients and fiber. We also discuss remaining knowledge gaps that should be addressed by research in humans and animals.

10.2 THE MOUTH

Influences of oral stimulation on appetite and food intake will only be briefly mentioned here, because they are discussed in-depth in Chapter 7 and Chapter 8 of this volume.

The mouth is a source of signals that may be explicitly perceived in terms of gustatory, textural, and (via airflow to nasal passageways) olfactory stimulus characteristics: quality, intensity, and hedonic value. Everyday experience and controlled research confirm the superficially trivial fact that people often eat more of better-liked foods when offered a choice, and that the presence of a highly liked food can stimulate its consumption in the absence of an energy deficit or perceived state of hunger.[3] It is reasonable to expect that these effects (and their anticipation) would primarily influence initiation of eating and intake within a meal (mainly affecting satiation), rather than lasting several hours through the postmeal period (less likely to affect postmeal satiety). This distinction is apparent, for example, in the work on effects of palatability on satiation and satiety by de Graaf et al.[4] Many studies have shown effects of sensory and hedonic qualities of foods on postmeal appetite ratings and behavior, although our view is that this evidence is inconsistent and relatively small in magnitude and duration.[5] Nevertheless, through learned associations, specific sensory qualities could potentially be exploited to convey the impression of a more filling product, or to reinforce the effects of more active satiety-inducing ingredients.

In addition to influencing intake within a meal, events in the mouth may also play a role as direct or indirect metabolic signals related to appetite and food intake. Direct effects could occur through stimulation of relevant oral receptor systems[6,7] that may trigger "downstream" GI and metabolic responses, such as pancreatic endocrine and exocrine secretions. Indirect effects would be signals arising secondarily through learned associations with specific sensory stimuli (perhaps even when these are present at levels below the perceptual threshold).[8] Although these effects of oral stimulation can be isolated and demonstrated experimentally, their actual relevance to ingestive behavior in the context of everyday eating remains to be clearly demonstrated.

10.3 THE STOMACH

Although the stomach is often treated as one single entity, perhaps even a simple mixing vat, its function is highly complex and should be regarded as multicompartmental. Chemical and mechanical properties of the ingesta are transduced in the gastric lumen through primary afferent neurons, coordinated via interneurons. The proximal stomach (fundus) accommodates food by reduction of its tone, followed by an increase in proximal and distal (antrum) stomach volume. The gastric motor function adapts to this fed state, and mixing and digestion are initiated. Nutrient emptying starts with the liquid phase, while solids are initially retained in the fundus. After a lag phase, solids empty selectively from the stomach, propelled toward the pylorus when the particle size is sufficiently reduced (to about 1 to 2 mm).[9]

Each of these steps in the gastric phase could potentially influence appetite and food intake. However, the magnitude and timing of each gastric step is dependent on meal composition parameters such as volume, consistency, energy value, and fat content, and all those parameters can influence appetite.[10–16] It should also be realized that it is not the stomach itself, but in actuality feedback from the small intestine, that determines the rate of gastric emptying (GE).

The exact nature of the gastric signals and their hierarchy of importance are unknown. Nevertheless, a relationship between gastric parameters (gastric distension, emptying, accommodation, compliance) and satiety-related measures (reported sensations of fullness, hunger, etc.) has been shown many times.[17–23]

The most potent gastric signals are probably those reflecting distension, and the amount, timing, and site of distension can all influence ingestive behavior. Early work from Geliebter et al.[20] indicated that meal intake was lower when a gastric balloon was inflated to a volume of 400 ml or more, and hunger ratings also decreased accordingly. In subsequent research it became clear that distension in the (less compliant) antral area is more important than in the fundal region.[21,22,24,25]

In addition to site and amount of distension, the timing is important. Oesch et al.[26] used an intragastric balloon to distend the fundus (by 0, 400, 600, or 800 ml) of volunteers for 10 minutes. Ten minutes after the balloon was deflated and taken out, subjects were invited to eat and drink as much as they wished for 60 minutes. During the gastric distension, scores for hunger were significantly reduced at a volume of 600 and 800 ml, while fullness scores were significantly increased only at 800 ml, with a trend for 600 ml. However, as soon as the distension was terminated, satiety scores returned to baseline. This might explain why subsequent food intake did not differ in relation to the preceding volumes of distension. In the antrum 300-ml distension had no effect on hunger feelings or food intake, presumably because the volume was lower than the 400-ml threshold as suggested by Geliebter et al.[20]

These types of studies can be criticized for their use of the balloon. The position of the balloon was not always well defined (the balloon intended for the

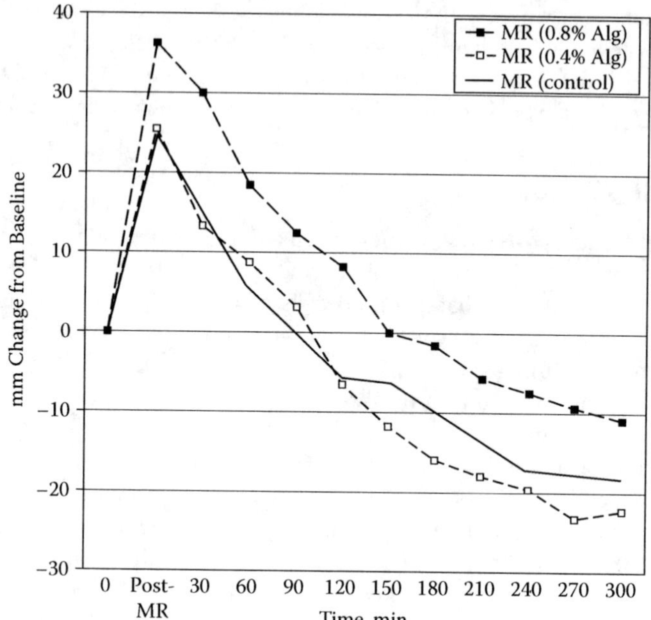

FIGURE 10.1 Effect of addition of 0.4% and 0.8% alginate to meal replacements (MR) on self-reported fullness (100 mm scale). (Data from Appleton, K., Hill, J., Haddeman, E., Rogers, P.J., and Mela, D.J., *Proc. Nutr. Soc.*, 2004, 63, 118A, abstract.)

fundus may have been placed in the antrum), and these techniques are invasive and uncomfortable. It has been shown that distension induced by this technique does not clearly simulate the intragastric distribution of a meal. Also, direct stimulation with a balloon may exaggerate relaxation of the stomach wall and interfere with normal gastric physiology.[27,28]

The most natural way of testing gastric distension is by the use of a meal. Rolls and Roe,[12] for instance, showed that — perhaps not surprisingly — increasing volume of gastrically infused food reduced hunger and food intake. However, by using a meal, both the gastric processes and duodenal feedback may play a role. Goetze et al.[29] used a noninvasive magnetic resonance imaging (MRI) technique and showed that perceptions of satiety and fullness are linearly associated with postprandial gastric volumes of meals (independent of macronutrient composition), although this research did not discriminate between antrum and fundus. We[30] distended the stomach in another way, by giving subjects meal replacement drinks containing a type of alginate, a fiber that gels in the stomach. Using MRI we were able to prove that the fiber did form lumps, and we found higher satiety ratings with the alginate meal compared to the control meal. This was confirmed in another trial, where two alginate concentrations were tested.[31] Only the drink where 0.8% alginate was added (see Figure 10.1) increased satiety significantly, pointing to a threshold effect. Note though that there are many different alginates, and these quantitative and qualitative results and their replication are highly dependent upon the chemical specification of the alginate source, as well as the food matrix in which they are used.

The alginate lumps in our experiments may have activated antral mechanoreceptors, although it is also possible that the lumps entrapped nutrients from the meal replacement drink (since carbohydrates and protein are water soluble). These nutrients might have increased subsequent satiety by selective and prolonged delivery to the small intestine.[32,33]

Marciani et al.[34] limited the effects of the lumps to the stomach by using agar beads differing in strength. They clearly showed that fullness increased with increasing gel strength of the beads and, as such, showed that the antral grinding forces are important determinants of fullness. It is not known if this difference between antrum and fundus is also related to differences in the characteristics or density of mechanoreceptors in these areas, although differences in the mechanical properties and neural innervations between antrum and fundus have been shown.[35,36] A gastric mechanosensor has recently been identified that could also be linked to feeding behavior.[37]

In addition to distension, gastric emptying might be an important determinant of ingestive behavior.[38] Some authors suggest that antral distension is more important than the overall rate of gastric emptying,[21,39] but this remains to be confirmed. It is likely that they both are important. Gastric emptying affects not only the amount of gastric distension, but also the rate of delivery to the small intestine and how that interacts with the stomach (see Section 10.6). The selective emptying of nutrients might be especially important in this regard.

It is not only the stomach that is commonly regarded as a single uniform entity, but the meals entering the stomach are also often regarded as such. However, a meal consists of many components that behave and might be handled differently in the stomach and, consequently, leave the stomach at different rates. For example, in the intragastric environment, separation of fat content can occur with different meals or emulsions, whereby fat and water undergo phase-separation into distinct upper (fat) and lower (water) layers. Consequently, the lower layer with less fat and much more water empties much faster than fat.[40] It can be hypothesized that such a water phase may not contain sufficient fat to stimulate the duodenal feedback that mediates a reduction in gastric emptying rate, as a phase-separating meal was shown to generate less production of the satiety hormone cholecystokinin (CCK) and less reported satiety than an emulsified meal that did not separate into two distinct phases.[41]

Another example of the complex gastric behavior and of the role of gastric emptying is the comparison of casein and whey, which have been characterized respectively as "slow" and "fast" proteins,[42] because casein forms a complex in the stomach and is proposed to be more slowly released. Indeed, Hall et al.[43] showed that a liquid drink containing 49 g of protein as whey (versus casein) emptied significantly faster and resulted in a 19% reduction in meal intake 90 minutes later. This was accompanied by a higher satiety and higher total amino acid plasma level and higher levels of the satiety hormones CCK and glucagon-like peptide-1 (GLP-1). However, a more recent trial[44] could not confirm any of these differences, possibly because of a different design or because of other (postabsorptive) properties of the protein counteracting the differences in gastric emptying. The inconsistent effects observed for different protein sources may also depend on the specific sourcing and isolation of the protein and prior processing or composition of the test food matrix.

Adding to effects of mechanical stimuli in the stomach, chemical stimuli might be important for ingestive behavior, but these have hardly been studied. For instance the role of gastric pH and acid secretion on satiety is unknown, although it can be speculated that a different pH affects meal behavior in the stomach (e.g., by affecting optimal enzyme activity[45] or emulsion stability[41,46]). There could also be effects on rates of digestion and consequent delivery of digestion products to the small intestine.[45,47] An example may be the digestion of fat in the stomach. The extent of fat hydrolysis taking place in the stomach is approximately 10 to 30% of fat ingested,[48] and this gastric predigestion facilitates fat digestion in the duodenum. As gastric lipase is most active around pH 3–4, the gastric pH can affect digestion[45,49] and consequently satiety. However, so far this is largely speculation.

10.3.1 Hormonal Mediators of Eating Behavior

While gastric distension evokes neural signals that are transmitted directly to the brain, humoral factors can also play a role in eating behavior. We describe two hormones, gastric leptin and ghrelin, that may act to suppress or stimulate food intake, respectively.[50–53]

Up to 25% of circulating *leptin* is derived from the stomach,[54] but research on gastric leptin production and characteristics is thus far mainly limited to animals. While leptin produced by the adipose tissue plays a role in the long-term regulation of energy balance and acts more systemically,[55] gastric leptin appears to serve as a short-term satiety signal, acting much more locally.[53] The interplay between gastric leptin and nongastric leptin warrants further study.

Ghrelin is a 28-amino-acid peptide mostly expressed in the stomach and the only hormone identified so far that stimulates food intake.[51] Ghrelin stimulates acid secretion and motility in the stomach, but also food intake and jejunal motility, and its marked preprandial elevation suggests it might be a hunger signal leading to meal initiation.[51,56]

Although ghrelin is mainly expressed by the stomach, it is not really responding to luminal contents in either stomach or small intestine, but to metabolic state and neural signals in the small intestine.[50] Osmolality and insulin surges are probably involved in this,[50] thus explaining why lipids, calorie for calorie, are much less effective in simulating ghrelin than carbohydrates and proteins.[50] Ghrelin release patterns may also be partly entrained by habitual meal patterns, so it peaks prior to when food intake would normally occur, and may contribute toward "conditioned hunger."

10.4 THE SMALL INTESTINE

We have described how gastric distension plays an important role in satiety and food intake, while in the small intestine, both distension and nutrient stimulation play a role. Small intestinal mechanoreceptors initiate motor mechanisms which slow gastric emptying,[57] but the impact of mechanical stimulation in the intestine is clearly less potent than the effects of nutrients, mediated via the abundant chemoreceptors.

Gastric emptying and delivery of nutrients to the small intestine are precisely controlled by negative feedback from nutrients in the duodenum. Several chemical and osmotic effects can be considered. It is known that a low pH,[58] as well as a high osmolality[59–61] or viscosity[62] in the small intestine, can delay gastric emptying, and delayed gastric emptying affects satiety. However, direct effects of, for instance, osmolality on satiety have hardly been studied in humans.[63–65] Effects of osmolality on ghrelin have been mentioned,[65] and it is known that vagal receptors exist that respond to osmolality,[66] but the exact mechanism and impact on satiety is largely unknown. Perhaps part of the effects can be explained by intestinal hypertonicity inducing GI symptoms like reflux.[67] The effects of a low intestinal pH on satiety have not been tested, although a recent study showed that addition of organic acids to solid foods can delay gastric emptying[68] and increase satiety.[69] The satiety effect observed in the latter study, however, may have been confounded by low palatability of the acid test products.

Effects of intestinal viscosity on satiety are largely unknown, because most research only studies the viscosity of the test products (before eating) or perhaps under gastric conditions.[30] Viscosity of the meal itself is often not directly reflected in the subsequent gastric or intestinal viscosity.[30,70] The differential effects of fibers on satiety may be partly explained by variation in their effects on gastric and/or intestinal viscosity,[71,72] but that has not been directly tested in humans.

Upon entry of nutrients, intestinal motility is changed from the propagative contractions of peristalsis of the fasted state to the nonpropagative pattern that slows intestinal transit in the fed state.[73] The movement of a meal through the digestive tract must be tightly controlled to ensure adequate time for assimilation. Motility of the small intestine determines the time that the contents of a meal are in contact with the digestive enzymes and absorptive mucosal layer. In a normal healthy bowel, the control process (the feedback mechanisms) takes place in the entire small intestine, divided anatomically into duodenum, jejunum, and ileum. The feedback from each area is known as the "duodenal brake," the "jejunal brake," and the "ileal brake," respectively.[74–76] Each of these "brakes" act as a neurohormonal feedback mechanism, activated when end-products of digestion (such as unesterified fatty acids [FA] after a fatty meal) become available, but the ileal brake is clearly the most potent.[77] The ileal brake delays both gastric and intestinal transit time and is primarily triggered by FA. For an overview of the ileal brake, we refer to Van Citters and Lin.[78] All of these brakes can affect satiety and food intake.

Studies in animals have shown that small intestinal feedback on gastric emptying, intestinal transit, and appetite is dependent on load and duration of nutrient delivery and the length and region of small intestine exposed to these nutrients. In humans, however, this has hardly been studied, especially in the ileal region. As fat appears to be the most potent trigger, this is the most studied nutrient in this respect.

The load of nutrients affects motility, satiety, and food intake, although there is probably a minimal threshold for each of these parameters.[79] Loads as small as about 2 kcal/min of triacylglycerides have been shown to suppress hunger and food intake,[80] while the minimum effective dose for unesterified FA appears to be much lower.[81] For instance, Little et al.[81] found that very low intraduodenal doses of lauric acid (0.1, 0.2, or 0.4 kcal/min) for 90 minute dose-dependently modulated antral and duodenal motility and GI hormone release, and effects on energy intake were apparent with the highest dose infused (0.4 kcal/min). In this study no effect on appetite scores were observed, although a similar dose produced a reduction in hunger in a separate experiment by the same group.[82]

In addition to load, duration of nutrient delivery is important.[83] Load and duration probably interact as well.[79] In normal conditions, load and length of intestine exposed are linked. In dogs[84] increasing total load increased the spread of both lipolysis and absorption of fat to and along the ileum: only 7% of a 15-g duodenal fat load reached the ileum, compared to 30% after a 60-g fat load. In rats it has been shown that suppression of food intake is only maximal when feedback is generated from both proximal and distal gut sensors,[85,86] while in dogs it has been observed that the larger the surface area triggered, the stronger the feedback signals.[32]

While load, duration, and length of intestine triggered are important for feedback control of motility and for satiety and food intake, it is evident that the intestinal region is of utmost importance. Studies in dogs[77] have shown that stimulation of the ileal brake is clearly most potent, but data in humans are limited.[87–89] Most studies so far have focused on infusion in the duodenal/jejunal region, and few on the ileal region. The ileal brake plays an important role in the physiologic regulation of gut function; especially at higher intakes, increases in postprandial ileal nutrient concentrations have been shown in humans,[90] and even low ileal nutrient concentrations can affect the transition from a fasted to a fed intestinal motility pattern.[73] Amounts as low as 1.2 g lipids delivered to the ileum slow down gastric emptying in humans.[91]

Unfortunately, human studies assessing the relationship between the ileal brake and food intake and satiety are scarce. Welch et al.[87] infused a liquid meal in the ileum (40 g fat, 370 kcal) for 90 minutes and observed a net reduction in food intake. After the start of the meal, fullness increased significantly during the ileal infusion, most probably due to a delayed gastric emptying.[87] As the ileal infusion did not suppress appetite before the meal, but did increase fullness during the meal, the authors concluded that the effect on satiety might be explained by the earlier attainment of a critical level of gastric distension due to the delay in gastric emptying, as opposed to a more direct influence of ileal fat on the satiety centers in the brain. This would then suggest that inhibition of food intake by ileal brake activation could be enhanced by providing a concurrent intragastric volume load.

Apart from reducing food intake during an *ad libitum* meal, activation of the ileal brake can also lead to a reduction in between-meal hunger. We[92] found that, compared to an oral lipid load, an ileal lipid load caused a significant reduction in between-meal hunger and subsequent food intake.

Fat is the most potent trigger of all intestinal braking mechanisms,[76,80,93,94] at least when it is directly infused into the small intestine. Protein and carbohydrate trigger the brakes, but to a lesser extent. Soluble fibers can also trigger the brakes by extending the spread of nutrients down the intestine and consequently stimulating the more potent ileal brake, although this has only been tested in dogs.[95]

Pilichiewicz et al.[83] performed an elegant study in which they tested how the combinations of load, duration, and region of small intestinal fat exposure might affect GI response, satiety, and meal intake. They infused lipids intraduodenally at 1.33 kcal/min for either 50 minutes (1.33/50) or for 150 minutes (1.33/150), or at 4 kcal/min for 50 minutes (4/50), versus a saline infusion for 150 minutes. Although they did not directly measure the distribution of lipolytic products along the gut, they presumed that the 4/50 would result in the release of lipolytic products in the jejunum for the first 50 minutes, followed by further release in the ileum (as this high dose exceeds proximal gut lipolytic and absorptive capacity). The 1.33 kcal/minute load would be digested and absorbed efficiently and therefore confined to the jejunum. There was no significant effect of any of the lipid infusions on appetite or energy intake, although prospective food consumption during 4/50 tended to be reduced as compared to the others, while food intake tended to be lower (–8%) with the 1.33/150 infusion. Gastric motility was mostly affected by the highest dose (4/50) and persisted even after cessation of the infusion.

10.4.1 Hormonal Mediators of Eating Behavior

The interaction of nutrients with specific receptors in the small (and also large) intestine triggers release of hormones, several of which play a major role in triggering changes in satiation, satiety, and food intake. In particular CCK,[55] GLP-1,[96,97] and peptide YY (PYY)[98,99] have been extensively characterized and their effects tested. However, other hormones like amylin, oxyntomodulin, and apo-lipoprotein A-IV might be equally important, but have not been studied to the same extent in humans. The site of release of these satiety hormones and their responsiveness to nutrients appears to be region specific: CCK is mostly proximal, GLP-1 and PYY more distal, while amylin is produced in the pancreas.

We will discuss shortly several hormones (but also refer to Chapters 9 and 10).

CCK is the most-studied satiety hormone,[55] both in humans and animals. CCK is primarily released from the duodenal and jejunal mucosa in response to nutrients, especially fatty acids of at least 12-carbon chain length,[80,100] and to a lesser extent proteins or amino acids. As with most satiety hormones, CCK acts via endocrine and/or neural mechanisms to affect many GI functions such as gut motility, gastric emptying, gall bladder contraction, and gastric acid secretion.

CCK has been shown to act to limit meal size under experimental conditions.[101,102] Exogenous CCK stimulates meal termination,[103,104] and CCK antagonists increase meal size,[105] suggesting that CCK is a natural endogenous satiation factor. Part of the satiation induced by CCK might result from inhibition of gastric emptying. CCK and gastric distension combine to limit food intake,[106] with signals probably being integrated by vagal-afferent fibers.

Amylin is produced in the pancreas and rises rapidly with meal onset, but has a brief duration of action. In addition to an inhibitory action on insulin and glucagon secretion, exogenous amylin leads to a dose-related reduction in meal size. Like many other hormones, it reduces meal size and duration without affecting intake in subsequent meals in rats.[107]

Most research on amylin has focused on animals (for an overview we refer to Lutz[107]). Most human research so far has tested the amylin analog pramlintide and found it to reduce gastric emptying and to have benefits for glycemic control and weight loss.[108] Chapman et al.[109] have recently found that pramlintide reduced food intake both in type 2 diabetics (–23%) and nondiabetic obese men (–16%), without a significant effect on self-reported hunger or fullness.[109] Satiety ratings, however, might have been confounded because the meal intake (before the satiety was rated) differed.

GLP-1 is one of the more distally produced hormones, hypothesized to mediate the ileal and colonic brake.[96,110] This proglucagon-derived peptide is released by the enteroendocrine L-cells in the distal small intestine and colon. Its release depends partly on direct contact between the luminal nutrients and the distal L-cells, predominantly in response to carbohydrates and fat.[111] GLP-1 increases during meal consumption, long before a significant amount of nutrients from that meal reaches the ileum, suggesting that neurohumoral triggers are also involved.

Intravenous infusions of GLP-1 have been shown to inhibit GE[112–114] and to relax the proximal stomach, stimulate phasic and tonic motility of the pylorus, and inhibit gastric acid and exocrine pancreatic secretion.[96,115] Furthermore, intravenous infusion of physiological amounts of GLP-1 leads to a 10% reduction in food intake[116] and promotes satiety[113,117,118] in humans.

As previously noted, maximal suppression of food intake appears to occur only when feedback is generated from both proximal and distal gut sensors, as shown in rats[85,86] and dogs.[32] This has not been formally tested in humans, except for Little et al.,[119] who showed that, when a larger intestinal segment was exposed to glucose (3.5 kcal/min for 60 minutes), effects on GLP-1 and ghrelin, but not CCK, were much more pronounced than when this same infusion was limited to a shorter segment. Unfortunately satiety was not measured in that study.

PYY is also involved in distal-to-proximal intestinal feedback and is also a candidate mediator of the effects of the ileal brake. PYY is a 36-amino-acid peptide, secreted by L-cells in the ileum and colon. PYY release is mainly triggered by fat in the ileum and colon, but may be stimulated by fat in the duodenum via CCK-dependent pathways.[120] PYY is released into the circulation about 15 minutes following food intake, and plasma levels peak after about 90 minutes and can remain elevated for several hours, depending on caloric content and composition of the meal.

PYY release (triggered by ileal fat perfusion) delays small intestinal transit,[76,121] while, as shown in dogs, immunoneutralization of PYY abolishes this delay.[122] The inhibitory effects of PYY on gastrointestinal motility have also been confirmed by intravenous infusion studies.[123] Batterham et al. demonstrated that intravenous infusions replicating (very high?) postprandial PYY3-36 concentrations lessened hunger and decreased *ad libitum* food intake by 36%, without affecting nausea, food palatability, or fluid intake.[98,99] The inhibitory effect of PYY on food intake in animals and humans has been discussed intensively.[124–126] Recently, the anorectic effect of PYY3-36 infusion has been confirmed in humans, but only at very high concentrations that cannot be regarded as physiological.[125]

As described above, Pilichiewicz et al.[83] showed that the effect of load, duration, and region of small intestinal nutrient exposure on food intake and satiety was not very clear and relatively small. In contrast, the effects on plasma CCK and PYY were much more pronounced, and these were clearly different in magnitude and duration among treatments (see Figure 10.2). This implies that production of these hormones depends on load, duration, and region of the small intestine exposed to the lipids, but that the relationship with satiety and food intake is much less straightforward.

When we infused lipids directly into the ileum at a rate of 0.54 kcal/min for 45 minutes, satiety scores increased significantly, and food intake decreased significantly (11%).[92] Small intestinal transit time was reduced, and CCK was elevated,

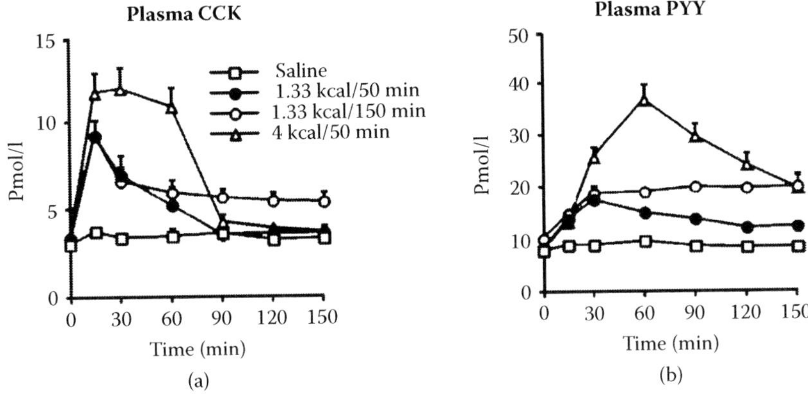

FIGURE 10.2 Plasma concentrations of CCK (A) and peptide YY (PYY; B) during intraduodenal infusion of 10% Intralipid at 1.33 kcal/min for 50 minutes, 1.33 kcal/min for 150 minutes, and 4 kcal/min for 50 minutes or saline for 150 minutes. CCK concentrations were significantly higher during 1.33/50 when compared with the others between 0 and 60 minutes and significantly higher during 1.33/150 when compared with the others between 90 and 150 minutes. PYY concentrations were significantly higher during 4/50 when compared with the others between 30 and 90 minutes and between 120 and 150 minutes; 4/50 and 1.33/150 were significantly higher when compared with the others. (From Pilichiewicz, A.N., Little, T.J., Brennan, I.M., et al., *Am. J. Physiol.*, 2006, 290, R668–R677. Reproduced with permission.)

while PYY was not affected. However, these effects were seen in comparison to oral intake of the same amount of lipids and not to duodenal infusion, and lipids were delivered with different timings.

The possibility that PYY acts more as a paracrine or neurocrine agent than as an endocrine agent (and as such plasma levels may not reflect the local effects of PYY) might explain the discrepancy between observed correlations with endogenous PYY and the effects of exogenous PYY in some studies. Until these issues are resolved, the role of PYY as the primary humoral mediator of the ileal brake, or perhaps the particular conditions in which its effects dominate, will remain unsettled.

Apolipoprotein A-IV (Apo A-IV) is synthesized in response to lipid in the intestine, and there is evidence that it may be involved in signaling fat content in the intestine to other organ systems,[127] inhibiting, for example, GE[128] and signaling satiety in the rat.[129,130]

After luminal hydrolysis of triacylglycerols (TAG), the resulting fatty acids (FA) and monoacylglycerols diffuse into enterocytes. Within the enterocytes, they are resynthesized into TAG, packaged into chylomicrons, and secreted into the lymph. Apo A-IV is a component of the surface coating of chylomicrons. When the release of chylomicrons into lymph is blocked by pluronic L81, an inhibitor of chylomicron formation and secretion, the satiating effects of intestinal lipids is attenuated.[131] Thus, transportation of TAG as chylomicrons into lymph is essential for at least a part of the inhibitory effect of intestinal lipids on gastric emptying and food intake.[131] Intra-arterial perfusion of lymph has been shown to inhibit gastric motility,[132] and further studies in rats indicate that Apo A-IV is the component in the lymph responsible for the effects on gastric emptying.[133] So far, the vast majority of research has concentrated on animals, and the importance of Apo A-IV in humans has to be clarified.

Oxyntomodulin is another satiety hormone originating from the distal small intestine, but it has hardly been studied in humans. This peptide is also cleaved from proglucagon, produced by L-cells and colocalized with PYY and GLP-1. It is released in proportion to ingested calories, and intravenous infusion immediately decreases hunger and meal intake.[134] Longer-term use leads to body weight loss, although part of that effect might be induced by increased energy expenditure.[56] Additional research is required to clarify its importance in human eating behavior.

10.5 THE COLON

The colon possesses an inhibitory mechanism like the ileal brake, but this colonic brake is less potent than other brakes.[110] It shows that colonic feedback inhibits proximal gut motility,[135,136] possibly via GLP-1 and PYY, but the relationship to food intake and satiety is unclear.

Actually very few studies have been performed on the role of the colon in satiety and food intake. Some fermentable carbohydrates have documented effects of increasing satiety,[137] and short-chain fatty acids (SCFA) (like acetate and propionate) might explain this, because they are produced by colonic fermentation. L-cells that produce several satiety hormones (for example, PYY and GLP-1) are also found in large concentrations in the colon.

Only a very limited number of studies have been performed on the effects of SCFA specifically, or prebiotics (potential substrates for microbial SCFA production), on food intake, satiety, or weight gain. In rats, daily ingestion of lactitol (a nondigestible, fermentable sugar alcohol) for 10 days lowered total food intake and weight gain over this period, while the authors observed no significant effect on satiety after 1 day of lactitol in humans, although suggestive trends were observed.[138]

There is some indirect evidence for satiety effects of fermentable substrates as well. Effects on GLP-1 and PYY have been studied with mixed results. Piche et al.[139] gave 20 g oligofructose per day for 7 days to patients with gastroesophageal reflux disease. Plasma concentrations of GLP-1 after a subsequent test meal were significantly higher after the oligofructose treatment compared to after a week of sucrose as placebo. CCK and PYY were not changed. In earlier studies colonic infusion of SCFA also did not change GLP-1 or PYY.[135,136,139] Fermentable carbohydrates and SCFA might influence satiety also via an effect on gastric emptying. This has been shown in humans.[136]

Studies to date would indicate that diets rich in resistant starch do not substantially affect satiety,[140] although a very recent study does suggest that 8 g oligofructose twice a day for 2 weeks affects satiety and food intake at the last day.[137] Underlying mechanisms were not explored in this study, although the same material affected satiety hormones in rats.[141]

There is also some indication that colonic distension affects GI motor function in humans,[142] but effects on satiety and food intake have not been directly tested. A recent finding[143] that gas and methane production (and possibly associated distension) is linked to GI motility is very intriguing, but warrants much more research in humans. Issues of side effects (for example, flatulence) at levels required to affect appetite will likely influence eventual food applications.

All in all, it can be concluded that the role of the colon in human satiety and food intake remains unclear since most data have been gathered in rodents. Confirmation in humans is needed.

10.6 INTEGRATION OF MULTIPLE GASTROINTESTINAL (GI) TARGETS

We have thus far discussed the effect of the GI tract by considering each segment independently, but obviously the effects from the different segments are integrated and interactive. Ingested nutrients induce signals of satiation and satiety by means of their physicochemical characteristics and digestion products, either directly or indirectly through effects on gastric or intestinal function (for example, by mechanical, chemical, or osmotic effects). Subsequently, these effects stimulate neural responses and the release of various peptide hormones influencing appetite and food intake. However, as the hormones affect the digestion process itself, a positive or negative feedback loop on satiety is introduced. For instance, CCK is stimulated by peptides resulting from protein digestion, but CCK also stimulates gastric acid secretion. An enhanced gastric acid secretion will affect the optimal pepsin activity,[144] which in turn either increases or decreases the production of smaller protein breakdown products, and that by itself then affects the stimulation of CCK.

Just as the effects from the different GI segments are integrated and interactive, the hormones produced by the GI tract interact as well, although the number of human studies testing these interactions is fairly limited.[145–147] One example is the possible interaction of GLP-1 and PYY. Because they are cosecreted by intestinal L-cells, an interaction seems obvious. However, while one study showed that the effects of simultaneous perfusion of both peptides on food intake in humans was larger than the sum of the individual contributions,[145] another study indicates that the release of GLP-1 may inhibit the release of PYY.[112]

Another example of possible interaction is that of PYY and Apo A-IV; PYY infusion, resulting in levels that are similar to those produced by ileal lipid infusion, has been shown to result in increased Apo A-IV secretion.[148]

Other examples of interactions are illustrated by the work of French and Cecil,[149] showing the interactions amongst oral, gastric, and duodenal effects on satiety. Studies that have combined intraduodenal lipid infusions with gastric distension show that this produces a greater reduction in food intake than when these two stimuli are separated.[79]

As described above, Oesch et al.[26] used intragastric balloon distension of the antrum (300 ml) for 20 minutes and combined this with a continuous duodenal infusion of either fat or saline. Antral distension decreased hunger feelings only when fat was infused. Food intake was also reduced by the fat infusion independent of antral distension. However, antral volume did not exceed 300 ml, which might have been too low to produce the full array of possible interactions.

Another example of the interaction between duodenal and gastric effects was tested by Oesch et al.[150] An oral protein preload alone significantly reduced the

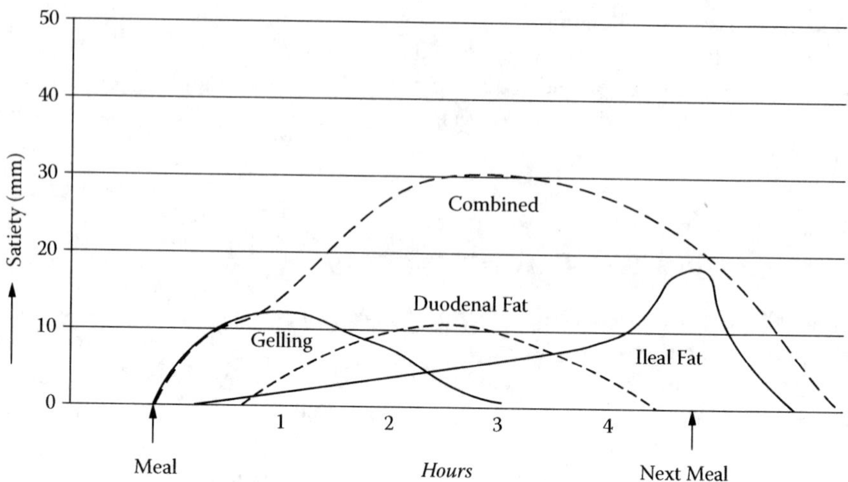

FIGURE 10.3 Theoretical effects of different discrete or combined GI targets on satiety.

amount of food eaten by 20%, and an intraduodenal fat infusion alone caused a 13% reduction, while the combination reduced food intake by 29%. They concluded that the effect was additive and not synergistic. However, because total energy was not the same in all conditions, this may not be a true example of interaction. Hunger was only reduced after the protein preload and not after the duodenal infusion.

Degen et al.[151] showed that the combined food intake-reducing effect of ileal stimulation (using exogenous GLP-1 infusion) and gastric distension (using a protein preload) was larger than the effect of each on its own. Also Kissileff et al.[106] showed that gastric distension plus intravenously administered CCK reduced test meal food intake by 200 g (from about 760 g), and this effect was only partly dependent on the reduced gastric emptying (induced by CCK). The 300-ml distension on its own had little effect (31 g), while CCK alone reduced food intake by 90 g. Fullness was significantly enhanced after distension, but less after CCK infusion. At the 300-ml distension, CCK showed no additional effect on fullness.

These examples of interaction show how the quantitative and qualitative impact of some potentially important GI influences on satiety and food may be over- or underestimated, or missed altogether, when studied in isolation. These interactions are likely to occur in natural eating conditions and can also be considered as possible targets for food or pharmacological interventions. Based on current literature on satiety and food intake and the time course of nutrient effects within the GI tract,[152] Figure 10.3 illustrates the theoretical timing and extent of GI effects on satiation and satiety. As an example of how this might be applied in manufactured foods, the gelling of alginate in the stomach can be used to increase gastric distension, and this distension can be expected to increase the satiety-enhancing effects of, for instance, duodenal fat delivery. If it is then also possible to achieve (later) ileal fat delivery, a further enhancement of the magnitude and duration of appetite-control effects could be accomplished.

What is proposed here is an approach whereby multiple different GI targets may each be modestly affected, and the combination could provide for additive or even synergistic and prolonged satiety signaling. In contrast to single-target strategies, this approach may also better address individual differences and prevent long-term adaptation, and might be a more feasible strategy to manipulate hunger and meal intake practically through foods. One such approach could include use of soluble fibers that delay gastric emptying and nutrient absorption, displace nutrients to the ileum, and might even increase satiety via by-products of colonic fermentation. Several challenges remain to confirm these ideas and realize them in practice.

10.7 RESEARCH WITH HUMAN SUBJECTS VERSUS ANIMAL MODELS

There are several research issues that would be best addressed by researchers working with animal models. Animals have long been used as a research stage (bioassay) between *in vitro* and human clinical trials, whereby active agents or stimuli seen in *in vitro* models can be screened in more detail. This naturally affords a cost-effective and feasible approach to consider factors such as bioavailability, biotransformation, and safety before testing in humans. However, it should be realized that certain aspects of GI physiology are species specific. Most aspects of human GI motility are probably best reflected in canine or pig models (with the exception of the ileal brake, which appears not to work in pigs[153]). For instance, ileal brake is mainly affected by lipids in dogs and humans, while proteins also play an important role in the ileal brake in rats. In particular, the role of the colon in human satiety and food intake should be tested in humans and not in rodents because of significant species differences in anatomy. Colonic effects in rodents can be influenced by the much greater relative size and weight of the first part of the rat's large intestine, and this may lead to exaggerated conclusions regarding potential effects in humans.[141]

We have described how multiple GI processes and hormones interact and are dependent on load, duration, and site of nutrient delivery. Animal models might be suitable to discriminate between the different GI processes. For instance, by using a meal, both the gastric processes and duodenal feedback may play a role, and these can be separated in animals much more easily by, for example, gastric cannulas or pyloric cuffs to limit the effect to small intestine or stomach. Other possibilities are the use of more potent or longer-acting blockers or agonists of hormone action.

We have described several feedback mechanisms that tend to reduce food intake and inhibit hunger, partly by prolongation of gastric emptying time and the transit time through the small intestine. However, it is uncertain whether this is purely an indirect effect, or also a direct effect of these brakes on the central satiety centers in the brain. Animal studies might elucidate this, while human studies combining intestinal intubation with fMRI techniques, though technically challenging and costly, might also help in testing for such a direct effect.

Animals, preferably pigs, can be used for targeted delivery of nutrients to specific areas of the GI tract. While intubation in humans is possible, animals can be used much more easily and frequently. However, considerable skill is needed to successfully implant cannulas at the required sites in small animals like rats or mice.

Very few studies have been performed in humans to assess hormonal interactions, so the relative importance of these is largely unknown. The availability of specific antagonists, for instance for GLP-1, enables new studies, especially in animals, investigating the role of individual satiety hormones and their interactions in food intake.

Furthermore, we (and the research literature) have primarily considered humoral factors as nutrient-induced effects, but neural mechanisms are certainly as important.[154,155] Vagal afferents transmit information from the gut to the brain, primarily to the nucleus of the solitary tract. For example, intestinal infusion with fatty acids and, to a lesser extent, triacylglycerols increases activity of vagal afferents in rats. After vagotomy the inhibitory effect of jejunal lipid infusion on food intake is markedly reduced.[154,155] The effects of PYY and GLP-1 on GI function and food intake are also attenuated after vagotomy.[156,157] This suggests a role of vagal afferents in the hormone-induced changes in GI motor and secretory function and their effects on food intake, and is a research issue that, for obvious reasons, would be best addressed by researchers working with animal models.

Lastly, animal models can also be applied to unravel long-term effects (e.g., adaptation, repeat exposure) of nutrients much more easily and cost effectively than testing with humans.

10.8 CONCLUSIONS

How important is the GI tract as a source of signals influencing satiety and food intake in humans? In reality, humans mostly consume meals at times that are convenient or habitual, and eating is most often initiated based on social influences and learned cues. Meal termination is often largely determined simply by initial serving size availability; we eat what we take (or are given) and stop when it is gone. Thus, it could be argued that much of behavior reflects automated routines and momentary environmental conditions. This is certainly true for the bulk of meal-eating under normal conditions. However, this does not mean that GI signals are irrelevant to everyday eating behavior. It is likely that the repeated experience of GI signals is a significant factor in the initial and continued entraining of habitual eating behaviors (e.g. self-selected portion sizes and meal timing). Furthermore, statistical analyses of normal eating patterns in humans suggest significant associations with feedback from GI signals.[158,159]

It is not possible to quantify the power of signals arising from the GI tract in meal termination or preventing opportunistic between-meal "snacking," because these are also integrated with postabsorptive metabolic events and longer-term adiposity signals like leptin. Nevertheless, it is clear that GI signals are capable of independently generating substantial inhibition of hunger feelings and eating motivation. The fact that infusion of nutrients into the small intestine reduces food intake much more than when these nutrients are given intravenously[160] shows the satiating power of the GI tract. Nevertheless this can be overridden by, for example, environmental conditions that stimulate so-called "nonhomeostatic" eating.[3]

Further research to clarify the potency of GI tract signals and the longer-term persistence of short-term effects would help to identify optimal targets and patterns of exposure that may help in suppressing or stimulating appetite and eating. The continuous (oral) ingestion of different macronutrients shows equivocal results with respect to compensation effects on meal intake, satiety, and GI function.[161–164] The effects of compensation after continuous infusion directly into the intestine have mostly been limited to animals,[165] and its implications therefore remain to be assessed in humans.

There is clearly much already known, and much still to be learned, about the role of the GI tract in appetite and food intake. There also remains a considerable opportunity for translating fundamental knowledge into clinical and consumer applications. Several of the examples described here indicate the advantage of multidisciplinary research teams that combine expertise in gastroenterology and ingestive behavior. The addition of expertise in food materials science (physical behavior and chemical characterization of food components and matrices) can provide additional understanding of the complex interactions between food and the body and help in taking research from the laboratory into the marketplace.

REFERENCES

1. Woods, S.C., Gastrointestinal satiety signals — I. An overview of gastrointestinal signals that influence food intake, *Am. J. Physiol. Gastrointest. Liver Physiol.,* 2004, 286, G7–G13.
2. Badman, M.K. and Flier, J.S., The gut and energy balance: visceral allies in the obesity wars, *Science,* 2005, 307, 1909–1914.
3. Mela, D.J., Eating for pleasure or just wanting to eat? Reconsidering sensory hedonic responses as a driver of obesity, *Appetite,* 2006, 47, 10–17.
4. De Graaf, C., De Jong, L.S., and Lambers, A.C., Palatability affects satiation but not satiety, *Physiol. Behav.,* 1999, 66, 681–688.
5. Sorensen, L.B., Moller, P., Flint, A., Martens, M., and Raben, A., Effect of sensory perception of foods on appetite and food intake: a review of studies on humans, *Int. J. Obes. Relat. Metab. Disord.,* 2003, 27, 1152–1166.
6. Laugerette, F., Passilly-Degrace, P., Patris, B., et al., CD36 involvement in orosensory detection of dietary lipids, spontaneous fat preference, and digestive secretions, *J. Clin. Invest.,* 2005, 115, 3177–3184.
7. Teff, K., Nutritional implications of the cephalic-phase reflexes: endocrine responses, *Appetite,* 2000, 34, 206–213.
8. Lorig, T.S., EEG and ERP studies of low-level odor exposure in normal subjects, *Toxicol. Ind. Health,* 1994, 10, 579–586.
9. Camilleri, M., Integrated upper gastrointestinal response to food intake, *Gastroenterology,* 2006, 131, 640–658.
10. Bell, E.A. and Rolls, B.J., Energy density of foods affects energy intake across multiple levels of fat content in lean and obese women, *Am. J. Clin. Nutr.,* 2001, 73, 1010–1018.
11. Doran, S., Jones K.L., Andrews, J.M., and Horowitz, M., Effects of meal volume and posture on gastric emptying of solids and appetite, *Am. J. Physiol.,* 1998, 44, R1712–R1718.
12. Rolls, B.J. and Roe, L.S., Effect of the volume of liquid food infused intragastrically on satiety in women, *Physiol. Behav.,* 2002, 76, 623–631.
13. Santangelo, A., Peracchi, M., Conte, D., Fraquelli, M., and Porrini, M., Physical state of meal affects gastric emptying, cholecystokinin release and satiety, *Br. J. Nutr.,* 1998, 80, 521–527.
14. Phillips, R.J. and Powley, T.L., Gastric volume rather than nutrient content inhibits food intake, *Am. J. Physiol.,* 1996, 40, R766–R779.

15. Hunt, J.N., Smith, J.L., and Jiang, C.L., Effect of meal volume and energy density on the gastric-emptying of carbohydrates, *Gastroenterology,* 1985, 89, 1326–1330.
16. Calbet, J.A.L. and MacLean, D.A., Role of caloric content on gastric emptying in humans, *J. Physiol.,* 1997, 498, 553–559.
17. Read, N., French, S., and Cunningham, K., The role of the gut in regulating food-intake in man, *Nutr. Rev.,* 1994, 52, 1–10.
18. Feinle, C., Grundy, D., and Read, N.W., Effects of duodenal nutrients on sensory and motor responses of the human stomach to distension, *Am. J. Physiol. Gastrointest. Liver Physiol.,* 1997, 36, G721–G726.
19. Feinle, C., Rades, T., Otto, B., and Fried, M., Fat digestion modulates gastrointestinal sensations induced by gastric distention and duodenal lipid in humans, *Gastroenterology,* 2001, 120, 1100–1107.
20. Geliebter, A., Gastric distension and gastric capacity in relation to food-intake in humans, *Physiol. Behav.,* 1988, 44, 665–668.
21. Hveem, K., Jones K.L., Chatterton, B.E., and Horowitz, M., Scintigraphic measurement of gastric emptying and ultrasonographic assessment of antral area: relation to appetite, *Gut,* 1996, 38, 816–821.
22. Jones, K.L., Doran, S.M., Hveem, K., et al., Relation between postprandial satiation and antral area in normal subjects, *Am. J. Clin. Nutr.,* 1997, 66, 127–132.
23. Clarkston, W.K., Pantano, M.M., Morley, J.E., Horowitz, M., Littlefield, J.M., and Burton, F.R., Evidence for the anorexia of aging: gastrointestinal transit and hunger in healthy elderly vs young adults, *Am. J. Physiol.,* 1997, 41, R243–R248.
24. Sturm, K., Parker, B., Wishart, J., et al., Energy intake and appetite are related to antral area in healthy young and older subjects, *Am. J. Clin. Nutr.,* 2004, 80, 656–667.
25. Mundt, M.W., Hausken, T., Smout, A.J.P.M., and Samsom, M., Relationships between gastric accommodation and gastrointestinal sensations in healthy volunteers. A study using the barostat technique and two- and three-dimensional ultrasonography, *Dig. Dis. Sci.,* 2005, 50, 1654–1660.
26. Oesch, S., Ruegg, C., Fischer, B., Degen, L., and Beglinger, C., Effect of gastric distension prior to eating on food intake and feelings of satiety in humans, *Physiol. Behav.,* 2006, 87, 903–910.
27. Zwart de, I.M., Haans, J.J.L., Verbeek, P., Eilers, P.H.C., Roos de, A., and Masclee, A.A.M., Gastric accommodation and motility are influenced by the barostat device: assessment with magnetic resonance imaging, *Am. J. Physiol. Gastrointest. Liver Physiol.,* 2007, 292, G208–G214.
28. Mundt, M.W., Hausken, T., and Samsom, M., Effect of intragastric barostat bag on proximal and distal gastric accommodation in response to liquid meal, *Am. J. Physiol. Gastrointest. Liver Physiol.,* 2002, 283, G681–G686.
29. Goetze, O., Steingoetter, A., Menne, D., et al., The effect of macronutrients on gastric volume responses and gastric emptying in humans: a magnetic resonance imaging study, *Am. J. Physiol. Gastrointest. Liver Physiol.,* 2007, 292, G11–G17.
30. Hoad, C.L., Rayment, P., Spiller, R.C., et al., In vivo imaging of intragastric gelation and its effect on satiety in humans, *J. Nutr.,* 2004, 134, 2293–2300.
31. Appleton, K., Hill, J., Haddeman, E., Rogers, P.J., and Mela, D.J., Addition of alginate fibre to a liquid meal replacer: effects on satiety and food intake, *Proc. Nutr. Soc.,* 2004, 63, 118A, abstract.
32. Lin, H.C., Doty, J.E., Reedy, T.J., and Meyer, J.H., Inhibition of gastric-emptying by sodium oleate depends on length of intestine exposed to nutrient, *Am. J. Physiol.,* 1990, 259, G1031–G1036.
33. Read, N.W., Aljanabi, M.N., Edwards, C.A., and Barber, D.C., Relationship between postprandial motor-activity in the human small-intestine and the gastrointestinal transit of food, *Gastroenterology,* 1984, 86, 721–727.

34. Marciani, L., Gowland, P.A., Fillery-Travis, A., et al., Assessment of antral grinding of a model solid meal with echo-planar imaging, *Am. J. Physiol. Gastrointest. Liver Physiol.*, 2001, 280, G844–G849.
35. Ladabaum, U., Koshy, S.S., Woods, M.L., Hooper, F.G., Owyang, C., and Hasler, W.L., Differential symptomatic and electrogastrographic effects of distal and proximal human gastric distension, *Am. J. Physiol. Gastrointest. Liver Physiol.*, 1998, 38, G418–G424.
36. Horowitz, M. and Dent, J., Disordered gastric-emptying — mechanical basis, assessment and treatment, *Baillieres Clin. Gastroenterol.*, 1991, 5, 371–407.
37. Walder, K., Cooper, A., Todd, S., Jowett, J., Blangero, J., and Collier, G., TRPV2 is a novel gut mechanosensor associated with obesity, *Obes. Rev.*, 2006, 7 (Suppl. 2), 42, abstract.
38. Peters, H.P.F., Haddeman, E., Mela, D.J., and Rayment, P., The effect of viscosifying and gelling fibres on satiety, fullness and gastric emptying of drinks, *Obes. Rev.*, 2006, 7 (Suppl. 2), 311, abstract.
39. Jones, K.L., O'Donovan, D., Horowitz, M., Russo, A., Lei, Y., and Hausken, T., Effects of posture on gastric emptying, transpyloric flow, and hunger after a glucose drink in healthy humans, *Dig. Dis. Sci.*, 2006, 51, 1331–1338.
40. Marciani, L., Wickham, M.S.J., Bush, D., et al., Magnetic resonance imaging of the behaviour of oil-in-water emulsions in the gastric lumen of man, *Br. J. Nutr.*, 2006, 95, 331–339.
41. Marciani, L., Wickham, M., and Singh, G., et al., Delaying gastric emptying and enhancing cholecystokinin release and satiety by using acid stable fat emulsions, *Gastroenterology*, 2006, 130, A227.
42. Boirie, Y., Dangin, M., Gachon, P., Vasson, M.P., Maubois, J.L., and Beaufrere, B., Slow and fast dietary proteins differently modulate postprandial protein accretion, *Proc. Natl. Acad. Sci. USA*, 1997, 94, 14930–14935.
43. Hall, W.L., Millward, D.J., Long, S.J., and Morgan, L.M., Casein and whey exert different effects on plasma amino acid profiles, gastrointestinal hormone secretion and appetite, *Br. J. Nutr.*, 2003, 89, 239–248.
44. Bowen, J., Noakes, M., Trenerry, C., and Clifton, P.M., Energy intake, ghrelin, and cholecystokinin after different carbohydrate and protein preloads in overweight men, *J. Clin. Endocrinol. Metab.*, 2006, 91, 1477–1483.
45. Carriere, F., Renou, C., Lopez, V., et al., The specific activities of human digestive lipases measured from the in vivo and in vitro lipolysis of test meals, *Gastroenterology*, 2000, 119, 949–960.
46. Evans, D.F. and Wennerström, H., *The Colloidal Domain: Where Physics, Chemistry, Biology and Technology Meet*, Wiley VCH, New York, 1999.
47. Layer, P. and Keller, J., Pancreatic enzymes: secretion and luminal nutrient digestion in health and disease, *J. Clin. Gastroenterol.*, 1999, 28, 3–10.
48. Caririere, F., Barrowman, J.A., Verger, R., and Laugier, R., Secretion and contribution to lipolysis of gastric and pancreatic lipases during a test meal in humans, *Gastroenterology*, 1993, 105, 876–888.
49. Chahinian, H., Snabe, T., Attias, C., Fojan, P., Petersen, S.B., and Carriere, F., How gastric lipase, an interfacial enzyme with a Ser-His-Asp catalytic triad, acts optimally at acidic pH, *Biochemistry*, 2006, 45, 993–1001.
50. Cummings, D.E., Ghrelin and the short- and long-term regulation of appetite and body weight, *Physiol. Behav.*, 2006, 89, 71–84.
51. Wren, A.M., Seal, L.J., Cohen, M.A., et al., Ghrelin enhances appetite and increases food intake in humans, *J. Clin. Endocrinol. Metab.*, 2001, 86, 5992–5995.
52. Druce, M.R., Wren, A.M., Park, A.J., et al., Ghrelin increases food intake in obese as well as lean subjects, *Int. J. Obes. Relat. Metab. Disord.*, 2005, 29, 1130–1136.

53. Pico, C., Oliver, P., Sanchez, J., and Palou, A., Gastric leptin: a putative role in the short-term regulation of food intake, *Br. J. Nutr.,* 2003, 90, 735–741.
54. Sobhani, I., Bado, A., Vissuzaine, C., et al., Leptin secretion and leptin receptor in the human stomach, *Gut,* 2000, 47, 178–183.
55. Geary, N., Endocrine controls of eating: CCK, leptin, and ghrelin, *Physiol. Behav.,* 2004, 81, 719–733.
56. Wynne, K., Park, A.J., Small, C.J., et al., Oxyntomodulin increases energy expenditure in addition to decreasing energy intake in overweight and obese humans: a randomised controlled trial, *Int. J. Obes. Relat. Metab. Disord.,* 2006, 30, 1729–1736.
57. Edelbroek, M., Horowitz, M., Dent, J., et al., Effects of duodenal distension on fasting and postprandial antropyloroduodenal motility in humans, *Gastroenterology,* 1994, 106, 583–592.
58. Lin, H.C., Doty, J.E., Reedy, T.J., and Meyer, J.H., Inhibition of gastric-emptying by acids depends on pH, titratable acidity, and length of intestine exposed to acid, *Am. J. Physiol.,* 1990, 259, G1025–G1030.
59. Vist, G.E. and Maughan, R.J., The effect of osmolality and carbohydrate content on the rate of gastric-emptying of liquids in man, *J. Physiol.,* 1995, 486, 523–531.
60. Shafer, R.B., Levine, A.S., Marlette, J.M., and Morley, J.E., Do calories, osmolality, or calcium determine gastric-emptying, *Am. J. Physiol.,* 1985, 248, R479–R483.
61. Rao, S.S.C., Safadi, R., Lu, C., and SchulzeDelrieu, K., Manometric responses of human duodenum during infusion of HCl, hyperosmolar saline, bile and oleic acid, *Neurogastroenterol. Motil.,* 1996, 8, 35–43.
62. Meyer, J.H., Gu, Y., Elashoff, J., Reedy, T., Dressman, J., and Amidon, G., Effects of viscosity and fluid outflow on postcibal gastric-emptying of solids, *Am. J. Physiol.,* 1986, 250, G161–G164.
63. Houpt, T.R., Baldwin, B.A., and Houpt, K.A., Effects of duodenal osmotic loads on spontaneous meals in pigs, *Physiol. Behav.,* 1983, 30, 787–795.
64. Houpt, T.R., Anika, S.M., and Houpt, K.A., Preabsorptive intestinal satiety controls of food-intake in pigs, *Am. J. Physiol.,* 1979, 236, R328–R337.
65. Tylee, T., Overduin, J., Frayo, R.S., and Cummings, D.E., Intestinal infusions of lactulose suppress ghrelin in a dose-dependent manner: role of intestinal osmolarity in prandial ghrelin regulation, *J. Investig. Med.,* 2004, 52, S92.
66. Mei, N. and Garnier, L., Osmosensitive vagal receptors in the small-intestine of the cat, *J. Auton. Nerv. Syst.,* 1986, 16, 159–170.
67. Salvia, G., De Vizia, B., Manguso, F., et al., Effect of intragastric volume and osmolality on mechanisms of gastroesophageal reflux in children with gastroesophageal reflux disease, *Am. J. Gastroenterol.,* 2001, 96, 1725–1732.
68. Ostman, E.M., Elmstahl, H.G.M.L., and Bjorck, I.M.E., Barley bread containing lactic acid improves glucose tolerance at a subsequent meal in healthy men and women, *J. Nutr.,* 2002, 132, 1173–1175.
69. Ostman, E., Granfeldt, Y., Persson, L., and Bjorck, I., Vinegar supplementation lowers glucose and insulin responses and increases satiety after a bread meal in healthy subjects, *Eur. J. Clin. Nutr.,* 2005, 59, 983–988.
70. Guerin, S., Ramonet, Y., LeCloarec, J., Meunier-Salaun, M.C., Bourguet, P., and Malbert, C.H., Changes in intragastric meal distribution are better predictors of gastric emptying rate in conscious pigs than are meal viscosity or dietary fibre concentration, *Br. J. Nutr.,* 2001, 85, 343–350.
71. Schneeman, B.O., Building scientific consensus: the importance of dietary fiber, *Am. J. Clin. Nutr.,* 1999, 69, 1.
72. vonSchonfeld, J., Evans, D.F., and Wingate, D.L., Effect of viscous fiber (Guar) on postprandial motor activity in human small bowel, *Dig. Dis. Sci.,* 1997, 42, 1613–1617.

73. Keller, J., Runzi, M., Goebell, H., and Layer, P., Duodenal and ileal nutrient deliveries regulate human intestinal motor and pancreatic responses to a meal, *Am. J. Physiol. Gastrointest. Liver Physiol.*, 1997, 35, G632–G637.
74. Shahidullah, M., Kennedy, T.L., and Parks, T.G., The vagus, the duodenal brake, and gastric emptying, *Gut*, 1975, 16, 331–336.
75. Lin, H.C., Zhao, X.T., and Wang, L.J., Inhibition of intestinal transit by fat in the proximal small intestine, *Dig. Dis. Sci.*, 1996, 41, 326–329.
76. Spiller, R.C., Trotman, I.F., Adrian, T.E., Bloom, S.R., Misiewicz, J.J., and Silk, D.B.A., Further characterization of the ileal brake reflex in man — effect of ileal infusion of partial digests of fat, protein, and starch on jejunal motility and release of neurotensin, enteroglucagon, and peptide YY, *Gut*, 1988, 29, 1042–1051.
77. Lin, H.C., Zhao, X.T., and Wang, L., Intestinal transit is more potently inhibited by fat in the distal (ileal brake) than in the proximal (jejunal brake) gut, *Dig. Dis. Sci.*, 1997, 42, 19–25.
78. Van Citters, G.W. and Lin, H.C., Ileal brake: neuropeptidergic control of intestinal transit, *Curr. Gastroenterol. Rep.*, 2006, 8, 367–373.
79. Castiglione, K.E., Read, N.W., and French, S.J., Food intake responses to upper gastrointestinal lipid infusions in humans, *Physiol. Behav.*, 1998, 64, 141–145.
80. Feinle, C., Christen, M., Grundy, D., et al., Effects of duodenal fat, protein or mixed-nutrient infusions on epigastric sensations during sustained gastric distension in healthy humans, *Neurogastroenterol. Motil.*, 2002, 14, 205–213.
81. Little, T.J., Feltrin, K.L., Horowitz, M., et al., Dose-related effects of lauric acid on antropyloroduodenal motility, gastrointestinal hormone release, appetite, and energy intake in healthy men, *Am. J. Physiol.*, 2005, 289, R1090–R1098.
82. Feltrin, K.L., Little, T.J., Meyer, J.H., et al., Effects of intraduodenal fatty acids on appetite, antropyloroduodenal motility, and plasma CCK and GLP-1 in humans vary with their chain length, *Am. J. Physiol.*, 2004, 287, R524–R533.
83. Pilichiewicz, A.N., Little, T.J., Brennan, I.M., et al., Effects of load, and duration, of duodenal lipid on antropyloroduodenal motility, plasma CCK and PYY, and energy intake in healthy men, *Am. J. Physiol.*, 2006, 290, R668–R677.
84. Lin, H.C., Zhao, X.T., and Wang, L.J., Fat absorption is not complete by midgut but is dependent on load of fat, *Am. J. Physiol. Gastrointest. Liver Physiol.*, 1996, 34, G62–G67.
85. Meyer, J.H., Hlinka, M., Tabrizi, Y., DiMaso, N., and Raybould, H.E., Chemical specificities and intestinal distributions of nutrient-driven satiety, *Am. J. Physiol.*, 1998, 44, R1293–R1307.
86. Meyer, J.H., Tabrizi, Y., DiMaso, N., Hlinka, M., and Raybould, H.E., Length of intestinal contact on nutrient-driven satiety, *Am. J. Physiol.*, 1998, 44, R1308–R1319.
87. Welch, I.M., Sepple, C.P., and Read, N.W., Comparisons of the effects on satiety and eating behavior of infusion of lipid into the different regions of the small-intestine, *Gut*, 1988, 29, 306–311.
88. Spiller, R.C., Trotman, I.F., Higgins, B.E. et al., The ileal brake — inhibition of jejunal motility after ileal fat perfusion in man, *Gut*, 1984, 25, 365–374.
89. Symersky, T., Kee, B.C., Haddeman, E., Peters, H.P.F., and Masclee, A., Low dose ileal oil perfusion increases satiety in humans, *Gastroenterology*, 2004, 126, A60.
90. Layer, P., Peschel, S., Schlesinger, T., and Goebell, H., Human pancreatic-secretion and intestinal motility — effects of ileal nutrient perfusion, *Am. J. Physiol.*, 1990, 258, G196–G201.
91. Read, N.W., Mcfarlane, A., Kinsman, R.I. et al., Effect of infusion of nutrient solutions into the ileum on gastrointestinal transit and plasma-levels of neurotensin and enteroglucagon, *Gastroenterology*, 1984, 86, 274–280.

92. Symersky, T., Kee, B., Haddeman, E., Peters, H., and Masclee, A., Ileal delivery of 3 grams of oil increases satiety, decreases meal intake and increases CCK but not PYY in humans, *Obes. Res.,* 2004, 12, A3.
93. Welch, I.M., Cunningham, K.M., and Read, N.W., Regulation of gastric-emptying by ileal nutrients in humans, *Gastroenterology,* 1988, 94, 401–404.
94. Chapman, I.M., Goble, E.A., Wittert, G.A., and Horowitz, M., Effects of small-intestinal fat and carbohydrate infusions on appetite and food intake in obese and nonobese men, *Am. J. Clin. Nutr.,* 1999, 69, 6–12.
95. Lin, H.C., Zhao, X.T., Chu, A.W., Lin, Y.P., and Wang, L.J., Fiber-supplemented enteral formula slows intestinal transit by intensifying inhibitory feedback from the distal gut, *Am. J. Clin. Nutr.,* 1997, 65, 1840–1844.
96. Schirra, J. and Goke, B., The physiological role of GLP-1 in human: incretin, ileal brake or more? *Regul. Pept.,* 2005, 128, 109–115.
97. Sinclair, E.M. and Drucker, D.J., Proglucagon-derived peptides: mechanisms of action and therapeutic potential, *Physiology,* 2005, 20, 357–365.
98. Batterham, R.L., Cowley, M.A., Small, C.J., et al., Gut hormone PYY3–36 physiologically inhibits food intake, *Nature,* 2002, 418, 650–654.
99. Batterham, R.L., Cohen, M.A., Ellis, S.M., et al., Inhibition of food intake in obese subjects by peptide YY3-36, *N. Engl. J. Med.,* 2003, 349, 941–948.
100. Stanley, S., Wynne, K., and Bloom, S., Gastrointestinal satiety signals — III. Glucagon-like peptide 1, oxyntomodulin, peptide YY, and pancreatic polypeptide, *Am. J. Physiol. Gastrointest. Liver Physiol.,* 2004, 286, G693–G697.
101. Beglinger, C. and Degen, L., Fat in the intestine as a regulator of appetite — role of CCK, *Physiol. Behav.,* 2004, 83, 617–621.
102. Ballinger, A., McLoughlin, L., Medbak, S., and Clark, M., Cholecystokinin is a satiety hormone in humans at physiological post-prandial plasma concentrations, *Clin. Sci. (Lond.),* 1995, 89, 375–381.
103. Muurahainen, N., Kissileff, H.R., Derogatis, A.J., and Pisunyer, F.X., Effects of cholecystokinin-octapeptide (CCK-8) on food-intake and gastric-emptying in man, *Physiol. Behav.,* 1988, 44, 645–649.
104. Kissileff, H.R., Pisunyer, F.X., Thornton, J., and Smith, G.P., C-Terminal octapeptide of cholecystokinin decreases food-intake in man, *Am. J. Clin. Nutr.,* 1981, 34, 154–160.
105. Beglinger, C., Degen, L., Matzinger, D., D'Amato, M., and Drewe, J., Loxiglumide, a CCK-A receptor antagonist, stimulates calorie intake and hunger feelings in humans, *Am. J. Physiol.,* 2001, 280, R1149–R1154.
106. Kissileff, H.R., Carretta, J.C., Geliebter, A., and Pi-Sunyer, F., Cholecystokinin and stomach distension combine to reduce food intake in humans, *Am. J. Physiol.,* 2003, 285, R992–R998.
107. Lutz, T.A., Amylinergic control of food intake, *Physiol. Behav.,* 2006, 89, 465–471.
108. Hollander, P., Maggs, D.G., Ruggles, J.A., et al., Effect of pramlintide on weight in overweight and obese insulin-treated type 2 diabetes patients, *Obes. Res.,* 2004, 12, 661–668.
109. Chapman, I., Parker, B., Doran, S., et al., Effect of pramlintide on satiety and food intake in obese subjects and subjects with type 2 diabetes, *Diabetologia,* 2005, 48, 838–848.
110. Wen, J., Phillips, S.F., Sarr, M.G., Kost, L.J., and Holst, J.J., PYY and GLP-1 contribute to feedback inhibition from the canine ileum and colon, *Am. J. Physiol. Gastrointest. Liver Physiol.,* 1995, 32, G945–G952.
111. Giralt, M. and Vergara, P., Glucagonlike peptide-1 (GLP-1) participation in ileal brake induced by intraluminal peptones in rat, *Dig. Dis. Sci.,* 1999, 44, 322–329.
112. Naslund, E., Bogefors, J., Skogar, S., et al., GLP-1 slows solid gastric emptying and inhibits insulin, glucagon, and PYY release in humans, *Am. J. Physiol.,* 1999, 46, R910–R916.

113. Naslund, E., Gutniak, M., Skogar, S., Rossner, S., and Hellstrom, P.M., Glucagon-like peptide 1 increases the period of postprandial satiety and slows gastric emptying in obese men, *Am. J. Clin. Nutr.,* 1998, 68, 525–530.
114. Nauck M.A., Niedereichholz, U., Ettler, R., et al., Glucagon-like peptide 1 inhibition of gastric emptying outweighs its insulinotropic effects in healthy humans, *Am. J. Physiol.,* 1997, 36, E981–E988.
115. Meier, J.J. and Nauck, M.A., Glucagon-like peptide 1(GLP-1) in biology and pathology, *Diabetes Metab. Res. Rev.,* 2005, 21, 91–117.
116. Verdich, C., Flint, A., Gutzwiller, J.P., et al., A meta-analysis of the effect of glucagon-like peptide-1 (7–36) amide on ad libitum energy intake in humans, *J. Clin. Endocrinol. Metab.,* 2001, 86, 4382–4389.
117. Naslund, E., Barkeling, B., King, N., et al., Energy intake and appetite are suppressed by glucagon-like peptide-1 (GLP-1) in obese men, *Int. J. Obes. Relat. Metab. Disord.,* 1999, 23, 304–311.
118. Flint, A., Raben, A., Astrup, A., and Holst, J.J., Glucagon-like peptide 1 promotes satiety and suppresses energy intake in humans, *J. Clin. Invest.,* 1998, 101, 515–520.
119. Little, T.J., Doran, S., Meyer, J.H., et al., The release of GLP-1 and ghrelin, but not GIP and CCK, by glucose is dependent upon the length of small intestine exposed, *Am. J. Physiol. Endocrinol. Metab.,* 2006, 291, E647–E655.
120. McFadden, D.W., Rudnicki, M., Kuvshinoff, B., and Fischer, J.E., Postprandial peptide YY release is mediated by cholecystokinin, *Surg. Gynecol. Obstet.,* 1992, 175, 145–150.
121. Pironi, L., Stanghellini, V., Miglioli, M., et al., Fat-induced ileal brake in humans — a dose-dependent phenomenon correlated to the plasma-levels of peptide-YY, *Gastroenterology,* 1993, 105, 733–739.
122. Lin, H.C., Zhao, X.T., Wang, L.J., and Wong, H., Fat-induced ileal brake in the dog depends on peptide YY, *Gastroenterology,* 1996, 110, 1491–1495.
123. Savage, A.P., Adrian, T.E., Carolan, G., Chatterjee, V.K., and Bloom, S.R., Effects of peptide YY (PYY) on mouth to cecum intestinal transit-time and on the rate of gastric-emptying in healthy-volunteers, *Gut,* 1987, 28, 166–170.
124. Boggiano, M.M., Chandler, P.C., Oswald, K.D., et al., PYY3–36 as an anti-obesity drug target, *Obes. Rev.,* 2005, 6, 307–322.
125. Degen, L., Oesch, S., Casanova, M., et al., Effect of peptide YY3–36 on food intake in humans, *Gastroenterology,* 2005, 129, 1430–1436.
126. Cummings, D.E. and Overduin, J., Gastrointestinal regulation of food intake, *J. Clin. Invest.,* 2007, 117, 13–23.
127. Rodriguez, M.D., Kalogeris, T.J., Wang, X.L., Wolf, R., and Tso, P., Rapid synthesis and secretion of intestinal apolipoprotein A-IV after gastric fat loading in rats, *Am. J. Physiol.,* 1997, 41, R1170–R1177.
128. Okumura, T., Fukagawa, K., Tso, P., Taylor, I.L., and Pappas, T.N., Apolipoprotein A-IV acts in the brain to inhibit gastric emptying in the rat, *Am. J. Physiol. Gastrointest. Liver Physiol.,* 1996, 33, G49–G53.
129. Tso, P., Chen, Q., Fujimoto, K., Fukagawa, K., and Sakata, T., Apolipoprotein A-IV: a circulating satiety signal produced by the small intestine, *Obes. Res.,* 1995, 3, S689–S695.
130. Fujimoto, K., Cardelli, J.A., and Tso, P., Increased apolipoprotein-A-IV in rat mesenteric lymph after lipid meal acts as a physiological signal for satiation, *Am. J. Physiol.,* 1992, 262, G1002–G1006.
131. Sakata, Y., Fujimoto, K., Ogata, S.I., et al., Postabsorptive factors are important for satiation in rats after a lipid meal, *Am. J. Physiol. Gastrointest. Liver Physiol.,* 1996, 34, G438–G442.

132. Glatzle, J., Wang, Y.H., Adelson, D.W., et al., Chylomicron components activate duodenal vagal afferents via a cholecystokinin A receptor-mediated pathway to inhibit gastric motor function in the rat, *J. Physiol.,* 2003, 550, 657–664.
133. Glatzle, J., Kalogeris, T.J., Zittel, T.T., Guerrini, S., Tso, P., and Raybould, H.E., Chylomicron components mediate intestinal lipid-induced inhibition of gastric motor function, *Am. J. Physiol. Gastrointest. Liver Physiol.,* 2002, 282, G86–G91.
134. Cohen, M.A., Ellis, S.M., le Roux, C.W., et al., Oxyntomodulin suppresses appetite and reduces food intake in humans, *J. Clin. Endocrinol. Metab.,* 2003, 88, 4696–4701.
135. Piche, T., Zerbib, F., des Varannes, S.B., et al., Modulation by colonic fermentation of LES function in humans, *Am. J. Physiol. Gastrointest. Liver Physiol.,* 2000, 278, G578–G584.
136. Ropert, A., Cherbut, C., Roze, C., et al., Colonic fermentation and proximal gastric tone in humans, *Gastroenterology,* 1996, 111, 289–296.
137. Cani, P.D., Joly, E., Horsmans, Y., and Delzenne, N.M., Oligofructose promotes satiety in healthy human: a pilot study, *Eur. J. Clin. Nutr.,* 2006, 60, 567–572.
138. Gee, J.M. and Johnson, I.T., Dietary lactitol fermentation increases circulating peptide YY and glucagon-like peptide-1 in rats and humans, *Nutrition,* 2005, 21, 1036–1043.
139. Piche, T., Bruley, S., des Varannes, S.B., et al., Colonic fermentation influences lower esophageal sphincter function in gastroesophageal reflux disease, *Gastroenterology,* 2003, 124, 894–902.
140. Nugent, A.P., Health properties of resistant starch, *Nutr. Bull.,* 2005, 30, 27–54.
141. Delzenne, N.M., Cani, P.D., Daubioul, C., and Neyrinck, A.M., Impact of inulin and oligofructose on gastrointestinal peptides, *Br. J. Nutr.,* 2006, 93, S157–S161.
142. Delgado-Aros, S., Chial, H.J., Camilleri, M., et al., Effects of a kappa-opioid agonist, asimadoline, on satiation and GI motor and sensory functions in humans, *Am. J. Physiol. Gastrointest. Liver Physiol.,* 2003, 284, G558–G566.
143. Pimentel, M., Lin, H.C., Enayati, P., et al., Methane, a gas produced by enteric bacteria, slows intestinal transit and augments small intestinal contractile activity, *Am. J. Physiol. Gastrointest. Liver Physiol.,* 2006, 290, G1089–G1095.
144. Foltmann, B., Gastric proteinases — structure, function, evolution and mechanism of action, *Essays Biochem.,* 1981, 17, 52–84.
145. Neary, N.M., Small, C.J., Druce, M.R., et al., Peptide YY3–36 and glucagon-like peptide-1(7–36) inhibit food intake additively, *Endocrinology,* 2005, 146, 5120–5127.
146. Yoshimichi, G., Tamashiro, K., Lo, C.M., et al., Interaction of CCK and apolipoprotein A-IV in the regulation of food intake, *Obes. Res.,* 2005, 13, A113.
147. Gutzwiller, J.P., Degen, L., Matzinger, D., Prestin, S., and Beglinger, C., Interaction between GLP-1 and CCK-33 in inhibiting food intake and appetite in men, *Am. J. Physiol.,* 2004, 287, R562–R567.
148. Kalogeris, T.J., Qin, X.F., Chey, W.Y., and Tso, P., PYY stimulates synthesis and secretion of intestinal apolipoprotein AIV without affecting mRNA expression, *Am. J. Physiol. Gastrointest. Liver Physiol.,* 1998, 38, G668–G674.
149. French, S.J. and Cecil, J.E., Oral, gastric and intestinal influences on human feeding, *Physiol. Behav.,* 2001, 74, 729–734.
150. Oesch, S., Degen, L., and Beglinger, C., Effect of a protein preload on food intake and satiety feelings in response to duodenal fat perfusions in healthy male subjects, *Am. J. Physiol.,* 2005, 289, R1042–R1047.
151. Degen, L., Oesch, S., Matzinger, D., et al., Effects of a preload on reduction of food intake by GLP-1 in healthy subjects, *Digestion,* 2006, 74, 78–84.
152. Camilleri, M., Brown, M.L., and Malagelada, J.R., Impaired transit of chyme in chronic intestinal pseudoobstruction — correction by cisapride, *Gastroenterology,* 1986, 91, 619–626.

153. Dobson, C.L., Hinchcliffe, M., Davis, S.S., Chauhan, S., and Wilding, I.R., Is the pig a good animal model for studying the human ileal brake? *J. Pharm. Sci.*, 1998, 87, 565–568.
154. Cox, J.E., Kelm, G.R., Meller, S.T., Spraggins, D.S., and Randich, A., Truncal and hepatic vagotomy reduce suppression of feeding by jejunal lipid infusions, *Physiol. Behav.*, 2004, 81, 29–36.
155. Cox, J.E., Tyler, W.J., Randich, A., Kelm, G.R., and Meller, S.T., Celiac vagotomy reduces suppression of feeding by jejunal fatty acid infusions, *Neuroreport*, 2001, 12, 1093–1096.
156. Abbott, C.R., Monteiro, M., Small, C.J., et al., The inhibitory effects of peripheral administration of peptide YY3–36 and glucagon-like peptide-1 on food intake are attenuated by ablation of the vagal-brainstem-hypothalamic pathway, *Brain Res.*, 2005, 1044, 127–131.
157. Imeryuz, N., Yegen, B.C., Bozkurt, A., Coskun, T., VillanuevaPenacarrillo, M.L., and Ulusoy, N.B., Glucagon-like peptide-1 inhibits gastric emptying via vagal afferent-mediated central mechanisms, *Am. J. Physiol. Gastrointest. Liver Physiol.*, 1997, 36, G920–G927.
158. de Castro, J.M., Stomach filling may mediate the influence of dietary energy density on the food intake of free-living humans, *Physiol. Behav.*, 2005, 86, 32–45.
159. de Castro, J.M., Physiological, environmental, and subjective determinants of food-intake in humans — a meal pattern-analysis, *Physiol. Behav.*, 1988, 44, 651–659.
160. Welch, I., Saunders, K., and Read, N.W., Effect of ileal and intravenous infusions of fat emulsions on feeding and satiety in human volunteers, *Gastroenterology*, 1985, 89, 1293–1297.
161. Castiglione, K.E., Read, N.W., and French, S.J., Adaptation to high-fat diet accelerates emptying of fat but not carbohydrate test meals in humans, *Am. J. Physiol.*, 2002, 282, R366–R371.
162. Park, M.I., Camilleri, M., O'Connor, H., et al., Effect of supplementing different macronutrients on gastric sensory and motor functions and appetite in normal weight, overweight, or obese humans, *Gastroenterology*, 2006, 130, A606.
163. Boyd, K.A., O'Donovan, D.G., Doran, S., et al., High-fat diet effects on gut motility, hormone, and appetite responses to duodenal lipid in healthy men, *Am. J. Physiol. Gastrointest. Liver Physiol.*, 2003, 284, G188–G196.
164. French, S.J., Murray, B., Rumsey, R.D.E., Fadzlin, R., and Read, N.W., Adaptation to high-fat diets — effects on eating behavior and plasma cholecystokinin, *Br. J. Nutr.*, 1995, 73, 179–189.
165. Cox, J.E., Tyler, W.J., Randich, A. et al., Suppression of food intake, body weight, and body fat by jejunal fatty acid infusions, *Am. J. Physiol.*, 2000, 278, R604–R610.

11 Postabsorptive Endocrine Factors Controlling Food Intake and Regulation of Body Adiposity: Animal Research

Mihai Covasa

CONTENTS

11.1 INTRODUCTION

Following food ingestion, the alimentary organs secrete a complex array of substances that play a role in meal termination. These signals use neural, paracrine, or endocrine pathways to convey information in an integrated manner to hindbrain or hypothalamic structures that control food intake and energy balance. They also play important roles in digestion and absorption, including gastrointestinal secretion, motility, and blood flow, as well as whole-organism physiological function. These signals are generated from gut compartments such as the stomach and intestine and primarily influence aspects of short-term control of food intake; however, they either directly, or indirectly, also influence long-term energy balance. Other peripheral secretory organs such as the pancreas, liver, adrenal glands, the gonads, and adipose tissue also produce numerous substances that have profound effects on food intake and energy balance. The picture is complicated by the fact that several hormones that act peripherally can also act in the brain or be produced by the brain, with seemingly different functions. Therefore, teasing out their endocrine effects can prove challenging. This chapter deals primarily with endocrine signals traditionally known to affect food intake and body weight. The roles of gut-derived and neuronally derived signals involved in food intake are discussed in Chapters 9, 10, and 13, respectively, of this book, but because some gut signals exert their action through an endocrine route, they will also be briefly discussed here.

11.2 GASTRIC AND INTESTINAL SIGNALS

The presence of food in the gastrointestinal lumen evokes the release of various substances from specialized gastric and intestinal enteroendocrine cells. Several types of endocrine cells have been identified as "nutrient sensors" due to their nutrient-sensitive chemoreceptors. They synthesize and release peptides in response to specific classes of macronutrients, but also respond to other regulatory molecules and neurotransmitters produced by adjacent cells. These peptides enter the extracellular fluid and act on local cells through a paracrine mode of action or enter the circulation and access hindbrain structures lying outside the brain–blood barrier.[1]

11.2.1 Gastrin-Releasing Peptides (GRP)

The stomach releases several peptides known to influence food intake and gastrointestinal (GI) function. GRP suppresses food intake, stimulates gastric acid secretion and GI motility, but inhibits gastric emptying. Administration of bombesin (BBS), a nonmammalian tetradecapeptide amphibian homolog of GRP and neuromedin B (NMB), also suppresses food intake after either peripheral or central administration.[2] In the rat, GRP/BBS-like peptide levels in the gut and brain increase postprandially, supporting GRP's role as an inhibitor of food intake.[3–5] Most of the experimental evidence points to a neural mechanism of action, with both upper gastrointestinal and central (hindbrain) GRP receptors mediating the bombesin-induced suppression of feeding. However, endogenous bombesin-like peptides can also provide endocrine afferent input by activating peripheral neural pathways leading to peptide release into the brain which, in turn, contributes to meal termination.[6] Alternatively, and less well documented, is the possibility that bombesin-like peptides act directly on the brain through an endocrine mechanism. Consistent with this, GRP receptor–deficient mice consume larger meals than their controls and become obese.[7]

11.2.2 Ghrelin

Ghrelin, released mainly by the X/A-like cells in the fundus of the stomach, is an endogenous ligand for the growth hormone secretagogue receptor localized in the gastric mucosa, intestine, and other peripheral and central nervous tissues.[8] The only currently known orexigenic gut hormone, ghrelin stimulates food intake and increases body energy stores. Its release is influenced, among other things, by meal composition and caloric load.[9,10] Both intracerebroventricular and peripheral administration of ghrelin induce hyperphagia and weight gain in rodents.[10,11] Ghrelin levels rise before and fall after a meal; however, whether the rise in circulating ghrelin triggers meal initiation is not known.[12,13] Among macronutrients, carbohydrate is the most potent in suppressing ghrelin levels, followed by protein and lipid.[1] The weak effect of lipid has been linked to overeating on a high-fat diet.[14] If elevated ghrelin levels drive overconsumption and weight gain, it follows that reduced ghrelin concentrations should do the reverse: inhibit food intake and cause weight loss. Indeed, gastrectomized mice have 80% less ghrelin and lose weight compared with intact mice.[15] When ghrelin levels are restored to normal, weight gain ensues. Furthermore, acute administration of ghrelin receptor antagonists, anti-ghrelin antibodies, or antisense oligonucleotides results in a reduced food intake and weight loss,[16–18] suggesting a physiological role for endogenous ghrelin, but the mechanisms that inhibit ghrelin release after a meal are not known.

In addition to its role in control of short-term food intake, ghrelin contributes to long-term body weight regulation. For example, rats chronically treated with ghrelin exhibit sustained overeating and weight gain,[10] and ghrelin administration has been shown to contribute to weight gain by stimulating adipogenesis and inhibiting activity of the sympathetic nervous system.[10,19] However, ghrelin knockout mice have the same food intake and body weight as wild-type mice, and knockout and wild-type mice respond similarly to exogenous ghrelin.[20,21] On the other hand, adult, but not young, mice with ghrelin or ghrelin receptor deletions become obese on a high-fat diet.[22,23] Together, these results illustrate the subtle, but complex nature of the knockout models, the interaction of ghrelin with other genes that might influence food intake, and the possible role of ghrelin in development.

It also is interesting that, unlike lean individuals, ghrelin levels in fasted obese subjects are reduced, while weight loss increases ghrelin concentrations.[13,24] Furthermore, postprandial ghrelin is not reduced in obese individuals. This lack of a "suppression pedal" may contribute to overeating and weight gain. The accumulation of body fat and a corresponding increase in leptin results in a gradual decrease in ghrelin levels.[25] Conversely, ghrelin is increased after weight loss due to anorexia or cachexia,[26,27] but not after bariatric surgery when ghrelin levels are low.[28,29] Therefore, ghrelin may play a role in long-term regulation of body weight, but circulating levels may also be influenced by metabolic status.

11.2.3 Gastric Leptin

The long-held view of the stomach as the "volume detector" of ingesta has undergone significant transformation during the past several years. With the recent discovery of the synthesis and secretion of ghrelin and leptin by the stomach, it has become clear that, in addition to its role in mechanoreception, the stomach is a rich source of humoral signals that participate in control of food intake and energy balance.[30] Leptin, the product of the *ob* gene, originally discovered in mature white adipocytes, has been isolated from gastric mucosa.[31] Epithelial endocrine and exocrine gastric cells (pepsinogen secreting chief cells and endocrine P cells) secrete significant amounts of leptin.[30] There are two main pools (exocrine and endocrine) of gastric leptin, which potentially have distinct functions. The exact role of gastric leptin has not been fully elucidated, but exocrine, luminal, gastric leptin can act on intestinal brush border leptin receptors to regulate several intestinal functions.[32] In addition, leptin has been reported to stimulate cholecystokinin (CCK) release, and CCK has been reported to increase leptin secretion in the duodenum; therefore the two hormones exaggerate and potentiate each other's activity.[33]

There is substantial evidence that circulating leptin (adipose-derived) inhibits food intake and reduces body weight.[34] It is unknown whether significant amounts of gastric leptin reach the systemic circulation to influence food intake, but very recently, Peters et al.[35] produced strong circumstantial evidence supporting a paracrine mode of action for gastrointestinal leptin. They demonstrated that leptin infusion into the celiac artery suppresses food intake, whereas a jugular infusion, which produced higher systemic plasma levels, did not change food intake. The effect on food intake by celiac arterial infusions was prevented by subdiaphragmatic vagotomy, and low doses of leptin infused into either intraceliac artery or jugular vein had no effect on food intake. This led to the suggestion that, similar to CCK, low, local concentrations of gastric leptin can access vagal afferents and reduce meal size,[35] but the contribution of gastric leptin to the main circulating pool of leptin and its impact on food intake and energy balance remain to be investigated.

11.2.4 Cholecystokinin (CCK)

The role of CCK as a gut hormone and its influence on satiation is discussed in Chapters 9 and 10. Here, the possible role of endocrine CCK is briefly discussed as well as its involvement in GI functions to facilitate digestion and absorption and, in doing so, to control caloric intake. CCK is released by the enteroendocrine I-type cells of duodenal and jejunal mucosa in response to intraluminal nutrients, in particular, long-chain fatty acids and unhydrolyzed or partially hydrolyzed proteins. There is substantial evidence from physiological, pharmacological, and molecular studies to support the notion that CCK octapeptide acts locally in a paracrine fashion to influence intake.[36] Although CCK-8 is the most active biological form, it is not the predominant endocrine form of CCK. It has been recently shown that CCK-58 is the major endocrine form of CCK in the rat, with 40% more CCK-58 than CCK-8 recovered from rat blood.[37] The presence of CCK-58 as a predominant endocrine form of CCK in the rat explains its strong effects on physiological functions such as pancreatic secretion, gall bladder contraction, and central and peripheral nerve activation.

How much intestinal CCK-58 is stored in tissue and how much is degraded to smaller forms that could, in turn, influence digestive functions and intake remains to be determined. CCK concentration rises immediately after a meal, reaching peak levels at approximately 30 minutes and lasting 3 to 5 hours.[38] In addition to its effect on meal size, CCK can also exert a postabsorptive effect by interacting with long-term adiposity signals such as leptin and insulin as well as with gonadal hormones such as estrogen.[39–41]

Data from a variety of species clearly demonstrate that endogenous, meal-elicited CCK acts at CCK-1 receptor sites as a physiological satiety agent. CCK reduces meal size; that is, it contributes to satiation. CCK may be considered to control food intake solely in the interest of GI function by reducing the rate of passage of nutrients to facilitate efficient and complete digestion. For example, when we adapted animals to low- or high-fat isoenergetic diets and measured pancreatic enzyme secretion using *in vitro* preparation assays, chronic ingestion of a high-fat diet decreased amylase secretion, but increased absorptive capacity for fat and increased secretion of lipase for fat digestion.[42] Changes like these enable an animal to take best advantage of a variable source of calories and represent a very simple system of an adaptive response to dietary changes. On the other hand, the satiating effects of CCK also could reduce calorie consumption in the interest of control or regulation of other systems, such as energy homeostasis. Although experiments using selective CCK receptor agonists and antagonists have not produced compelling evidence that CCK directly contributes to the control of body fat, there are several reports in the literature indicating that at least some genetically obese rodents might have a reduced sensitivity to CCK and other satiation signals from the gastrointestinal tract. For example, several investigators have reported that Zucker fatty rats exhibit reduced satiation in response to exogenous CCK, compared to lean controls[43,44] and exhibit a reduced responsiveness by other systems that also are controlled by CCK.[45,46] Since the Zucker rat has a missence mutation of the leptin receptor gene, it seems probable that the impaired satiation response to CCK is a result of, rather than an inducer of, obesity. On the other hand, the dulling of satiation signals during obesity may interfere with mechanisms to limit food intake and weight gain and thereby contribute to the refractory nature of the condition. For example, the Otsuka Long Evans Tokushima Fatty rat, (OLETF), which lack CCK-1 receptors, overeat and become obese.[47] Not surprisingly, these rats do not reduce their food intake in response to exogenous CCK,[47,48] and they have deficits in the satiation response to intestinal infusion of some, but not all, nutrients.[48]

11.2.5 Peptide YY (PYY)

PYY is produced by intestinal endocrine L-cells in the presence of intraluminal nutrients, with higher concentrations being secreted by the terminal ileum and colon, and lower concentrations by the duodenum and jejunum.[49,50] It is also produced by endocrine cells of the stomach and pancreas and is present in CNS neurons.[51–53] PYY inhibits several GI functions such as gastric emptying and secretion, GI motility, gall bladder emptying, and pancreatic and intestinal secretion.[54–57] After a meal, two major forms of PYY are released into the circulation — PYY(1-36) and PYY(3-36)

— with PYY(3-36) being the most potent in suppressing food intake.[58] PYY(3-36) secretion is influenced by caloric load and the composition of the meal[59] with long-chain fatty acids being the most potent secretagogue, and glucose and peptone being less potent inducers of PYY(3-36) release.[60,61]

Initial studies of systemic PYY(3-36) influencing food intake and body weight in rodents produced inconsistent results.[62] Subsequent studies, however, have now confirmed that PPY(3-36) produces a sustained suppression of food intake and adiposity in rodents,[58,63,64] but it should also be noted that some investigators have shown that PYY(3-36) produces conditioned taste aversion, which may contribute to the drop in food intake.[65,66]

PYY is also thought to play a role in energy homeostasis. PYY knockout mice exhibit obesity which can be corrected by PYY replacement.[67] In addition, rats that are resistant to obesity (DR) when fed a high-fat diet have higher circulating PYY as well as increased PYY intestinal mRNA levels compared to rats that become obese (DIO) on a high-fat diet.[68] These results suggest that impaired release of PYY in DIO rats consuming a palatable diet may contribute to the development of obesity. However, a recent study showed that, although increased dietary fat may increase PYY release, there is no difference in PYY enteroendocrine cell number, tissue content, or fasted serum PYY levels between DIO and DR rats maintained on a medium high-fat diet.[69] These observations do not, however, exclude the possibility that postprandial PYY release might be different in DR and DIO rats, similar to the difference that has been reported for obese versus lean humans.[28] Recently, Chelikani et al.[70] reported that obese rats are more sensitive than lean rats to the anorexic effects of PYY(3-36). Intermittent intraperitoneal administration of PYY(3-36) reduced caloric intake, body weight, and adiposity in DIO rats. It is not known whether a similar drug delivery paradigm could suppress food intake and body weight in obese humans, but these findings, in conjunction with the fact that obese individuals retain sensitivity to the drug, make PYY a promising therapeutic tool.

11.2.6 Pancreatic Polypeptide (PP)

PP belongs to the family of peptides that includes neuropeptide Y (NPY) and PYY. It is produced mainly by the endocrine pancreas, although the exocrine pancreas, colon, and rectum also secrete PP.[71,72] It is released in response to a meal,[71] and like PYY(3-36), PP reduces food intake and body weight when administered peripherally.[73–75] The suppression of food intake occurs immediately after administration and continues for up to 24 hours.[76] The mechanisms by which PP affects food intake appear to be different from those of PYY(3-36).[77] PP seems to act at peripheral sites to suppress feeding by increasing gastric motility,[78] but others have reported a reduction in food intake independent of changes in gastric motility.[78] PP's effects on feeding are vagally mediated,[74] but it may also penetrate the incomplete blood–brain barrier to act in the brain.[79] Finally, it may interact with several other peptides involved in the control of food intake.

PP may also influence long-term energy balance. In animals, chronic administration of PYY in ob/ob mice reduce body weight[73] without the development of resistance. In humans, PP concentrations are diminished in obese Prader-Willi syndrome patients, and PP treatment suppresses food intake in these individuals.[80,81] A reduced postprandial PP response has also been reported in morbidly obese patients,[82] while anorexics have elevated rates of PP release.[83] In contrast, Kosha et al. reported that, although the change in PP concentrations following a meal was negatively associated with weight gain in Pima Indians, there was also a positive correlation between fasting PP levels and weight change.[84] Thus, the role of PP in suppressing food intake and weight gain in humans is not completely understood.

11.2.7 Glucagon-Like Peptide 1 (GLP-1)

GLP-1, a posttranslational product of the preproglucagon gene is secreted from intestinal endocrine L-cells, located mainly in the distal ileum and colonic mucosa, although GLP-1 producing cells are scattered along all segments of the small intestine,[85–87] pancreas, and brain.[88,89] Nutrients, particularly fats and carbohydrates, coming in contact with the apical surface or basolateral neural and vascular elements of the L-cells are potent triggers of GLP-1 release.[90] Other nutrients such as proteins, their hydrolysates, and fiber also release GLP-1.[91,92] After a meal, GLP-1 is secreted in a biphasic mode, with a short rapid rise in release (10 to 15 minutes) followed by a second longer release (30 to 60 minutes) that gradually declines within 3 hours.[91] This has resulted in the postulation that there are two different mechanisms of GLP-1 action: the early phase associated with a direct or indirect neural or endocrine signaling, and the second, longer phase associated with direct cell stimulation by the products of nutrient digestion.[93]

It is now well established that systemic or central administration of GLP-1 reduces food intake, gastric emptying, and body weight.[94–96] These actions are mediated by receptors (GLP-1R) present in pancreas, intestine, brain, and vagal afferents.[87,97–99] Studies using the GLP-1 antagonist exendin(9-39) have confirmed the role of endogenous GLP-1 in suppressing food intake, gastric emptying, and energy balance. For example, intravenous infusion of exendin(9-39) completely blocked the inhibitory effects of GLP-1 infusion on feeding and gastric emptying in rats.[100,101] Likewise, intracerebroventricular administration of the GLP-1 receptor antagonist increased food intake, body weight, and adiposity in rats.[96,102,103] In the rat, intravenous administration of a dose of GLP-1 that raises GLP concentration to a level similar to that observed after ingestion of food suppressed food intake and gastric emptying.[58,101] Whether a postprandial increase in plasma GLP-1 is sufficient to inhibit intake and gastric emptying remains to be tested directly. Initial studies suggested that GLP-1 inhibits food intake by reducing gastric emptying (increasing gastric distention);[101] however, it is now recognized that inhibition of food intake by GLP-1 can also occur independent of a change in gastric emptying.[58] The source, the site, and the exact mechanisms of GLP-1 actions are not fully elucidated. Both GLP-1 and its receptor antagonist can permeate the blood–brain barrier and access hypothalamic and hindbrain structures containing GLP-1 receptors known to control food intake.[104,105] However, due to rapid degradation in the systemic circulation (<2 minutes), the effect of peripheral GLP-1 in the brain is uncertain. In addition, several distinct brain neurons synthesize their own GLP-1,[106,107] and GLP-1 can act on vagal afferents to suppress intake and gastric emptying.[100] Thus, whether the satiating effects of peripheral GLP-1 are linked to the central anorectic effects of GLP-1 is still uncertain.

In contrast to its physiological importance in feeding, the role of GLP-1 in obesity is less clear. In obese humans, GLP-1 concentrations are decreased and are normalized by weight loss.[108] Treatment of obese humans with GLP-1 reduces calorie intake and body weight.[109] Therefore, although mice lacking GLP-1 receptors exhibit normal food intake and body weight,[110] GLP-1 remains a viable candidate for treatment of human obesity and type-2 diabetes.

11.3 PANCREATIC AND ADIPOSITY SIGNALS

11.3.1 INSULIN

Insulin is an anabolic hormone that has substantial effects on both carbohydrate and lipid metabolism and significant influences on protein and mineral metabolism. For example, insulin promotes synthesis of glycogen and fatty acids in the liver and inhibits the breakdown of fat in adipose tissue by inhibiting the intracellular lipase that hydrolyzes triglycerides to release fatty acids. It also facilitates entry of glucose into adipocytes, and within those cells, glucose can be used to synthesize triglyceride. By these mechanisms, insulin promotes accumulation of triglyceride in fat cells.[111–115] Circulating basal concentrations of insulin change inversely with insulin sensitivity of peripheral tissues. Total body fat, and visceral fat specifically, are key determinants of whole-body insulin sensitivity.[116] Insulin secretion increases rapidly after a meal,[117] whereas there is a delayed elevation of leptin levels following meal ingestion.[118]

Like leptin, basal insulin concentrations vary directly with changes in adiposity,[119] increasing during positive energy balance and decreasing during negative energy balance. There is a substantial amount of evidence supporting the role of insulin as a major peripheral signal involved in the control of food intake and energy stores.[120] Insulin penetrates the blood–brain barrier via a saturable, receptor-mediated process, at a rate that is proportional to circulating insulin concentrations.[121] While little or no insulin is produced in the brain itself,[121,122] centrally administered insulin acts as a potent anorexigenic signal, decreasing food intake and body weight. Similarly, intracerebroventricular administration of an insulin mimetic in rats dose-dependently reduces food intake and body weight and changes the expression of hypothalamic genes known to regulate food intake and body weight.[123] When administered orally to mice made obese on a high-fat diet, the mimetic also inhibits weight gain and adiposity and prevents development of insulin resistance.[123] Conversely, down-regulation of insulin receptor proteins in the medial arcuate nucleus of the hypothalamus (ARC), using an antisense RNA directed against the insulin receptor precursor protein, results in hyperphagia and increased fat mass.[124] Several experiments testing the effects of systemic insulin on food intake have been complicated by the fact that increasing circulating insulin causes hypoglycemia, which in itself potently stimulates food intake. Experiments in which glucose levels have been controlled in the face of elevated plasma insulin levels have indeed shown a reduction in food intake in both rodents and baboons.[125,126] Thus data from studies in which insulin has been applied peripherally or centrally are consistent with the insulin system acting as an endogenous controller of appetite.

11.3.2 Leptin

The existence of a peripheral factor(s) that would convey the availability of energy stores to the brain was hypothesized[127] and demonstrated through parabiosis experiments.[128] This was confirmed by the discovery of the hormone product of the *ob* gene leptin.[129] The name is derived from the Greek *leptos* meaning thin, as leptin was shown to inhibit feeding and reduce body weight and adipose deposits in lean[130] and leptin-deficient mice.[130,131] Subsequently, the receptors for leptin, the products of the *db* gene, were cloned and shown to be localized mainly in the hypothalamus,[132] with high levels of expression in the arcuate nucleus.[133] The leptin receptor (Ob-R) is a member of the cytokine I receptor family;[132] six splice variants have been described all sharing a common extracellular domain.[132] The long form of Ob-R has a 302-amino acid cytoplasmic domain, is thought to be the main signal transduction splice variant,[134] and is highly expressed in hypothalamic nuclei known to regulate food intake and energy homeostasis.[135]

Leptin is a 16-kDa protein hormone produced and released primarily by white adipose tissue,[129] but it is also found in the pituitary,[136] hypothalamus,[137] placenta,[138] and stomach.[30] It is well established that leptin serves as an endocrine signal involved in the control of energy and body weight homeostasis by relaying information primarily to the hypothalamus on the availability of fat stores.[139] Both peripheral and central administration of leptin decrease food intake and reduce body weight in rodents,[130] supporting its role as a feedback signal in regulation of energy balance, but others have suggested that a decrease in leptin serves as a signal of reduced energy stores and that its primary role is to mediate adaptive responses to fasting.[140]

Despite the experimental evidence supporting a role for leptin in the regulation of energy balance, circulating leptin levels are significantly higher in obese than lean individuals.[141] Thus, in a majority of individuals obesity is associated with leptin resistance, and leptin administration has little beneficial effect on weight management, with the exception of few patients with mutations in the *ob* gene.[142] Central leptin resistance is probably caused by saturated or defective transport of leptin through the blood–brain barrier[143] in conjunction with decreased responsiveness of neuronal targets of leptin in diet-induced obesity.[144] Decreased hypothalamic responsiveness to leptin leads to hyperphagia, which perpetuates positive energy intake.[145] In the periphery, hyperleptinemia leads to gradual leptin resistance, resulting in a decrease in glucose uptake and glycogen synthesis, and an increase in intracellular lipid deposits, causing insulin resistance.[146,147]

Although circulating concentrations of leptin are largely determined by the size of body fat stores, leptin secretion is also stimulated by several postabsorptive factors. Diurnal leptin secretion rhythms are linked to meal timing in human subjects,[118] and circulating leptin concentrations rise after a meal in rats,[148] possibly in response to the postprandial peak in insulin secretion[149] or the postabsorptive rise in energy substrates, because *in vitro* studies have demonstrated that glucose and amino acids stimulate leptin secretion from adipocytes.[32] In addition to the response to individual meals, there is a rapid drop in leptin expression in food-deprived humans and rodents, and the decrease is proportionally larger than the change in body fat mass, suggesting an association between energy status and leptin production.[150,151] Interestingly, there have been several demonstrations of a synergistic relation between CCK and leptin, such that leptin exaggerates the satiety effects of CCK,[39,41,152] providing an opportunity for signals of long-term energy balance to influence short-term control of food intake.

11.4 CHANGES IN THE ENDOCRINE MILIEU: IMPAIRED SATIATION AND BODY WEIGHT REGULATION

Most factors described in this chapter share the following characteristics: they are secreted by peripheral tissues and organs; they reduce food intake when administered exogenously; they are secreted in response to nutrients; and they interact with nutrients to reduce intake. For these peptides, the signal that ultimately causes satiety may be generated in the peripheral nervous system and relayed to the brain where it is integrated with other information to determine meal size. In many cases, defects in release, or functionality, of the peptides change short-term food intake, increasing food intake and ultimately obesity. Over the past two decades the proposition that deficits in response to satiation peptides may lead to hyperphagia and obesity has become an important focus of investigation. There is now mounting evidence for synergistic interactions between some of these peptides to control feeding behavior. These interactions provide an opportunity to integrate input from short-term, meal-related signals into the long-term control of energy balance.

11.4.1 Dietary Manipulations and the Endocrine Milieu

Digestive function adapts to the composition of the diet that is consumed, with a majority of evidence coming from studies testing the effects of chronic consumption of dietary fat. Physiological, cellular, and molecular aspects of the adaptation of intestinal transport have been described.[153] For example, adaptation leads to more efficient absorption of dietary fat,[153] increased production of hydrolytic enzymes and transporters, and increased lipid absorption.[154–156] Physical adaptations of the small intestine to dietary fat include hypertrophy, shortening and thickening of microvilli, an increase in the number of enterocytes per villus, and an increase in mucosal protein content.[155,157] There is also an increased release of CCK and pancreatic exocrine secretions in response to intraduodenal fat in rats adapted to a high-fat diet compared to rats fed a low-fat diet.[156] Collectively, these adaptive alimentary changes to chronic fat consumption may promote a more efficient utilization of energy from the diet and may also lead to the storage of energy in the form of adipose tissue.

Experimental evidence indicates that responses to gastrointestinal satiation signals change considerably in response to the dietary and endocrine milieu. Rats adapted to a high-fat diet become less sensitive to both exogenous[158,159] and endogenous CCK[48,160,161] and exhibit short-term hyperphagia compared to rats maintained on low-fat isoenergetic diet.[159] These results are consistent with human subjects adapted to a high-fat diet reporting greater hunger during a duodenal lipid infusion than subjects receiving the same infusion but adapted to a low-fat diet.[162] There was also a significant increase in the average daily food consumption and an increase in body weights of the subjects adapted to the high-fat diet. Postprandial CCK levels are higher in humans and animals fed a high-fat diet, but increased production of gut peptides in response to dietary manipulations and their effects on food intake and energy balance are not limited to CCK. For example, GLP-1 is decreased in both the ileum and colon of mice maintained on a high-fat diet compared to those on low-fat diet.[163]

In some conditions an increase in food intake may be secondary to receptor overstimulation and down-regulation, but this assumption has never been put to the test. It is known that gut-derived peptides, such as CCK and GLP-1, act through G-protein–coupled receptors, and sustained agonism of G-protein–coupled receptors can induce receptor down-regulation and tolerance.[164,165] This could explain the more robust and consistent effects of some peptides on food intake and weight loss with an intermittent pattern of delivery. For example, continuous infusion of PYY(3-36) produces a transient decrease in food intake,[62,166,167] while intermittent infusion of PYY(3-36) produces a sustained reduction in daily food intake.[70] These observations provide an example of the ability of the digestive system to respond to constant challenges. However, this ability to adapt in order to efficiently meet its primordial functions (digestion and absorption) may also facilitate excess caloric intake and weight gain. On the other hand, there are opportunities for developing new therapeutic strategies by manipulating the delivery pattern of satiety factors. As noted above, intermittent drug administration has been shown to produce a prolonged reduction in food intake and adiposity in the rat model, but it remains to be determined whether intermittent infusion of anorexigenic substances (either alone or in combination) can be used successfully in obese individuals.

11.4.2 Weight Manipulations and the Endocrine Milieu

Increases as well as decreases in body weight are associated with gastrointestinal endocrine adaptive changes. With the rapid increase in the number of morbidly obese patients in the absence of an effective behavioral treatment for obesity, bariatric surgery has become one of the most popular procedures used to induce weight loss. The finding that, following surgery, patients experience substantial (30 to 60%) and sustained weight loss (for up to 5 years)[168] in the absence of a compensatory increase in appetite[169] has generated a lot of interest in determining possible factors responsible for weight loss. Bariatric surgery imposes a restriction on the volume of food that can be ingested and leads to malabsorption of nutrients, but numerous studies have also documented changes in gastrointestinal endocrine function.[28] Ghrelin has been intensely studied because bariatric surgery causes a dramatic drop in ghrelin concentrations,[170] which contrasts with the increase in ghrelin that is observed following nonsurgical weight loss.[13] The decrease in ghrelin concentration was thought to contribute to the suppression of food intake and weight loss following bariatric surgery; however, it has since been demonstrated that nutrient delivery to the jejunum effectively stimulates ghrelin secretion, which questions the notion that gastric restriction is responsible for reduced ghrelin levels.[14,171] After bariatric surgery there also is a significant increase in the concentration of several other intestinal hormones, most notably those derived from intestinal proglucagon such as PYY(3-36) and GLP-1.[28,172]

For example, rats undergoing gastric bypass surgery lost 33% of their body weight, while PYY levels almost tripled (273%) compared with controls.[29] This was presumably due to the increased delivery of nutrients stimulating distal PYY-secreting cells. The elevated levels of PYY would inhibit gastric transit, motility, and emptying and facilitate hypophagia and weight loss. Elevated levels of PYY(3-36) and GLP-1 have also been found in the rat ileal transposition model, which is not associated with malabsorption,[169] suggesting that the peptides could also be responsible for hypophagia and postsurgical weight loss in this mode.[173,174] The most intriguing finding following bariatric surgery is the immediate dramatic improvement of glucose tolerance that precedes substantial weight loss.[175] This has been attributed to increased secretion of incretins such as CCK and GLP-1.[176,177] Other hormones secreted by the stomach and upper intestine in response to nutrient delivery may also influence food intake, weight loss, and insulin sensitivity.

11.5 CONCLUSIONS AND FUTURE DIRECTIONS FOR RESEARCH

The systems that control food intake and energy balance are both elegant and complex. No one single hormone can be identified as the sole influence on intake. It has become increasingly obvious that effective therapy for weight loss can only be achieved by targeting more than one hormone or pathway. Therefore, studying the interactions between different signals acting at various sites is essential. Neuroanatomical, immunhistochemical, and molecular studies in animal or *in vitro* models have provided a host of evidence demonstrating cellular colocalization and corelease of various hormones in response to a meal or nutrient. For example, GLP-1 and PYY(3-36) are cosecreted in the L-cells in response to a meal, and simultaneous administration of exendin-4 and PYY(3-36) produces an additive inhibitory effect on food intake,[64] indicating a high degree of interaction between these hormones. Numerous other hormones also interact at different levels of the gut–brain neuroaxis. For example, CCK interacts with gut hormones, such as GLP-1, 5-HT, and with long-term adiposity signals, such as leptin and insulin, to enhance suppression of food intake. Similarly, ghrelin interacts with leptin and insulin, and it has been suggested that ghrelin may stimulate food intake, in part, by attenuating the inhibitory effects of GLP-1 and PYY(3-36). Therefore, a systematic examination of interactions of low doses of two or more peptides will be useful in determining the most effective combination for inhibiting food intake. Since high doses of some inhibitory hormones are aversive, the combination of low doses of multiple drugs could also prove useful from this perspective. In the opposite situation, concomitant removal of multiple peptides in animal models could help to identify their impact on feeding. Due to the complexity of the system, it is clear that a significant amount of work is needed to establish the physiological role and mechanism of action of these hormones in determining meal initiation and termination and body-weight regulation.

11.5.1 Animal Models and Translational Research

There is no doubt that the use of animal models combined with recent molecular progress has propelled the field of ingestive behavior to new levels of sophistication.

Recently, the rate of identification of new molecules that could potentially be involved in controlling food intake has outpaced research characterizing their physiological role. Despite this scientific progress the epidemic of obesity still exists. Most studies have examined metabolic changes in animals in which obesity is preexisting and of genetic origin, but dietary-induced obesity models offer the possibility of evaluating changes in animals during the progression of weight gain caused by overeating. This type of study would identify the most appropriate timing and therapy for prevention of obesity and would aid development of long-term intervention studies in humans that combine dietary intervention with measures of the physiologic indicators discussed in this chapter.

Gene knockout animals have proven valuable in identifying the importance of specific gene products in controlling food intake and body weight. On the other hand, interpretation of data from these studies has been complicated by the fact that disruption of one particular gene may affect not only the synthesis of its product, but also of other protein products involved in food intake (for example, ghrelin knockout mice have impaired obestatin secretion, and PYY knockout mice also lack the PP gene). In addition, significant phenotypical and behavioral differences can exist between knockout and spontaneous mutations of a similar gene. For example, the natural mutant CCK-1 receptor deficient rat becomes obese and diabetic, while the CCK knockout mouse is lean and normoglycemic.[178] Thus, teasing out the differences between natural and engineered animal models, although a daunting process, is of critical importance.

Finally, animal and *in vitro* models could be used to design more effective drugs (delay degradation and improve half-life) that mimic the endogenous release of the hormone. This is important, since most hormones degrade rapidly in the circulation.

11.5.2 Hormonal Endocrine Changes in Obesity: Cause or Effect

It is clear that the obese state is associated with changes in hormone release induced by food intake, but it remains uncertain how obesity influences hormone concentrations or changes in sensitivity to the hormones that might exacerbate the obese condition. It has been suggested that obese individuals have a reduced sensitivity to satiation mechanisms, but a systematic investigation has not been completed. Although there has been considerable progress in understanding how gastrointestinal and other humoral feedback signals participate in satiation, very little attention has been paid to the possibility that an alteration in the response to the gastrointestinal signals may result in disordered phagia and body weight gain. Likewise, relatively little attention has been paid to the consequences of obesity, which could contribute to maintenance or exacerbation of the obese state. Finally, bariatric surgery has provided an opportunity to understand changes in gastrointestinal peptides that result from weight loss. Development of animal models for bariatric surgery that would permit investigation of the long-term consequences of the surgery should also be high on the agenda.

11.5.3 An Integrated Approach

The average Western diet provides 49% of energy intake from carbohydrate, 35% from fat, and 16% from protein.[179] Gut hormones are released in response to specific nutrients; hence they could mediate the differential satiation produced by protein, fat, and carbohydrate. Studies examining hormone profiles in response to a mixed meal reflective of a typical human diet could play an important role not only in understanding the regulation of digestive processes, but also in identifying adaptive responses to a range of luminal cues and dietary components.

Another aspect of gut-, pancreas-, and adiposity-derived hormones that is not well defined is their impact on food intake during development. A limited number of animal studies have shown that several of these hormones play a role in the development of metabolic pathways and compensatory signals that allow for the maintenance of normal body weight and sensitivity to ingested nutrients.[180] Since most of these studies would be difficult to conduct with human subjects at different developmental stages, it will be important to develop models that can translate animal data to humans. Similarly, obesity is associated with the development of peripheral tissue resistance or altered responsiveness to various peptides, justifying the need for studies that establish an efficacious drug delivery protocol and others that investigate the role of these peptides in the development, or maintenance, of the obese-prone or obese-resistant phenotype. Thus, an integrated approach using both human and animal models will add significantly to our knowledge on the control of food intake and regulation of body weight.

REFERENCES

1. Cummings, D.E., Foster-Schubert, K.E., and Overduin, J., Ghrelin and energy balance: focus on current controversies, *Curr. Drug Targets,* 6, 153–169, 2005.
2. Gibbs, J., Kulkosky, P.J., and Smith, G.P., Effects of peripheral and central bombesin on feeding behavior of rats, *Peptides,* 2 (Suppl. 2), 179–183, 1981.
3. Kateb, C.C. and Merali, Z., A single meal elicits regional changes in bombesin-like peptide levels in the gut and brain, *Brain Res.,* 596, 10–16, 1992.
4. Jensen, J. and Holmgren, S., The gastrointestinal canal, in *Comparative Physiology and Evolution of the Autonomic Nervous System,* Nilsson, S. and Holmgren, S., Eds., Harwood Academic Publishers, Switzerland, 1994, pp. 119–167.
5. Jensen, J.A., Carroll, R.E., and Benya, R.V., The case for gastrin-releasing peptide acting as a morphogen when it and its receptor are aberrantly expressed in cancer, *Peptides,* 22, 689–699, 2001.
6. Ladenheim, E.E. et al., Hindbrain GRP receptor blockade antagonizes feeding suppression by peripherally administered GRP, *Am. J. Physiol.,* 271, R180–R184, 1996.
7. Ladenheim, E.E. et al., Disruptions in feeding and body weight control in gastrin-releasing peptide receptor deficient mice, *J. Endocrinol.,* 174, 273–281, 2002.
8. Huda, M.S., Wilding, J.P., and Pinkney, J.H., Gut peptides and the regulation of appetite, *Obes. Rev.,* 7, 163–182, 2006.
9. Sakata, I. et al., Postnatal changes in ghrelin mRNA expression and in ghrelin-producing cells in the rat stomach, *J. Endocrinol.,* 174, 463–471, 2002.
10. Tschop, M., Smiley, D.L., and Heiman, M.L., Ghrelin induces adiposity in rodents, *Nature,* 407, 908–913, 2000.
11. Wren, A.M. et al., Ghrelin enhances appetite and increases food intake in humans, *J. Clin. Endocrinol. Metab.,* 86, 5992, 2001.
12. Callahan, H.S. et al., Postprandial suppression of plasma ghrelin level is proportional to ingested caloric load but does not predict intermeal interval in humans, *J. Clin. Endocrinol. Metab.,* 89, 1319–1324, 2004.

13. Tschop, M. et al., Circulating ghrelin levels are decreased in human obesity, *Diabetes,* 50, 707–709, 2001.
14. Overduin, J. et al., Role of the duodenum and macronutrient type in ghrelin regulation, *Endocrinology,* 146, 840–850, 2005.
15. Dornonville de la Cour, C. et al., Ghrelin treatment reverses the reduction in weight gain and body fat in gastrectomised mice, *Gut,* 54, 907–913, 2005.
16. Nakazato, M. et al., A role for ghrelin in the central regulation of feeding, *Nature,* 409, 194–198, 2001.
17. Asakawa, A. et al., Antagonism of ghrelin receptor reduces food intake and body weight gain in mice, *Gut,* 52, 947–952, 2003.
18. Bagnasco, M. et al., Endogenous ghrelin is an orexigenic peptide acting in the arcuate nucleus in response to fasting, *Regul. Pept.,* 111, 161–167, 2003.
19. Matsumura, K. et al., Central ghrelin modulates sympathetic activity in conscious rabbits, *Hypertension,* 40, 694–699, 2002.
20. Sun, Y., Ahmed, S., and Smith, R.G., Deletion of ghrelin impairs neither growth nor appetite, *Mol. Cell. Biol.,* 23, 7973–7983, 2003.
21. Wortley, K.E. et al., Genetic deletion of ghrelin does not decrease food intake but influences metabolic fuel preference, *Proc. Natl. Acad. Sci. USA,* 101, 8227–8232, 2004.
22. Wortley, K.E. et al., Absence of ghrelin protects against early-onset obesity, *J. Clin. Invest.,* 115, 3573–3578, 2005.
23. Zigman, J.M. et al., Mice lacking ghrelin receptors resist the development of diet-induced obesity, *J. Clin. Invest.,* 115, 3564–3572, 2005.
24. Shiiya, T. et al., Plasma ghrelin levels in lean and obese humans and the effect of glucose on ghrelin secretion, *J. Clin. Endocrinol. Metab.,* 87, 240–244, 2002.
25. Rosicka, M. et al., Serum ghrelin levels in obese patients: the relationship to serum leptin levels and soluble leptin receptors levels, *Physiol. Res.,* 52, 61–66, 2003.
26. Otto, B. et al., Weight gain decreases elevated plasma ghrelin concentrations of patients with anorexia nervosa, *Eur. J. Endocrinol.,* 145, 669–673, 2001.
27. Nagaya, N. et al., Elevated circulating level of ghrelin in cachexia associated with chronic heart failure: relationships between ghrelin and anabolic/catabolic factors, *Circulation,* 104, 2034–2038, 2001.
28. le Roux, C.W. et al., Attenuated peptide YY release in obese subjects is associated with reduced satiety, *Endocrinology,* 147, 3–8, 2006.
29. Suzuki, S. et al., Changes in GI hormones and their effect on gastric emptying and transit times after Roux-en-Y gastric bypass in rat model, *Surgery,* 138, 283–290, 2005.
30. Bado, A. et al., The stomach is a source of leptin, *Nature,* 394, 790–793, 1998.
31. Berthoud, H.R., A new role for leptin as a direct satiety signal from the stomach, *Am. J. Physiol. Regul. Integr. Comp. Physiol.,* 288, R796–R797, 2005.
32. Cammisotto, P.G. et al., Regulation of leptin secretion from white adipocytes by insulin, glycolytic substrates, and amino acids, *Am. J. Physiol. Endocrinol. Metab.,* 289, E166–E171, 2005.
33. Guilmeau, S., Buyse, M., and Bado, A., Gastric leptin: a new manager of gastrointestinal function, *Curr. Opin. Pharmacol.,* 4, 561–566, 2004.
34. Coll, A.P., Farooqi, I.S., and O'Rahilly, S., The hormonal control of food intake, *Cell,* 129, 251–262, 2007.
35. Peters, J.H., Simasko, S.M., and Ritter, R.C., Modulation of vagal afferent excitation and reduction of food intake by leptin and cholecystokinin, *Physiol. Behav.,* 89, 477–485, 2006.
36. Ritter, R.C., Increased food intake and CCK receptor antagonists: beyond abdominal vagal afferents, *Am. J. Physiol. Regul. Integr. Comp. Physiol.,* 286, R991–R993, 2004.

37. Reeve, J.R., Jr., et al., CCK-58 is the only detectable endocrine form of cholecystokinin in rat, *Am. J. Physiol. Gastrointest. Liver Physiol.,* 285, G255–G265, 2003.
38. Liddle, R.A. et al., Cholecystokinin bioactivity in human plasma, Molecular forms, responses to feeding, and relationship to gallbladder contraction, *J. Clin. Invest.,* 75, 1144–1152, 1985.
39. Matson, C.A. et al., Cholecystokinin and leptin act synergistically to reduce body weight, *Am. J. Physiol. Regul. Integr. Comp. Physiol.,* 278, R882–R890, 2000.
40. Matson, C.A., Reid, D.F., and Ritter, R.C., Daily CCK injection enhances reduction of body weight by chronic intracerebroventricular leptin infusion, *Am. J. Physiol. Regul. Integr. Comp. Physiol.,* 282, R1368–R1373, 2002.
41. Emond, M. et al., Central leptin modulates behavioral and neural responsivity to CCK, *Am. J. Physiol.,* 276, R1545–R1549, 1999.
42. Brenner, L. et al., Dietary adaptation increases digestive capacity and decreases satiety responses to macronutrients, *Society for Neuroscience Abstract Viewer, Itinerary Planner,* 1997.
43. Niederau, C. et al., CCK-resistance in Zucker obese versus lean rats, *Regul. Pept.,* 70, 97–104, 1997.
44. McLaughlin, C.L. and Baile, C.A., Decreased sensitivity of Zucker obese rats to the putative satiety agent cholecystokinin, *Physiol. Behav.,* 25, 543–548, 1980.
45. McLaughlin, C.L., Peikin, S.R., and Baile, C.A., Decreased pancreatic exocrine response to cholecystokinin in Zucker obese rats, *Am. J. Physiol.,* 242, G612–G619, 1982.
46. Maggio, C.A., Greenwood, M.R., and Vasselli, J.R., The satiety effects of intragastric macronutrient infusions in fatty and lean Zucker rats, *Physiol. Behav.,* 31, 367–372, 1983.
47. Moran, T.H. et al., Disordered food intake and obesity in rats lacking cholecystokinin A receptors, *Am. J. Physiol.,* 274, R618–R625, 1998.
48. Covasa, M. and Ritter, R.C., Attenuated satiation response to intestinal nutrients in rats that do not express CCK-A receptors, *Peptides,* 22, 1339–1348, 2001.
49. Ekblad, E. and Sundler, F., Distribution of pancreatic polypeptide and peptide YY, *Peptides,* 23, 251–261, 2002.
50. Bottcher, G. et al., Peptide YY: a neuropeptide in the gut. Immunocytochemical and immunochemical evidence, *Neuroscience,* 55, 281–290, 1993.
51. Bottcher, G. et al., Peptide YY in the mammalian pancreas: immunocytochemical localization and immunochemical characterization, *Regul. Pept.,* 43, 115–130, 1993.
52. Miyachi, Y. et al., The distribution of polypeptide YY-like immunoreactivity in rat tissues, *Endocrinology,* 118, 2163–2167, 1986.
53. Ekman, R. et al., Peptide YY-like immunoreactivity in the central nervous system of the rat, *Regul. Pept.,* 16, 157–168, 1986.
54. Adrian, T.E. et al., Effect of peptide YY on gastric, pancreatic, and biliary function in humans, *Gastroenterology,* 89, 494–499, 1985.
55. Tatemoto, K., Isolation and characterization of peptide YY (PYY), a candidate gut hormone that inhibits pancreatic exocrine secretion, *Proc. Natl. Acad. Sci. USA,* 79, 2514–2518, 1982.
56. Hoentjen, F., Hopman, W.P., and Jansen, J.B., Effect of circulating peptide YY on gallbladder emptying in humans, *Scand. J. Gastroenterol.,* 36, 1086–1091, 2001.
57. Korner, J. et al., Effects of Roux-en-Y gastric bypass surgery on fasting and postprandial concentrations of plasma ghrelin, peptide YY, and insulin, *J. Clin. Endocrinol. Metab.,* 90, 359–365, 2005.
58. Chelikani, P.K., Haver, A.C., and Reidelberger, R.D., Intravenous infusion of peptide YY(3-36) potently inhibits food intake in rats, *Endocrinology,* 146, 879–888, 2005.

59. Adrian, T.E. et al., Human distribution and release of a putative new gut hormone, peptide YY, *Gastroenterology,* 89, 1070–1077, 1985.
60. Taylor, I.L., Distribution and release of peptide YY in dog measured by specific radioimmunoassay, *Gastroenterology,* 88, 731–737, 1985.
61. McFadden, D.W. et al., Postprandial peptide YY release is mediated by cholecystokinin, *Surg. Gynecol. Obstet.,* 175, 145–150, 1992.
62. Tschop, M. et al., Physiology: does gut hormone PYY3-36 decrease food intake in rodents? *Nature,* 430, 162–165, 2004.
63. Cox, J.E. and Randich, A., Enhancement of feeding suppression by PYY(3-36) in rats with area postrema ablations, *Peptides,* 25, 985–989, 2004.
64. Talsania, T. et al., Peripheral exendin-4 and peptide YY(3-36) synergistically reduce food intake through different mechanisms in mice, *Endocrinology,* 146, 3748–3756, 2005.
65. Chelikani, P.K., Haver, A.C., and Reidelberger, R.D., Dose-dependent effects of peptide YY(3-36) on conditioned taste aversion in rats, *Peptides,* 27, 3193–3201, 2006.
66. Halatchev, I.G. and Cone, R.D., Peripheral administration of PYY(3-36) produces conditioned taste aversion in mice, *Cell Metab.,* 1, 159–168, 2005.
67. Batterham, R.L. et al., Critical role for peptide YY in protein-mediated satiation and body-weight regulation, *Cell Metab.,* 4, 223–233, 2006.
68. Yang, N. et al., Interaction of dietary composition and PYY gene expression in diet-induced obesity in rats, *J. Huazhong Univ. Sci. Technolog. Med. Sci.,* 25, 243–246, 2005.
69. Hyland, N.P., Pittman, Q.J., and Sharkey, K.A., Peptide YY containing enteroendocrine cells and peripheral tissue sensitivity to PYY and PYY(3-36) are maintained in diet-induced obese and diet-resistant rats, *Peptides,* 28, 1185–1190, 2007.
70. Chelikani, P.K., Haver, A.C., and Reidelberger, R.D., Intermittent intraperitoneal infusion of peptide YY(3-36) reduces daily food intake and adiposity in obese rats, *Am. J. Physiol. Regul. Integr. Comp. Physiol.,* 293, R39–R46, 2007.
71. Adrian, T.E. et al., Distribution and release of human pancreatic polypeptide, *Gut,* 17, 940–944, 1976.
72. Larsson, L.I., Sundler, F., and Hakanson, R., Immunohistochemical localization of human pancreatic polypeptide (HPP) to a population of islet cells, *Cell Tissue Res.,* 156, 167–171, 1975.
73. Asakawa, A. et al., Mouse pancreatic polypeptide modulates food intake, while not influencing anxiety in mice, *Peptides,* 20, 1445–1448, 1999.
74. Asakawa, A. et al., Characterization of the effects of pancreatic polypeptide in the regulation of energy balance, *Gastroenterology,* 124, 1325–1336, 2003.
75. Malaisse-Lagae, F. et al., Pancreatic polypeptide: a possible role in the regulation of food intake in the mouse. Hypothesis, *Experientia,* 33, 915–917, 1977.
76. Hazelwood, R.L., The pancreatic polypeptide (PP-fold) family: gastrointestinal, vascular, and feeding behavioral implications, *Proc. Soc. Exp. Biol. Med.,* 202, 44–63, 1993.
77. Moran, T.H., Pancreatic polypeptide: more than just another gut hormone? *Gastroenterology,* 124, 1542–1544, 2003.
78. Katsuura, G., Asakawa, A., and Inui, A., Roles of pancreatic polypeptide in regulation of food intake, *Peptides,* 23, 323–329, 2002.
79. Whitcomb, D.C., Taylor, I.L., and Vigna, S.R., Characterization of saturable binding sites for circulating pancreatic polypeptide in rat brain, *Am. J. Physiol.,* 259, G687–G691, 1990.
80. Zipf, W.B. et al., Blunted pancreatic polypeptide responses in children with obesity of Prader-Willi syndrome, *J. Clin. Endocrinol. Metab.,* 52, 1264–1266, 1981.

81. Berntson, G.G. et al., Pancreatic polypeptide infusions reduce food intake in Prader-Willi syndrome, *Peptides,* 14, 497–503, 1993.
82. Lieverse, R.J. et al., Significant satiety effect of bombesin in lean but not in obese subjects, *Int. J. Obes. Relat. Metab. Disord.,* 18, 579–583, 1994.
83. Uhe, A.M. et al., Potential regulators of feeding behavior in anorexia nervosa, *Am. J. Clin. Nutr.,* 55, 28–32, 1992.
84. Koska, J. et al., Pancreatic polypeptide is involved in the regulation of body weight in pima Indian male subjects, *Diabetes,* 53, 3091–3096, 2004.
85. Mortensen, K. et al., GLP-1 and GIP are colocalized in a subset of endocrine cells in the small intestine, *Regul. Pept.,* 114, 186–196, 2003.
86. Theodorakis, M.J. et al., Human duodenal enteroendocrine cells: source of both incretin peptides, GLP-1 and GIP, *Am. J. Physiol. Endocrinol. Metab.,* 290, E550–E559, 2006.
87. Eissele, R. et al., Glucagon-like peptide 1 immunoreactivity in gastroentero-pancreatic endocrine tumors: a light- and electron-microscopic study, *Cell Tissue Res.,* 276, 571–579, 1994.
88. Larsen, P.J. et al., Distribution of glucagon-like peptide-1 and other preproglucagon-derived peptides in the rat hypothalamus and brainstem, *Neuroscience,* 77, 257–270, 1997.
89. Merchenthaler, I., Lane, M., and Shughrue, P., Distribution of pre-pro-glucagon and glucagon-like peptide-1 receptor messenger RNAs in the rat central nervous system, *J. Comp. Neurol.,* 403, 261–280, 1999.
90. Brubaker, P.L., The glucagon-like peptides: pleiotropic regulators of nutrient homeostasis, *Ann. N.Y. Acad. Sci.,* 1070, 10–26, 2006.
91. Herrmann, C. et al., Glucagon-like peptide-1 and glucose-dependent insulin-releasing polypeptide plasma levels in response to nutrients, *Digestion,* 56, 117–226, 1995.
92. Elliott, R.M. et al., Glucagon-like peptide-1 (7-36) amide and glucose-dependent insulinotropic polypeptide secretion in response to nutrient ingestion in man: acute post-prandial and 24-h secretion patterns, *J. Endocrinol.,* 138, 159–166, 1993.
93. Roberge, J.N. and Brubaker, P.L., Secretion of proglucagon-derived peptides in response to intestinal luminal nutrients, *Endocrinology,* 128, 3169–3174, 1991.
94. Meier, J.J. et al., Normalization of glucose concentrations and deceleration of gastric emptying after solid meals during intravenous glucagon-like peptide 1 in patients with type 2 diabetes, *J. Clin. Endocrinol. Metab.,* 88, 2719–2725, 2003.
95. Davis, H.R., Jr., et al., Effect of chronic central administration of glucagon-like peptide-1 (7-36) amide on food consumption and body weight in normal and obese rats, *Obes. Res.,* 6, 147–156, 1998.
96. Schick, R.R. et al., Peptides that regulate food intake: glucagon-like peptide 1-(7-36) amide acts at lateral and medial hypothalamic sites to suppress feeding in rats, *Am. J. Physiol. Regul. Integr. Comp. Physiol.,* 284, R1427–R1435, 2003.
97. Bullock, B.P., Heller, R.S., and Habener, J.F., Tissue distribution of messenger ribonucleic acid encoding the rat glucagon-like peptide-1 receptor, *Endocrinology,* 137, 2968–2978, 1996.
98. Dunphy, J.L., Taylor, R.G., and Fuller, P.J., Tissue distribution of rat glucagon receptor and GLP-1 receptor gene expression, *Mol. Cell. Endocrinol.,* 141, 179–186, 1998.
99. Thorens, B., Expression cloning of the pancreatic beta cell receptor for the gluco-incretin hormone glucagon-like peptide 1, *Proc. Natl. Acad. Sci. USA,* 89, 8641–8645, 1992.
100. Imeryuz, N. et al., Glucagon-like peptide-1 inhibits gastric emptying via vagal afferent-mediated central mechanisms, *Am. J. Physiol.,* 273, G920–G927, 1997.

101. Tolessa, T. et al., Inhibitory effect of glucagon-like peptide-1 on small bowel motility, Fasting but not fed motility inhibited via nitric oxide independently of insulin and somatostatin, *J. Clin. Invest.,* 102, 764–774, 1998.
102. Meeran, K. et al., Repeated intracerebroventricular administration of glucagon-like peptide-1-(7-36) amide or exendin-(9-39) alters body weight in the rat, *Endocrinology,* 140, 244–250, 1999.
103. Turton, M.D. et al., A role for glucagon-like peptide-1 in the central regulation of feeding, *Nature,* 379, 69–72, 1996.
104. Kastin, A.J., Akerstrom, V., and Pan, W., Interactions of glucagon-like peptide-1 (GLP-1) with the blood-brain barrier, *J. Mol. Neurosci.,* 18, 7–14, 2002.
105. Kastin, A.J. and Pan, W., Peptide transport across the blood-brain barrier, *Prog. Drug Res.,* 61, 79–100, 2003.
106. Han, V.K. et al., Cellular localization of proglucagon/glucagon-like peptide I messenger RNAs in rat brain, *J. Neurosci. Res.,* 16, 97–107, 1986.
107. Jin, S.L. et al., Distribution of glucagonlike peptide I (GLP-I), glucagon, and glicentin in the rat brain: an immunocytochemical study, *J. Comp. Neurol.,* 271, 519–532, 1988.
108. Verdich, C. et al., The role of postprandial releases of insulin and incretin hormones in meal-induced satiety — effect of obesity and weight reduction, *Int. J. Obes. Relat. Metab. Disord.,* 25, 1206–1214, 2001.
109. Naslund, E. et al., Energy intake and appetite are suppressed by glucagon-like peptide-1 (GLP-1) in obese men, *Int. J. Obes. Relat. Metab. Disord.,* 23, 304–311, 1999.
110. Scrocchi, L.A. et al., Glucose intolerance but normal satiety in mice with a null mutation in the glucagon-like peptide 1 receptor gene, *Nat. Med.,* 2, 1254–1258, 1996.
111. Barak, Y. et al., PPAR gamma is required for placental, cardiac, and adipose tissue development, *Mol Cell.,* 4, 585–595, 1999.
112. Reue, K. et al., Adipose tissue deficiency, glucose intolerance, and increased atherosclerosis result from mutation in the mouse fatty liver dystrophy (fld) gene, *J. Lipid Res.,* 41, 1067–1076, 2000.
113. Seppala-Lindroos, A. et al., Fat accumulation in the liver is associated with defects in insulin suppression of glucose production and serum free fatty acids independent of obesity in normal men, *J. Clin. Endocrinol. Metab.,* 87, 3023–3028, 2002.
114. Kim, J.K. et al., Mechanism of insulin resistance in A-ZIP/F-1 fatless mice, *J. Biol. Chem.,* 275, 8456–8460, 2000.
115. Shimomura, I. et al., Insulin resistance and diabetes mellitus in transgenic mice expressing nuclear SREBP-1c in adipose tissue: model for congenital generalized lipodystrophy, *Genes Dev.,* 12, 3182–3194, 1998.
116. Woods, S.C., Decke, E., and Vasselli, J.R., Metabolic hormones and regulation of body weight, *Psychol. Rev.,* 81, 26–43, 1974.
117. Polonsky, K.S., Given, B.D., and Van Cauter, E., Twenty-four-hour profiles and pulsatile patterns of insulin secretion in normal and obese subjects, *J. Clin. Invest.,* 81, 442–448, 1988.
118. Schoeller, D.A. et al., Entrainment of the diurnal rhythm of plasma leptin to meal timing, *J. Clin. Invest.,* 100, 1882–1887, 1997.
119. Bagdade, J.D., Bierman, E.L., and Porte, D., Jr., The significance of basal insulin levels in the evaluation of the insulin response to glucose in diabetic and nondiabetic subjects, *J. Clin. Invest.,* 46, 1549–1557, 1967.
120. Benoit, S.C. et al., Insulin and leptin as adiposity signals, *Recent Prog. Horm. Res.,* 59, 267–285, 2004.
121. Woods, S.C. et al., Insulin and the blood–brain barrier, *Curr. Pharm. Des.,* 9, 2003.
122. Banks, W.A., The source of cerebral insulin, *Eur. J. Pharmacol.,* 490, 795–800, 2004.

123. Air, E.L. et al., Small molecule insulin mimetics reduce food intake and body weight and prevent development of obesity, *Nat. Med.,* 8, 179–183, 2002.
124. Obici, S. et al., Decreasing hypothalamic insulin receptors causes hyperphagia and insulin resistance in rats, *Nat. Neurosci.,* 5, 566–572, 2002.
125. Woods, S.C. et al., Chronic intracerebroventricular infusion of insulin reduces food intake and body weight of baboons, *Nature,* 282, 503–505, 1979.
126. Nicolaidis, S. and Rowland, N., Metering of intravenous versus oral nutrients and regulation of energy balance, *Am. J. Physiol.,* 231, 661–668, 1976.
127. Kennedy, G.C., The role of depot fat in the hypothalamic control of food intake in rats, *Proc. R. Soc. Lond. B Biol. Sci.,* 140, 578–592, 1953.
128. Hervey, G.R., The effects of lesions in the hypothalamus in parabiotic rats, *J. Physiol.,* 145, 336–352, 1959.
129. Zhang, Y. et al., Positional cloning of the mouse obese gene and its human homologue, *Nature,* 372, 425–432, 1994.
130. Halaas, J.L. et al., Weight-reducing effects of the plasma protein encoded by the obese gene, *Science,* 269, 543–546, 1995.
131. Pelleymounter, M.A. et al., Effects of the obese gene product on body weight regulation in ob/ob mice, *Science,* 269, 540–543, 1995.
132. Tartaglia, L.A. et al., Identification and expression cloning of a leptin receptor, OB-R, *Cell,* 83, 1263–1271, 1995.
133. Schwartz, M.W. et al., Identification of targets of leptin action in rat hypothalamus, *J. Clin. Invest.,* 98, 1101–1106, 1996.
134. Lee, G.H. et al., Abnormal splicing of the leptin receptor in diabetic mice, *Nature,* 379, 632–634, 1996.
135. Vaisse, C. et al., Leptin activation of Stat3 in the hypothalamus of wild-type and ob/ob mice but not db/db mice, *Nature, Genetics* 14, 95–97, 1996.
136. Jin, L. et al., Leptin and leptin receptor expression in normal and neoplastic human pituitary: evidence of a regulatory role for leptin on pituitary cell proliferation, *J. Clin. Endocrinol. Metab.,* 84, 2903–2911, 1999.
137. Morash, B. et al., Leptin gene expression in the brain and pituitary gland, *Endocrinology,* 140, 5995–5998, 1999.
138. Hoggard, N. et al., Leptin and leptin receptor mRNA and protein expression in the murine fetus and placenta, *Proc. Natl. Acad. Sci. USA,* 94, 11073–11078, 1997.
139. Cowley, M.A. et al., Leptin activates anorexigenic POMC neurons through a neural network in the arcuate nucleus, *Nature,* 411, 480–484, 2001.
140. Ahima, R.S. et al., Role of leptin in the neuroendocrine response to fasting, *Nature,* 382, 250–252, 1996.
141. Considine, R.V. et al., Serum immunoreactive-leptin concentrations in normal-weight and obese humans, *N. Engl. J. Med.,* 334, 292–295, 1996.
142. Farooqi, S. et al., ob gene mutations and human obesity, *Proc. Nutr. Soc.,* 57, 471–475, 1998.
143. Caro, J.F. et al., Decreased cerebrospinal-fluid/serum leptin ratio in obesity: a possible mechanism for leptin resistance, *Lancet,* 348, 156–161, 1996.
144. Levin, B.E., Dunn-Meynell, A.A., and Banks, W.A., Obesity-prone rats have normal blood-brain barrier transport but defective central leptin signaling before obesity onset, *Am. J. Physiol. Regul. Integr. Comp. Physiol.,* 286, R143–R150, 2004.
145. Munzberg, H. and Myers, M.G., Jr., Molecular and anatomical determinants of central leptin resistance, *Nat. Neurosci.,* 8, 566–570, 2005.
146. Liu, Y.L., Emilsson, V., and Cawthorne, M.A., Leptin inhibits glycogen synthesis in the isolated soleus muscle of obese (*ob/ob*) mice, *FEBS Lett.,* 411, 351–355, 1997.
147. Unger, R.H., The hyperleptinemia of obesity-regulator of caloric surpluses, *Cell,* 117, 145–146, 2004.

148. Harris, R.B. et al., Early and late stimulation of ob mRNA expression in meal-fed and overfed rats, *J. Clin. Invest.*, 97, 2020–2026, 1996.
149. Lee, M.J. and Fried, S.K., Multilevel regulation of leptin storage, turnover, and secretion by feeding and insulin in rat adipose tissue, *J. Lipid Res.*, 47, 1984–1993, 2006.
150. Weigle, D.S. et al., Effect of fasting, refeeding, and dietary fat restriction on plasma leptin levels, *J. Clin. Endocrinol. Metab.*, 82, 561–565, 1997.
151. Buckley, C.A. and Schneider, J.E., Food hoarding is increased by food deprivation and decreased by leptin treatment in Syrian hamsters, *Am. J. Physiol. Regul. Integr. Comp. Physiol.*, 285, R1021–R1029, 2003.
152. Matson, C.A. et al., Synergy between leptin and cholecystokinin (CCK) to control daily caloric intake, *Peptides,* 18, 1275–1278, 1997.
153. Thomson, A.B., Keelan, M., and Wild, G.E., Nutrients and intestinal adaptation, *Clin. Invest. Med.*, 19, 331–345, 1996.
154. Singh, A. et al., Adaptive changes of the rat small intestine in response to a high fat diet, *Biochim. Biophys. Acta,* 260, 708–715, 1972.
155. Balint, J.A., Fried, M.B., and Imai, C., Ileal uptake of oleic acid: evidence for adaptive response to high fat feeding, *Am. J. Clin. Nutr.*, 33, 2276–2280, 1980.
156. Spannagel, A.W. et al., Adaptation to fat markedly increases pancreatic secretory response to intraduodenal fat in rats, *Am. J. Physiol.*, 270, G128–G130, 1996.
157. Goda, T. and Takase, S., Effect of dietary fat content on microvillus in rat jejunum, *J. Nutr. Sci. Vitaminol. (Tokyo),* 40, 127–136, 1994.
158. Covasa, M. and Ritter, R.C., Rats maintained on high-fat diets exhibit reduced satiety in response to CCK and bombesin, *Peptides,* 19, 1407–1415, 1998.
159. Savastano, D.M. and Covasa, M., Adaptation to a high-fat diet leads to hyperphagia and diminished sensitivity to cholecystokinin in rats, *J. Nutr.*, 135, 1953–1959, 2005.
160. Covasa, M. and Ritter, R.C., Reduced sensitivity to the satiation effect of intestinal oleate in rats adapted to high-fat diet, *Am. J. Physiol.*, 277, R279–R285, 1999.
161. Covasa, M., Grahn, J., and Ritter, R.C., Reduced hindbrain and enteric neuronal response to intestinal oleate in rats maintained on high-fat diet, *Auton. Neurosci.*, 84, 8–18, 2000.
162. Boyd, K.A. et al., High-fat diet effects on gut motility, hormone, and appetite responses to duodenal lipid in healthy men, *Am. J. Physiol. Gastrointest. Liver Physiol.*, 284, G188–G196, 2003.
163. Anini, Y. and Brubaker, P.L., Role of leptin in the regulation of glucagon-like peptide-1 secretion, *Diabetes,* 52, 252–259, 2003.
164. Salva, P.S. et al., TNF-alpha, IL-8, soluble ICAM-1, and neutrophils in sputum of cystic fibrosis patients, *Pediatr. Pulmonol.*, 21, 11–19, 1996.
165. Grady, E.F., Bohm, S.K., and Bunnett, N.W., Turning off the signal: mechanisms that attenuate signaling by G protein-coupled receptors, *Am. J. Physiol.*, 273, G586–G601, 1997.
166. Pittner, R.A. et al., Effects of PYY[3-36] in rodent models of diabetes and obesity, *Int. J. Obes. Relat. Metab. Disord.*, 28, 963–971, 2004.
167. Vrang, N. et al., PYY(3-36) reduces food intake and body weight and improves insulin sensitivity in rodent models of diet-induced obesity, *Am. J. Physiol. Regul. Integr. Comp. Physiol.*, 291, R367–R371, 2006.
168. Brolin, R.E., Bariatric surgery and long-term control of morbid obesity, *JAMA,* 288, 2793–2796, 2002.
169. Strader, A.D. et al., Weight loss through ileal transposition is accompanied by increased ileal hormone secretion and synthesis in rats, *Am. J. Physiol. Endocrinol. Metab.*, 288, E447–E453, 2005.
170. Cummings, D.E. et al., Plasma ghrelin levels after diet-induced weight loss or gastric bypass surgery, *N. Engl. J. Med.*, 346, 1623–1630, 2002.

171. Williams, D.L. and Cummings, D.E., Regulation of ghrelin in physiologic and pathophysiologic states, *J. Nutr.,* 135, 1320–1325, 2005.
172. Borg, C.M. et al., Progressive rise in gut hormone levels after Roux-en-Y gastric bypass suggests gut adaptation and explains altered satiety, *Br. J. Surg.,* 93, 210–215, 2006.
173. Naslund, E., Hellstrom, P.M., and Kral, J.G., The gut and food intake: an update for surgeons, *J. Gastrointest. Surg.,* 5, 556–567, 2001.
174. Naslund, E. et al., Importance of small bowel peptides for the improved glucose metabolism 20 years after jejunoileal bypass for obesity, *Obes. Surg.,* 8, 253–260, 1998.
175. Polyzogopoulou, E.V. et al., Restoration of euglycemia and normal acute insulin response to glucose in obese subjects with type 2 diabetes following bariatric surgery, *Diabetes,* 52, 1098–1103, 2003.
176. Pories, W.J. and Albrecht, R.J., Etiology of type II diabetes mellitus: role of the foregut, *World J. Surg.,* 25, 527–531, 2001.
177. Guidone, C. et al., Mechanisms of recovery from type 2 diabetes after malabsorptive bariatric surgery, *Diabetes,* 55, 2025–2031, 2006.
178. Bi, S. et al., Differential body weight and feeding responses to high-fat diets in rats and mice lacking cholecystokinin 1 receptors, *Am. J. Physiol. Regul. Integr. Comp. Physiol.,* 293, R55–R63, 2007.
179. Henderson, L., *The National Diet and Nutrition Survey: Adults Aged 19 to 64 Years.* Office for National Statistics, London, 2003.
180. Grove, K.L. and Cowley, M.A., Is ghrelin a signal for the development of metabolic systems? *J. Clin. Invest.,* 115, 3393–3397, 2005.

12 Role of Postabsorptive Endocrine Factors on Human Feeding and Regulation of Body Adiposity

Karen L. Teff and Chirag Kapadia

CONTENTS

12.1 INTRODUCTION

The architecture of meal ingestion is one of a complex, structured pattern with a domino-like series of physiological consequences. From the first experience of hunger motivating the acquisition of food, through the sensory experience of the ingested food prior to and during mastication, to the subsequent digestion, absorption, and metabolism of nutrients, a vast array of neural and hormonal responses are initiated, each dependent on a preceding response. Furthermore, the patterning and magnitude of physiological responses to food ingestion are dependent on the composition and macronutrient content of the diet. Together, these responses contribute to the energy status of the organism and establish a feedback system which regulates body adiposity. A discussion of postabsorptive endocrine influences on feeding behavior must take into account that the postabsorptive effects are a consequence of both preabsorptive and absorptive processes occurring in response to the composition of the diet. This chapter will focus specifically on those postprandial endocrine responses that have been shown to have the most significant effects on subsequent food intake and regulation of body adiposity in humans.

12.2 GENERAL PARADIGM FOR THE ROLE OF POSTPRANDIAL ENDOCRINE FACTORS IN BODY WEIGHT REGULATION

Endocrine factors released in response to ingested dietary components act as metabolic signals to both central nervous system and peripheral tissue sites (such as the portal vein), relaying information on energy status and body adiposity. Although it is not within the scope of this chapter to review the brain mechanisms involved in inhibiting and stimulating eating behavior and the overall regulation of body weight, it is important to delineate the working model by which postprandial hormonal responses could potentially regulate and modulate food intake. In general, it is thought that insulin and leptin are the primary long-term regulators of body weight.[1,2] Both hormones are highly correlated with body adiposity and, in humans, with body mass index.[3,4] Insulin and leptin, released peripherally by the pancreas and adipose tissue, respectively, are actively transported across the blood–brain barrier.[5] They exert their effects on body adiposity regulation by binding to specific brain regions and eliciting the release of other peptides and neurotransmitters to inhibit feeding behavior. Insulin and leptin also modulate responsivity of the brain to other neural and endocrine factors considered to be acute regulators of meal-to-meal feeding. Examples of short-term meal-to-meal regulators known to inhibit food intake, which are under modulatory control by leptin and to a lesser extent insulin, are cholecystokinin[6] and glucagon-like peptide (GLP).[7,8] Superimposed on these hormonal signals are metabolic fuels, such as glucose[9] and free fatty acids,[10] which have been shown to interact with neurons in the central nervous system (CNS). Thus, the quantity and dietary composition of a meal, as reflected by the postabsorptive metabolic profile, are recognized by the brain and subsequently influence behavior and metabolism through efferent neural and hormonal pathways. This establishes a prototypic feedback loop with dietary components, endocrine factors, and neural stimuli as the afferents, the brain and portal vein as the sensor sites, and neural and hormonal responses as the effectors.

12.3 FACTORS INFLUENCING POSTPRANDIAL ENDOCRINE RESPONSES

Within the context of the feedback loop described above, postabsorptive endocrine factors act as signals to the CNS on the energy status of the organism. Therefore, the magnitude of increase, and potentially the rate and length of time a hormone is elevated, may convey important information to the brain. The magnitude of hormonal response to a meal is dependent on the quantity of food consumed, the dietary composition of the ingested food, and the endocrine and energy status of the individual consuming the meal. Macronutrient composition of the meal is a primary determinant of which hormones are secreted, as well as the rate and magnitude of hormonal response. A good example of the differential effects of macronutrients is provided by a comparison between the effects of fat versus carbohydrate. The presence of fat in a meal delays gastric emptying, thereby slowing nutrient absorption and blunting rises in hormonal responses.[11] Fat is less of a potent insulin secretagogue than glucose, but is more effective in stimulating the release of other peptides, such as glucagon-like peptide[12] and cholecystokinin,[13] a neurally mediated intestinal peptide involved in acute meal-to-meal regulation. Thus, each macronutrient elicits a unique metabolic profile capable of relaying the energy status of the individual to the central nervous system and potentially influencing satiety to varying degrees. In addition, within each category of macronutrient, different types of fat, protein, or carbohydrate can influence postprandial hormonal release. Finally, the energy and adiposity status of the individual also exert significant influences on the magnitude of the postabsorptive endocrine profile. Insulin sensitivity, the degree of body adiposity, and neural responsivity further determine the magnitude and temporal patterning of hormonal release and subsequent behavioral responses.

12.4 LIMITATIONS OF INVESTIGATING MECHANISMS OF BODY ADIPOSITY REGULATION IN HUMANS

In humans, validation of the mechanisms and pathways involved in the regulation of body adiposity is limited to primarily two approaches: (1) measurement of endogenous compounds prior to or simultaneously with food intake, and (2) exogenous administration of a biological compound and subsequent monitoring of ingestive behavior. Both methods are scientifically flawed; the first provides only correlative associations, and the second involves the nonphysiological administration of a compound. In contrast, in mice, the availability of specific knock-out and knock-in techniques provide targeted physiological manipulations. The vast majority of human experimentation investigating food intake and body adiposity regulation involves studies in which participants are given acute dietary challenges. In many studies, subjects are administered a dietary challenge in the form of what is termed a "preload," a controlled meal or snack with a defined caloric and macronutrient content. The subsequent food intake of the subjects is then monitored surreptitiously at the next meal.[14–16,18] In fewer experiments, metabolic responses are measured simultaneously with food intake, permitting correlative evaluation of the relationship between hormonal release and food intake.[17,18] While some studies have monitored food intake over longer periods, such as 24 or 48 hours,[19,20] even this length of time is short, considering the emerging data, which suggests body weight is regulated over 4- to 5-day periods.[21] Thus, while this type of study design can shed light on the metabolic and endocrine responses to meal challenges, particularly acute regulators of meal-to-meal intake, it probably provides little insight into how body adiposity is regulated over the long-term.

Contributing to the problems of investigating the mechanisms of body adiposity regulation is the difficulty of accurate and precise measurement of food intake in humans. In free-living situations, assessment of dietary intake is dependent on food diaries, which are notoriously flawed with underreporting and other inadequacies. Conversely, measurement of food consumption within laboratory or hospital conditions is more precise, but may not reflect typical food patterns observed in normal conditions. Particularly important with respect to human experimentation are the psychological, social, cultural, and learned factors, unique to present day *Homo sapiens,* which may override the basic physiological mechanisms regulating body adiposity and food intake behavior. Currently our understanding of how the psychological factors interact at the biological level is still very limited, and their incorporation into human biological models is, at this point, still theoretical. In the remaining sections of this chapter, we will examine four individual hormones with respect to how their release is determined by dietary composition and individual energy status and, in turn, how they regulate food intake and energy homeostasis in humans.

12.5 INSULIN

Acute insulin secretion in response to meal ingestion is largely dependent on the macronutrient composition of the meal. In general, carbohydrates are the most potent stimulators of insulin release, followed by protein, which is a mild insulin secretagogue. Fat, which is rarely eaten independently of either protein or carbohydrate, does not elicit insulin secretion,[22] but significantly attenuates the rate of rise and magnitude of postprandial insulin levels in response to carbohydrate and protein meals by slowing gastric emptying. Within classes of macronutrients, individual sugars as well as amino acids have differential abilities to elicit insulin secretion. For example, arginine is a particularly effective stimulator of insulin release compared to other amino acids,[23] while glucose is the most potent carbohydrate stimulus of insulin secretion. In contrast, fructose is a weak elicitor of insulin release, and ingestion of fructose-containing products results in only modest elevations in plasma insulin.[24] As discussed below, the potency of a dietary component to stimulate insulin has important implications for the role of these hormones in the regulation of body adiposity.

In 1981, Porte and Woods proposed a model in which insulin was hypothesized to be a long-term regulator of body weight.[25] This model was based on data showing that peripheral levels of insulin were highly correlated with body weight and could gain access into the CNS to reduce body weight.[25,26] Furthermore, it was demonstrated that insulin administered directly into the central nervous system could inhibit food intake in lean but not obese rats,[26] demonstrating central resistance to the satiating effects of insulin in obesity. This feedback loop originally proposed for insulin has become the prototypic model for peripherally released circulating factors that act in the CNS to regulate body adiposity.[27] Evidence for the hypothesis that insulin tends to decrease food take and protect against body weight gain in humans is provided by a prospective study in Pima Indians,[28] in which 97 nondiabetic subjects underwent a series of tests to evaluate insulin sensitivity and secretion. It was found that insulin release during a meal-tolerance test, an oral glucose-tolerance test, as well as first phase insulin during an intravenous glucose tolerance test, were all inversely correlated to weight gain: the greater the insulin secretion in response to the challenge, the less weight gain. The authors hypothesized that circulating insulin gained access to the brain, thereby decreasing food intake.

Conversely, hyperinsulinemia has been touted as a stimulator of food intake and subsequent weight gain. In fact, many diets purported to result in weight loss claim that avoidance of foods which induce rapid and large rises in plasma insulin is essential to their efficacy. Two such diets are the Atkins diet and the low-glycemic index diet. These diets prescribe very different dietary regimens, but both result in low levels of postprandial insulin. While the Atkins diet recommends avoiding almost all carbohydrates, emphasizing protein and fat intake,[29–31] the low-glycemic index diet involves the avoidance of only those carbohydrate foods that are rapidly digested and absorbed and thus result in high glucose levels (high-glycemic index foods).[32–34] High-glycemic index foods include not only the expected culprits, such as candy, but other, unexpected items, such as whole wheat bread, pasta, carrots, fruit, and potatoes.[35] Surprisingly, many calorically dense foods that have both fat and carbohydrate, for example chips or muffins, can be categorized as having lower glycemic indexes, since the presence of the dietary fat blunts the rise of plasma glucose.[36]

The idea that high postprandial insulin levels stimulate food intake is based on two types of studies: those reporting that acute administration of insulin increases food intake,[37–39] and others that provide evidence that type 1 diabetic humans often gain weight at the onset of insulin treatment.[40] In type 1 diabetic humans, the increased weight gain is probably multifactorial, and although not definitive, one hypothesis suggests that the switch in metabolism from a catabolic to anabolic state, combined with the rapid increases in plasma insulin from exogenous insulin delivery following periods of insulin deficiency may lead to increased fat deposition.[41] In contrast, the reported increases in food intake following acute insulin administration in animals are typically due to an induction of hypoglycemia, also elicited by exogenous insulin administration.[38,42]

Rebound hypoglycemia which occurs only rarely in nondiabetic individuals, is a known initiator of food intake and, to a large extent, lies at the crux of the controversy surrounding the relationship of insulin to body weight. Proponents of low-glycemic index diets suggest that high postprandial levels of glucose, with their coincident high levels of insulin, result in hypoglycemia and subsequent food intake.[43] During hypoglycemia, the release of the counterregulatory hormones glucagon and cortisol, as well as the neurohormone norepinephrine, raises levels of plasma glucose and free fatty acids by increasing gluconeogenesis and lipolysis, respectively.[44] Sustained increases in free fatty acids in the portal vein contribute to the etiology of insulin resistance, the precipitating pathophysiology of many metabolic diseases including diabetes, hypertension, and cardiovascular disease. Thus, it has been postulated that the metabolic consequences of repeated episodes of hypoglycemia contribute to insulin resistance and metabolic disease.[33,43] However, the likelihood of repetitive hypoglycemic episodes under normal dietary conditions is questionable since humans typically ingest mixtures of macronutrients at most meals, and the presence of dietary fat delays nutrient absorption, blunts peak insulin levels, and prevents rebound hypoglycemia. Thus, the mechanisms presently proposed to be responsible for the relationship between high-glycemic index diets and disease are probably incorrect. Nevertheless, despite reports showing no association,[45–47] some epidemiological studies do demonstrate a correlation between high-glycemic index diets and metabolic disease, including obesity and diabetes.[48–50] One interpretation of this controversy is that high-glycemic index diets may be a surrogate marker for diets that are generally of poor nutritional content: highly caloric, high-fat diets.

Sweetened, carbonated soda is consistently correlated with various indices of metabolic disease in large epidemiological studies.[50–52] Calorie-containing sodas, as well as sweetened fruit juice and fruit drinks, often contain large quantities of liquid carbohydrate, which is rapidly absorbed and could potentially elicit hypoglycemia if prolonged increases in insulin release were to occur. However, the presence of fructose in many of these beverages, either by itself or in the form of high-fructose corn syrup (55% fructose and 45% glucose), attenuates the large increases in plasma insulin that would typically occur following ingestion of liquid carbohydrate. Figure 12.1 illustrates the differential insulin responses to meals containing 60% of total kilocalorie intake from either carbohydrate or fat sources (left graph), and the insulin responses to fixed mixed-nutrient meals ingested with high-fructose or high-glucose beverages contributing to 30% of the caloric intake (right graph). These data were derived from two separate within-subject design experiments, both conducted over a 24-hour period.[24,53] One compared the effect of ingesting high-carbohydrate meals versus high fat-meals, and another compared the effect of meals accompanied by either a high-fructose beverage or a high-glucose beverage. In Figure 12.1, the data from the two experiments are crossed over. As can be seen in the middle graph, insulin release after a high-fat meal is almost identical to insulin release after a mixed-nutrient meal ingested with a high-fructose beverage. Thus, from the perspective of insulin release, ingestion of fructose, a carbohydrate, is very similar to ingestion of dietary fat. To summarize, the magnitude of insulin release is dependent on the quantity and quality of ingested food as well as the energy status of the individual. The hormone is highly responsive to changes in dietary intake and, as discussed below, also contributes to the regulation of leptin secretion. Based on current data, insulin probably plays a critical role in the regulation of body adiposity.

12.6 LEPTIN

The adipokine hormone leptin is synthesized and secreted by adipocytes within adipose tissue. At the time of discovery of leptin and the absence of the leptin gene in genetically obese mice,[27] it was believed that a similar gene mutation would be observed in obese humans. However, surprisingly, measurement of the leptin protein in obese humans revealed that increased, not decreased, levels of leptin were evident.[54] Based on these data and those in diet-induced obese animals,[55] the concept of leptin-resistance at the level of the central nervous system was proposed[56] such that obesity animals and humans were unresponsive to these elevated levels of circulating leptin. Furthermore, it was hypothesized that the increased levels of leptin associated with obesity were either unable to cross the blood–brain barrier, due to impaired transport, or were interacting with impaired receptors in brain-impaired transport,[57,58] leading to a lack of satiety and increased food intake. We now know that only a handful of obese individuals exhibit genetic mutations of leptin receptors,[59,60] and although administration of exogenous leptin to these individuals is highly effective in restoring normal body weight,[61] leptin administration to leptin-resistant individuals is only modestly therapeutic, if at all.[62] More recently, it has

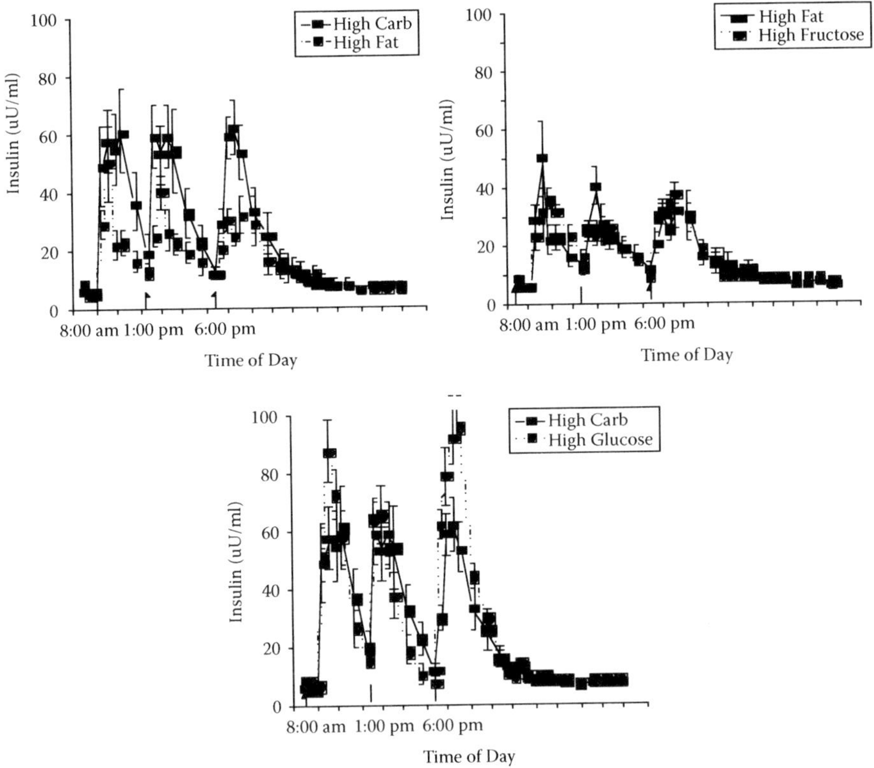

FIGURE 12.1 *Left Graph*: Mean plasma insulin levels (mean ± S.E, n = 19) over a 24-hour period in normal weight healthy women following ingestion of breakfast, lunch, and dinner (indicated by arrows) in which the total kilocalorie content consisted of either 60% fat (dashed line, round symbol) or 60% carbohydrate (solid line, square symbol). *Right Graph*: Mean plasma insulin levels (mean + S.E., n = 13) over a 24-hour period following ingestion of a mixed nutrient meal with a high fructose-containing beverage contributing 30% of total kilocalorie intake (dashed line, round symbol) compared to insulin levels following ingestion of the high fat meal shown in left graph (solid line, square symbol). *Bottom Graph*: Mean plasma insulin levels (mean + S.E., n = 13) over a 24-hour period following ingestion of mixed nutrient meal with a high glucose-containing beverage contributing 30% of total kilocalorie intake (dashed line, round symbol) compared to insulin levels following ingestion of the high carbohydrate meal shown in the left graph (solid line, square symbol). (Taken from data derived from Teff, K.L., Elliott, S.S., Tschop, M., Kieffer, T.J., Rader, D., Heiman, M., Townsend, R.R., Keim, N.L., and Havel, P.J., Dietary fructose reduces circulating insulin and leptin, attenuates postprandial suppression of ghrelin, and increases triglycerides in women, *J. Clin. Endocrinol. Metab.*, 89, 2963–2972, 2004; Havel, P.J., Townsend, R.C.L., and Teff, K., High-fat meals reduce 24-hour circulating leptin concentrations in women, *Diabetes*, 48, 334–341, 1999. With permission.)

been proposed that decreased leptin levels are of greater biological significance than elevated levels, since declines in leptin indicate decreased body adiposity and stimulate food intake.[63] Of particular interest to this book is how the scientific theory on the role of leptin in the regulation of body adiposity evolved with bidirectional flow of information and discoveries between basic and clinical experimentation.

Plasma leptin levels are highly correlated with body adiposity,[64] and fasting levels derived from morning samples are primarily a reflection of body fat. In humans, leptin is secreted in a circadian manner, with nadirs occurring in the morning and levels peaking between midnight and 2:00 a.m.,[65] although the mechanisms regulating the rise and fall are still unknown. Leptin synthesis and secretion is dependent on insulin-mediated glucose metabolism,[66] so that increasing glucose availability and metabolism increases leptin levels. Prolonged intravenous infusion of glucose increases insulin and leptin levels,[19,67] and dietary manipulations that significantly affect glucose and insulin levels can also influence circulating levels of leptin. We have found that circulating levels of leptin can be altered by dietary manipulations by approximately 25 to 30%. For example, a diet composed of 60% fat reduces 24-hour circulating levels of leptin by 30% compared to an equicaloric high-carbohydrate diet (Figure 12.2, left graph).[68] An almost identical attenuation of leptin secretion is evident when 30% of dietary carbohydrate is provided by fructose compared to glucose (Figure 12.2, middle graph).[24] The blunting of leptin secretion in response to fat and fructose is due to the decrease in insulin secretion elicited by both of these dietary components (Figure 12.1). Both dietary fat and fructose lower circulating levels of insulin and leptin compared to meals high in carbohydrates or mixed-nutrient meals served with high-glucose beverages. Furthermore, the reduction in leptin may be exacerbated by postprandial triglycerides released in response to both fat and fructose,[24] because triglycerides have been shown to inhibit leptin transport across the blood–brain barrier.[69] The resulting lower availability of leptin following high-fructose or high-fat diets may then contribute to decreased satiety and increased food intake.

Individual responsivity to the effects of reduced leptin availability on satiety may be phenotypic or dependent on individual psychological profiles. We found that increasing dietary fructose over a 24-hour period increased food intake, specifically fat intake, but only in individuals identified as restrained eaters (those individuals who consciously restrict their diet). In contrast, nonrestrained eaters ingested the same amount of food whether the diet was supplemented with glucose or fructose.[24] Conversely, the effects of increases in plasma leptin on food intake can be subtle even in lean, insulin-sensitive individuals. In a recent study,[19] we infused intravenously either saline (control condition) or glucose into lean subjects for a period of 48 hours, during which time we monitored their food intake without their knowledge. The glucose infusion significantly increased plasma glucose, plasma insulin, and circulating leptin levels. Despite no overall significant decreases in 48-hour food intake during the glucose infusion condition, a highly significant inverse correlation between plasma leptin levels and cumulative food intake over the 48-hour period was found (Figure 12.3, upper-right graph). This relationship between food intake and leptin levels was not significant under saline conditions (Figure 12.3, upper-left graph) and was only unveiled when leptin was increased by the glucose infusion. No statistically significant relationship was observed between insulin and food intake (bottom graphs). However, hunger levels as rated by visual analogue scales were also significantly correlated with plasma leptin (data not shown). These results suggest that the physiological increase in plasma leptin induced by the glucose infusion was recognized by the brain and altered food intake, but to a very small degree, not detectable in cumulative food intake over the 48-hour period in this small group

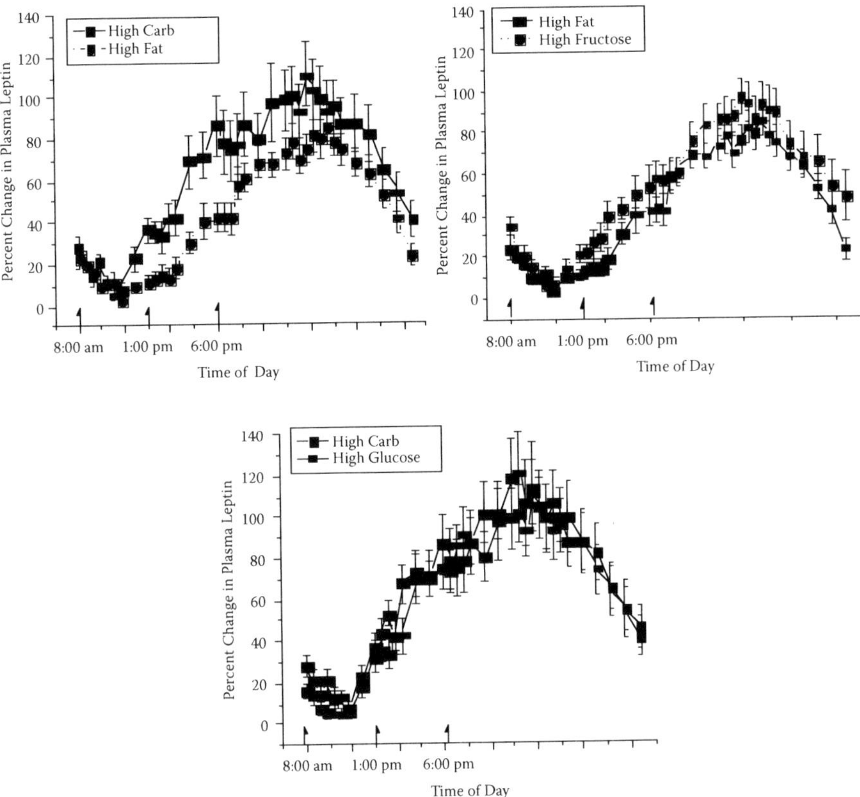

FIGURE 12.2 *Left Graph*: Mean plasma leptin levels (mean ± S.E, n = 19) expressed as a percent of nadir over a 24-hour period in normal weight healthy women following ingestion of breakfast, lunch, and dinner (time indicated by arrows) in which the total kilocalorie content consisted of either 60% fat (dashed line, round symbol) or 60% carbohydrate (solid line, square symbol). *Right Graph*: Mean plasma leptin levels (mean ± S.E, n = 13) expressed as a percent of nadir over a 24-hour period following ingestion of a mixed nutrient meal with a high fructose-containing beverage contributing 30% of total kilocalorie intake (dashed line, round symbol) compared to insulin levels following ingestion of the high fat meal shown in left graph (solid line, square symbol). *Bottom Graph*: Mean plasma leptin levels expressed as a percent of nadir over a 24-hour period following ingestion of mixed nutrient meal with a high glucose-containing beverage contributing 30% of total kilocalorie intake (dashed line, round symbol) compared to insulin levels following ingestion of the high carbohydrate meal shown in left graph (solid line, square symbol). (Taken from data derived from Teff, K.L., Elliott, S.S., Tschop, M., Kieffer, T.J., Rader, D., Heiman, M., Townsend, R.R., Keim, N.L., and Havel, P.J., Dietary fructose reduces circulating insulin and leptin, attenuates postprandial suppression of ghrelin, and increases triglycerides in women, *J. Clin. Endocrinol. Metab.*, 89, 2963–2972, 2004; Havel, P.J., Townsend, R.C.L., and Teff, K., High-fat meals reduce 24-hour circulating leptin concentrations in women, *Diabetes*, 48, 334–341, 1999. With permission.)

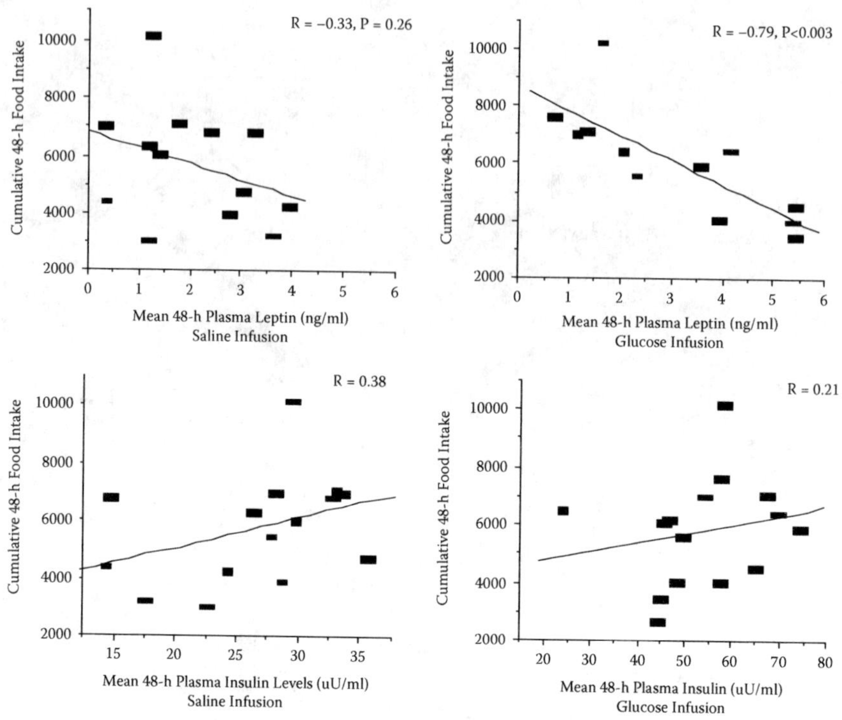

FIGURE 12.3 Mean of plasma leptin levels collected over a 48-hour period (*x*-axis) correlated with total food intake (*y*-axis) over a 48-hour period during saline infusion (upper left graph). Mean of plasma leptin levels collected over a 48-hour period (*x*-axis) correlated with total food intake (*y*-axis) over a 48-hour period during glucose infusion (upper right graph). Mean of plasma insulin levels collected over a 48-hour period (*x*-axis) correlated with total food intake (*y*-axis) over a 48-hour period during saline infusion (lower left graph). Mean of plasma insulin levels collected over a 48-hour period (*x*-axis) correlated with total food intake (*y*-axis) over a 48-hour period during glucose infusion (lower left graph). (Taken from Teff, K.L., Petrova, M., Havel, P.J., and Townsend, R.R., 48-hour glucose infusion in humans: Effect on hormonal responses, hunger and food intake, *Physiol. Behav.*, 90, 733–743, 2007. With permission.)

of subjects. Significant decreases in food intake may have been observed if the experimental treatment were administered over a longer period of time. Previous human studies have demonstrated correlations between either food intake or hunger and leptin, but these were in obese individuals on calorically restricted diets.[70,71] Our study was the first to demonstrate a correlation in free-feeding normal-weight humans who were not energy restricted.

12.7 GUT HORMONES: GLUCAGON-LIKE PEPTIDE-1 (GLP-1) AND PEPTIDE YY (PYY)

In the early 1960s, based on experiments demonstrating that ingested glucose elicited greater insulin release than matched levels of glucose infused intravenously, it was recognized that hormones released from the gut (referred to as "incretins") enhanced insulin secretion.[72] We now know that a vast array of peptides are released from the stomach and intestine during food ingestion. Many of these play an important role in modulating postprandial responses of insulin and leptin by influencing the rate of gastric emptying,[73] stimulating insulin release,[74] or enhancing insulin sensitivity.[75] Many gut peptides also act as anorexigenic peptides independently of insulin or leptin[76] and are transported across the blood–brain barrier to bind with receptors in the central nervous system. It is not within the scope of this chapter to discuss the effects of all the gut hormones known to influence food intake. Instead, we will concentrate on GLP-1 and PYY. GLP-1 is one of the most potent insulin secretagogues and for which there is evidence for a role in the regulation of food intake (particularly in humans). Peptide YY (PYY), a relatively newly recognized hormone surrounded by significant controversy, is also dependent on postabsorptive stimulation.

Both GLP-1 and peptide YY are products of the glucagon gene. They are secreted from the enteroendocrine L cells of the gut mucosa, which are located primarily in the distal intestine, but also in the proximal gut. GLP is released in a biphasic manner, with the early phase occurring within minutes, and a late phase occurring within 60 to 120 minutes after a meal. Given that the majority of the L cells are located in the distal small intestine, and that the peak of the GLP-1 and PYY responses begin before the majority of the L cells have been exposed to ingested nutrients,[77,78] it is likely that the early phase of release is neurally mediated, while the second phase is nutrient-stimulated. Lipids and simple carbohydrates are the most potent stimulators of GLP-1,[79] while protein meals do not appear to be particularly effective.[80] GLP-1 may influence food intake through both direct and indirect effects. One of the indirect effects is through modulation of insulin release, as it is one of the most potent stimulators of insulin biosynthesis and secretion known.[81] Together with another incretin hormone, GIP (gastrin inhibitory peptide), the two peptides account for at least half of the postmeal insulin response.[77] In addition, GLP-1 may influence insulin sensitivity through regulation of plasma glucose levels, both by inhibiting glucagon secretion and by decreasing hepatic glucose production.[75,82] GLP-1 also enhances glucose disposal through independent, noninsulin-mediated effects in the periphery.[82]

GLP-1 exerts its direct effects on food intake through peripheral and central receptors in the stomach and brain, respectively. In the gastrointestinal tract, physiological levels of GLP-1 slow gastric emptying and enhance satiety, an effect mediated via the autonomic nervous system, particularly the vagus nerve.[83,84] Peripherally released GLP-1 can cross the blood–brain barrier,[85] but in addition, the peptide is synthesized in the CNS,[86] and GLP-1 receptors are found in the hypothalamus and the nucleus of the tractus solitarius (NTS).[87] Both centrally produced and circulating GLP-1 may act in these areas to induce changes in feeding behavior, activity, and energy expenditure. In animal models, central administration of GLP-1 reduces acute caloric intake,[88] increases energy expenditure, and decreases weight gain when given chronically.[89] There is also good evidence of the physiologic and clinical significance of these effects in humans. Peripheral administration in humans at higher than physiologic levels of GLP-1 inhibits food intake in normal, obese, and diabetic subjects,[90–92] though peripheral infusions at lower levels are ineffective.[84] Consistent with these findings, a recent meta-analysis concluded that the effect of GLP-1 on *ad libitum* energy intake in humans is dose dependent.[93] In terms of energy expenditure, there is evidence that higher fasting plasma concentrations of GLP-1 are associated with higher resting energy expenditure in humans.[94,95] Obese subjects appear to have decreased GLP-1 secretion in some studies,[96] but this finding has been disputed by other studies.[94,97] Thus, GLP-1 has both peripheral and central effects on satiety. The peripheral effects are likely mediated via effects on gastric emptying; the central effects are likely mediated in a multifactorial fashion, and include input to the NTS from the vagal nerve, direct effects of circulating GLP-1, and central GLP-1 production and receptor binding. GLP-1 also appears to have the effect of increasing energy expenditure. These effects, along with its effects on insulin secretion, have made GLP-1 a gut peptide of unusual therapeutic potential. GLP-1 analogues are presently on the market as adjuvant therapies for type 2 diabetes and inhibitors of DPP-IV, the enzyme that degrades GLP-1 in plasma, are in phase 3 trials. Current therapeutic uses of GLP-1 receptor agonists, and compounds that prevent GLP-1 degradation, are covered well in a recent review.[98]

12.8 PYY

Peptide tyrosine-tyrosine ($PYY_{1\text{-}36}$) is cosecreted with GLP-1 from intestinal L cells and is cleaved by DPP-IV, resulting in $PYY_{3\text{-}36}$. PYY concentrations are proportional to meal energy content, with higher levels in response to high-calorie meals, particularly those with a high fat content.[99,100] Gut motility and gastric, pancreatic, and intestinal secretions are inhibited by PYY via vagal and perhaps also via direct effects.[101] Like GLP-1, PYY crosses the blood–brain barrier, in what appears to be a nonsaturable mechanism,[102] and binds to receptors in the hypothalamus and dorsal hind brain. PYY was initially reported to be abnormally low in obese humans, but recent data has challenged that conclusion.[103] Similarly, initial reports noted that PYY, infused at physiologic concentrations, induced satiety.[104] However, since that time, efforts to replicate these findings have shown no effects at physiologic concentrations, though effects at higher than physiologic dosing have been seen.[76,103] Presently, the role of PYY in the regulation of body adiposity and its potential as a therapeutic agent are not well established.

12.9 CONCLUSIONS AND FUTURE DIRECTIONS

Great advances have been made in the identification and measurement of biologically active compounds, and these will continue to grow with the sequencing of the human genome. However, understanding how these biological factors interact and contribute to the regulation of body adiposity within a physiological context will be a challenging enterprise. To date, we have been limited by our approaches toward studying eating behavior, which have been primarily nonecological in both animals and humans. Measurement of the quantity of a single food ingested by a rat isolated in a cage may have limited relevance to a human eating in a complex social environment. Short-term studies, whether they involve the acute administration of a peptide to a mouse or a dietary preload to a human followed by evaluation of meal-to-meal intake, reveal little of how long-term regulation of fat stores takes place during daily life. More sophisticated approaches to studying ingestive behavior in both animals and humans need to be developed. As a first step, application of approaches used for the study of psychiatric disease and addictive behavior may aid in broadening our view of how behavior can be studied. Utilizing innovative behavioral measurements may reveal phenotypes unique to ingestive behavior which may be driven by differential underlying physiological responses. Ultimately, this may lead to the development of individualized weight loss regimes that are more effective than those currently available. In addition, novel technologies are required to enhance our capabilities to measure and monitor food intake and energy expenditure in humans under normal living conditions. Thus, our approach to, and methods for, the study of the physiological mechanisms governing ingestive behavior must become as sophisticated as our methods for the analysis of the biological factors. To achieve this, greater interaction between basic and clinical scientists and between different scientific disciplines will be required. Long-term studies conducted within ecologically and physiologically relevant contexts are needed.

REFERENCES

1. Schwartz, M., Woods, S., Porte, D.J., Seeley, R., and Baskin, D., Central nervous system control of food intake, *Nature,* 404, 661–671, 2000.
2. Baskin, D.G., Figlewicz, L.D., Seeley, R.J., Woods, S.C., Porte, D., Jr., and Schwartz, M.W., Insulin and leptin: dual adiposity signals to the brain for the regulation of food intake and body weight, *Brain Res.,* 848, 114–123, 1999.
3. Bagdade, J.D., Bierman, E.L., and Porte, D., Jr., Influence of obesity on the relationship between insulin and triglyceride levels in endogenous hypertriglyceridemia, *Diabetes,* 20, 664–672, 1971.
4. Considine, R., Sinha, M., Heiman, M., Kriauciunas, A., Stephens, T., Nyce, M., Ohannesian, J., and Marco, C., Serum immunoreactive-leptin concentrations in normal-weight and obese humans, *N. Engl. J. Med.,* 334, 292–295, 1996.
5. Woods, S.C., Benoit, S.C., and Clegg, D.J., The brain-gut-islet connection, *Diabetes,* 55 (Suppl. 2), S114–S121, 2006.
6. Emond, M., Schwartz, G.J., Ladenheim, E.E., and Moran, T.H., Central leptin modulates behavioral and neural responsivity to CCK, *Am. J. Physiol.,* 276, R1545–R1549, 1999.
7. Anini, Y. and Brubaker, P.L., Role of leptin in the regulation of glucagon-like peptide-1 secretion, *Diabetes,* 52, 252–259, 2003.
8. Fehmann, H., Peiser, C., Bode, H., Stamm, M., Staats, P., Hedetoft, C., Lang, R., and Goke, B., Leptin: a potent inhibitor of insulin secretion, *Peptides,* 18, 1267–1273, 1997.
9. Levin, B.E., Dunn-Meynell, A.A., and Routh, V.H., CNS sensing and regulation of peripheral glucose levels, *Int. Rev. Neurobiol.,* 51, 219–258, 2002.
10. Obici, S., Feng, S., Morgan, K., Stein, D., Karkanias, G., and Rossetti, L., Central administration of oleic acid inhibits glucose production and food intake, *Diabetes,* 51, 271–275, 2002.
11. Ercan, N., Nutall, F.Q., and Gannon, M.C., Effect of added fat on the plasma glucose and insulin response to ingested potato given in various combinations as two meals in normal individuals, *Diabetes Care,* 17, 1453–1459, 1994.
12. Meier, J.J. and Nauck, M.A., Glucagon-like peptide 1 (GLP-1) in biology and pathology, *Diabetes Metab. Res. Rev.,* 21, 91–117, 2005.
13. Konturek, J.W., Thor, P., Maczka, M., Stoll, R., Domschke, W., and Konturek, S.J., Role of cholecystokinin in the control of gastric emptying and secretory response to a fatty meal in normal subjects and duodenal ulcer patients, *Scand. J. Gastroenterol.,* 29, 583–590, 1994.

14. Rolls, B.J., Kim, S., McNelis, A.L., Fischman, M.W., Foltin, R.W., and Moran, T.H., Time course of effects of preloads high in fat or carbohydrate on food intake and hunger ratings in humans, *Am. J. Physiol.,* 260, R756–R763, 1991.
15. Rolls, B.J., Laster, L.J., and Summerfelt, A., Hunger and food intake following consumption of low-calorie foods, *Appetite,* 13, 115–127, 1989.
16. Guss, J.L. and Kissileff, H.R., Microstructural analyses of human ingestive patterns: from description to mechanistic hypotheses, *Neurosci. Biobehav. Rev.,* 24, 261–268, 2000.
17. Nolan, L.J., Guss, J.L., Liddle, R.A., Pi-Sunyer, F.X., and Kissileff, H.R., Elevated plasma cholecystokinin and appetitive ratings after consumption of a liquid meal in humans, *Nutrition,* 19, 553–557, 2003.
18. Anderson, G.H. and Woodend, D., Effect of glycemic carbohydrates on short-term satiety and food intake, *Nutr. Rev.,* 61, S17–S17, 2003.
19. Teff, K.L., Petrova, M., Havel, P.J., and Townsend, R.R., 48-h glucose infusion in humans: effect on hormonal responses, hunger and food intake, *Physiol. Behav.,* 90, 733–743, 2007.
20. Dubuc, G., Phinney, S., Stern, J., and Havel, P., Changes of serum leptin and endocrine and metabolic parameters after 7 days of energy restriction in men and women, *Metabolism,* 47, 1–7, 1998.
21. de Castro, J.M., Eating behavior: lessons from the real world of humans, *Nutrition,* 16, 800–813, 2000.
22. Gannon, M.C., Nuttall, F.Q., Westphal, S.A., and Seaquist, E.R., The effect of fat and carbohydrate on plasma glucose, insulin, C- peptide, and triglycerides in normal male subjects, *J. Am. Coll. Nutr.,* 12, 36–41, 1997.
23. Palmer, J., Walter, R., and Ensinck, J., Arginine-stimulated acute phase of insulin and glucagon secretion. 1. in normal man, *Diabetes,* 24, 735–740, 1975.
24. Teff, K.L., Elliott, S.S., Tschop, M., Kieffer, T.J., Rader, D., Heiman, M., Townsend, R.R., D'Alessio, D., and Havel, P.J., Dietary fructose reduces circulating insulin and leptin, attenuates postprandial suppression of ghrelin, and increases triglycerides in women, *J. Clin. Endocrinol. Metab.,* 89, 2963–2972, 2004.
25. Porte, D., Jr. and Woods, S.C., Regulation of food intake and body weight by insulin, *Diabetologia,* 20 (Suppl.), 274–280, 1981.
26. Ikeda, H., West, D.B., Pustek, J.J., Figlewicz, D.P., Greenwood, M.R., Porte, D., Jr., and Woods, S.C., Intraventricular insulin reduces food intake and body weight of lean but not obese Zucker rats, *Appetite,* 7, 381–386, 1986.
27. Zhang, Y., Proenca, R., Maffei, M., Barone, M., Leopold, L., and Friedman, J.M., Positional cloning of the mouse obese gene and its human homologue, *Nature,* 372, 425–432, 1994.
28. Schwartz, M.W., Boyko, E.J., Kahn, S.E., Ravussin, E., and Bogardus, C., Reduced insulin secretion: an independent predictor of body weight gain, *J. Clin. Endocrinol. Metab.,* 80, 1571–1576, 1995.
29. Cunningham, W. and Hyson, D., The skinny on high-protein, low-carbohydrate diets, *Prev. Cardiol.,* 9, 166–171, 2006.
30. McAuley, K.A., Hopkins, C.M., Smith, K.J., McLay, R.T., Williams, S.M., Taylor, R.W., and Mann, J.I., Comparison of high-fat and high-protein diets with a high-carbohydrate diet in insulin-resistant obese women, *Diabetologia,* 48, 8–16, 2005.
31. Foster, G.D., Wyatt, H.R., Hill, J.O., McGuckin, B.G., Brill, C., Mohammed, B.S., Szapary, P.O., Rader, D.J., Edman, J.S., and Klein, S., A randomized trial of a low-carbohydrate diet for obesity, *N. Engl. J. Med.,* 348, 2082–2090, 2003.
32. Frost, G., Brynes, A.E., Bovill-Taylor, C., and Dornhorst, A., A prospective randomized trial to determine the efficacy of a low glycaemic index diet given in addition to healthy eating and weight loss advice in patients with coronary heart disease, *Eur. J. Clin. Nutr.,* 58, 121–127, 2004.

33. Ludwig, D., The glycemic index: physiologic mechanisms relating to obesity, diabetes, and cardiovascular disease, *JAMA,* 287, 2414–2423, 2002.
34. Jenkins, D.J., Wolever, T.M., and Talyor, R.H., Glycemic index of food: a physiological basis for carbohydrate exchange, *Am. J. Clin. Nutr.,* 34, 364, 1981.
35. Brand-Miller, J., Pang, E., and Broomhead, L., The glycaemic index of foods containing sugars: comparison of foods with naturally-occurring versus added sugars, *Br. J. Nutr.,* 73, 613–623, 1995.
36. Foster-Powell, K., Holt, S.H., and Brand-Miller, J.C., International table of glycemic index and glycemic load values: 2002, *Am. J. Clin. Nutr.,* 76, 5–56, 2002.
37. Flatt, P.R., Bailey, C.J., Gray, C., and Swanston-Flatt, S.K., Metabolic effects of radiation induced rat insulinoma at pancreatic, hepatic and subscapular transplantation sites, *Comp. Biochem. Physiol. A,* 85, 183–186, 1986.
38. Hudson, B. and Ritter, S., Hindbrain catecholamine neurons mediate consummatory responses to glucoprivation, *Physiol. Behav.,* 82, 241–250, 2004.
39. Dewan, S., Gillett, A., Mugarza, J.A., Dovey, T.M., Halford, J.C., and Wilding, J.P., Effects of insulin-induced hypoglycaemia on energy intake and food choice at a subsequent test meal, *Diabetes Metab. Res. Rev.,* 20, 405–410, 2004.
40. Purnell, J.Q. and Weyer, C., Weight effect of current and experimental drugs for diabetes mellitus: from promotion to alleviation of obesity, *Treat. Endocrinol.,* 2, 33–47, 2003.
41. Larger, E., Weight gain and insulin treatment, *Diabetes Metab.,* 31, 4S51–4S56, 2005.
42. Sanders, N.M., Figlewicz, D.P., Taborsky, G.J., Jr., Wilkinson, C.W., Daumen, W., and Levin, B.E., Feeding and neuroendocrine responses after recurrent insulin-induced hypoglycemia, *Physiol. Behav.,* 87, 700–706, 2006.
43. Roberts, S.B., High-glycemic index foods, hunger, and obesity: is there a connection? *Nutr. Rev.,* 58, 163–169, 2000.
44. Cryer, P., Hierarchy of physiological responses to hypoglycemia: relevance to clinical hypoglycemia in type 1 (insulin dependent) diabetes mellitus, *Horm. Metab. Res.,* 29, 92–96, 1997.
45. Meyer, K.A., Kushi, L.H., Jacobs, D.R., Stavin, J., Sellers, T.A., and Folsom, A.R., Carbohydrates, dietary fiber, and incident type 2 diabetes in older women, *Am. J. Clin. Nutr.,* 71, 921–930, 2000.
46. Mayer-Davis, E.J., Dhawan, A., Liese, A.D., Teff, K., and Schulz, M., Towards understanding of glycaemic index and glycaemic load in habitual diet: associations with measures of glycaemia in the Insulin Resistance Atherosclerosis Study, *Br. J. Nutr.,* 95, 397–405, 2006.
47. Alfenas, R.C. and Mattes, R.D., Influence of glycemic index/load on glycemic response, appetite, and food intake in healthy humans, *Diabetes Care,* 28, 2123–2129, 2005.
48. Hodge, A.M., English, D.R., O'Dea, K., and Giles, G.G., Glycemic index and dietary fiber and the risk of type 2 diabetes, *Diabetes Care,* 27, 2701–2706, 2004.
49. Salmeron, J., Asherio, M., Rimm, E.B., Colditz, G.A., Wing, A.L., and Wilett, W.C., Dietary fiber, glycemic load, and risk of NIDDM in men, *Diabetes Care,* 20, 545–550, 1997.
50. Schulze, M.B., Manson, J.E., Ludwig, D., Colditz, G., Stampfer, M., Wilett, W.C., and Hu, F.B., Sugar-sweetened beverages, weight gain, and incidence of type 2 diabetes in young and middle-aged women, *JAMA,* 292, 927–934, 2004.
51. Ludwig, D., Peterson, K., and Gortmaker, S., Relation between consumption of sugar-sweetened drinks and childhood obesity: a prospective, observational analysis, *Lancet,* 357, 505–508, 2001.
52. Willett, W., Mansson, J., and Liu, S., Glycemic index, glycemic load, and risk of type 2 diabetes, *Am. J. Clin. Nutr.,* 76, 274S–280S, 2002.
53. Havel, P., Chaump, L., and Teff, K., High fat meals reduce 24-hour circulating leptin concentrations in women, *Diabetes,* 48, 334–341, 1999.

54. Considine, R. and Caro, J., Leptin: genes, concepts and clinical perspective, *Horm. Res.,* 46, 249–256, 1996.
55. Frederich, R.C., Hamann, A., Anderson, S., Lollmann, B., Lowell, B.B., and Flier, J.S., Leptin levels reflect body lipid content in mice: evidence for diet-induced resistance to leptin action, *Nat. Med.,* 1, 1311–1314, 1995.
56. Caro, J., Kolaczynski, J., Nyce, M., Ohannesian, I., Goldman, W., Lynn, R., and Zhang, P., Decreased cerebrospinal-fluid/serum leptin ratio in obesity: a possible mechanism for leptin resistance, *Lancet,* 348, 159–161, 1996.
57. Banks, W.A., Leptin transport across the blood-brain barrier: implications for the cause and treatment of obesity, *Curr. Pharm. Des.,* 7, 125–133, 2001.
58. Hileman, S.M., Pierroz, D.D., Masuzaki, H., Bjorbaek, C., El Haschimi, K., Banks, W.A., and Flier, J.S., Characterization of short isoforms of the leptin receptor in rat cerebral microvessels and of brain uptake of leptin in mouse models of obesity, *Endocrinology,* 143, 775–783, 2002.
59. Yeo, G.S., Farooqi, I.S., Aminian, S., Halsall, D.J., Stanhope, R.G., and O'Rahilly, S., A frameshift mutation in MC4R associated with dominantly inherited human obesity, *Nat. Genet.,* 20, 111–112, 1998.
60. Montague, C.T., Farooqi, I.S., Whitehead, J.P., Soos, M.A., Rau, H., Wareham, N.J., Sewter, C.P., Digby, J.E., Mohammed, S.N., Hurst, J.A., Cheetham, C.H., Earley, A.R., Barnett, A.H., Prins, J.B., and O'Rahilly, S., Congenital leptin deficiency is associated with severe early-onset obesity in humans, *Nature,* 387, 903–908, 1997.
61. Gibson, W.T., Farooqi, I.S., Moreau, M., DePaoli, A.M., Lawrence, E., O'Rahilly, S., and Trussell, R.A., Congenital leptin deficiency due to homozygosity for the Delta133G mutation: report of another case and evaluation of response to four years of leptin therapy, *J. Clin. Endocrinol. Metab.,* 89, 4821–4826, 2004.
62. Hukshorn, C.J., Saris, W.H., Westerterp-Plantenga, M.S., Farid, A.R., Smith, F.J., and Campfield, L.A., Weekly subcutaneous pegylated recombinant native human leptin (PEG-OB) administration in obese men, *J. Clin. Endocrinol. Metab.,* 85, 4003–4009, 2000.
63. Ahima, R.S., Saper, C.B., Flier, J.S., and Elmquist, J.K., Leptin regulation of neuroendocrine systems, *Front. Neuroendocrinol.,* 21, 263–307, 2000.
64. Maffei, M., Halaas, J., Ravussin, E., Pratley, R., Lee, G., Zhang, Y., Fei, H., Kim, S., Lallone, R., and Ranganathan, S., Leptin levels in human and rodent: measurement of plasma leptin and ob RNA in obese and weight reduced subjects, *Nat. Med.,* 1, 1155–1161, 1995.
65. Sinha, M., Ohannesian, J., Heiman, M., Kriauciunas, A., and Stephens, T., Nocturnal rise of leptin in lean, obese, and non-insulin-dependent diabetes mellitus subjects, *J. Clin. Invest.,* 97, 1344–1347, 1996.
66. Mueller, W.M., Gregoire, F.M., Stanhope, K.L., Mobbs, C.V., Mizuno, T.M., Warden, C.H., Stern, J.S., and Havel, P.J., Evidence that glucose metabolism regulates leptin secretion from cultured rat adipocytes, *Endocrinology,* 139, 551–558, 1998.
67. Utriainen, T., Malmstrom, R., Makimattila, S., and Yki-Jarvinen, H., Supraphysiological hyperinsulinemia increases plasma leptin concentrations after 4 h in normal subjects, *Diabetes,* 45, 1364–1366, 1996.
68. Havel, P.J., Townsend, R.C.L., and Teff, K., High-fat meals reduce 24-h circulating leptin concentrations in women, *Diabetes,* 48, 334–341, 1999.
69. Banks, W.A., Coon, A.B., Robinson, S.M., Moinuddin, A., Shultz, J.M., Nakaoke, R., and Morley, J.E., Triglycerides induce leptin resistance at the blood-brain barrier, *Diabetes,* 53, 1253–1260, 2004.
70. Heini, A.F., Lara-Castro, C., Kirk, K.A., Considine, R.V., Caro, J.F., and Weinsier, R.L., Association of leptin and hunger-satiety ratings in obese women, *Int. J. Obes. Relat. Metab. Disord.,* 22, 1084–1087, 1998.

71. Keim, N., Stern, J., and Havel, P., Relation between circulating leptin concentrations and appetite during a prolonged, moderate energy deficit in women, *Amer. J. Clin. Nutr.*, 68, 794–801, 1998.
72. Creutzfeldt, W. and Ebert, R., New developments in the incretin concept, *Diabetologia*, 28, 565–573, 1985.
73. Nauck, M.A., Niedereichholz, U., Etler, R., Holst, J.J., Orskov, C., Ritzel, R., and Schmiegel, W.H., Glucagon-like peptide 1 inhibition of gastric emptying outweights its insulinotropic effects in healthy humans, *Am. J. Physiol.*, 273, E981–E988, 1997.
74. Ahren, B., Gut peptides and type 2 diabetes mellitus treatment, *Curr. Diab. Rep.*, 3, 365–372, 2003.
75. D'Alessio, D., Vahl, T., and Prigeon, R., Effects of glucagon-like peptide 1 on the hepatic glucose metabolism, *Horm. Metab. Res.*, 36, 837–841, 2004.
76. Degen, L., Oesch, S., Matzinger, D., Drewe, J., Knupp, M., Zimmerli, F., and Beglinger, C., Effects of a preload on reduction of food intake by GLP-1 in healthy subjects, *Digestion,* 74, 78–84, 2006.
77. Deleon, D., Crutchlow, M., Ham, J., and Stoffers, D., Role of GLP-1 in the pathogenesis and treatment of diabetes mellitus, *Int. J. Biochem. Cell. Biol.*, 38, 845–859, 2006.
78. Hermann, C., Goke, R., Richter, G., Fehmann, H., Arnold, R., and Goke, B., Glucagon-like peptide-1 and glucose-dependent insulin-releasing polypeptide plasma levels in response to nutrients, *Digestion,* 56, 117–126, 1995.
79. Holst, J., Glucagon-like peptide 1 (GLP-1): an intestinal hormone, signalling nutritional abundance, with an unusual therapeutic potential, *Trends Endocrinol. Metab.*, 10, 229–235, 1999.
80. Morgan, L., Elliott, R., Tredger, J., Nightingale, J., and Marks, V., GLP-1 secretion in response to nutrients in man, *Digestion,* 54, 374–376, 1993.
81. Fehmann, H., Goke, R., and Goke, B., Cell and molecular biology of the incretin hormones glucagon-like peptide-1 and glucose-dependent insulin releasing polypeptide, *Endocrine Rev.*, 16, 390–410, 1995.
82. Hvidberg, A., Nielsen, M., Hilstead, J., Orskov, C., and Holst, J., Effect of glucagons-like peptide 1 on hepatic glucose production in healthy man, *Metabolism,* 43, 104–108, 1994.
83. Flint, A., Raben, A., Astrup, A., and Holst, J., Glucagon-like peptide-1 promotes satiety and suppressses energy intake in humans, *J. Clin. Invest.*, 101, 515–520, 1998.
84. Flint, A., Raben, A., Ersboll, A., Holst, J., and Astrup, A., The effect of physiologic levels of glucagon-like peptide-1 on appetite, gastric emptying, energy and substrate metabolism in obesity, *Int. J. Obes.*, 25, 781–792, 2001.
85. Kastin, A.J., Akerstrom, V., and Pan, W., Interactions of glucagon-like peptide-1 (GLP-1) with the blood-brain barrier, *J. Mol. Neurosci.*, 18, 7–14, 2002.
86. Frezza, E.E., Wachtel, M.S., and Chiriva-Internati, M., The multiple faces of glucagon-like peptide-1-obesity, appetite, and stress: what is next? A review, *Dig. Dis. Sci.*, 52, 643–649, 2007.
87. Stanley, S., Wynne, K., and Bloom, S., Gastrointestinal satiety signals III. Glucagon-like peptide 1, oxyntomodulin, peptide YY, and pancreatic polypeptide, *Am. J. Physiol. Gastrointest. Liver Physiol.*, 286, G693–G697, 2004.
88. Turton, M.D., O'Shea, D., Gunn, I., Beak, S.A., Edwards, C.M., Meeran, K., Choi, S.J., Taylor, G.M., Heath, M.M., Lambert, P.D., Wilding, J.P., Smith, D.M., Ghatei, M.A., Herbert, J., and Bloom, S.R., A role for glucagon-like peptide-1 in the central regulation of feeding, *Nature,* 379, 69–72, 1996.
89. Meeran, K., O'Shea, D., Edwards, C.M., Turton, M.D., Heath, M.M., Gunn, I., Abusnana, S., Rossi, M., Small, C.J., Goldstone, A.P., Taylor, G.M., Sunter, D., Steere, J., Choi, S.J., Ghatei, M.A., and Bloom, S.R., Repeated intracerebroventricular administration of glucagon-like peptide-1-(7–36) amide or exendin-(9–39) alters body weight in the rat, *Endocrinology,* 140, 244–250, 1999.

90. Gutzwiller, J., Drewe, J., and Goke, B., Glucagon-like-peptide-1 promotes satiety and reduces food intake in patients with diabetes mellitus type 2, *Am. J. Physiol.,* 276, R1541–R1544, 1999.
91. Gutzwiller, J., Goke, B., and Drewe, J., Glucagon-like peptide-1: a potent regulator of food intake in humans, *Gut,* 44, 81–86, 1999.
92. Toft-Nielsen, M., Madsbad, S., and Holst, J., Continous subcutaneous infusion of GLP-1 lower plasma glucose and reduces appetite in Type 2 diabetic patients, *Diabetes Care,* 22, 1137–1143, 1999.
93. Verdich, C., Toubro, S., Buemann, B., Lysgard, M.J., Juul, H.J., and Astrup, A., The role of postprandial releases of insulin and incretin hormones in meal-induced satiety--effect of obesity and weight reduction, *Int. J. Obes. Relat. Metab. Disord.,* 25, 1206–1214, 2001.
94. Ranganath, L.R., Beety, J.M., Morgan, L.M., Wright, J.W., Howland, R., and Marks, V., Attenuated GLP-1 secretion in obesity: cause or consequence? *Gut,* 38, 916–919, 1996.
95. Perez-Tilve, D., Nogueiras, R., Mallo, F., Benoit, S.C., and Tschoep, M., Gut hormones ghrelin, PYY, and GLP-1 in the regulation of energy balance [corrected] and metabolism, *Endocrine,* 29, 61–71, 2006.
96. Iritani, N., Sugimoto, T., Fukuda, H., Komiya, M., and Ikeda, H., Oral triacylglycerols regulate plasma glucagon-like peptide-1(7–36) and insulin levels in normal and especially in obese rats, *J. Nutr.,* 129, 46–50, 1999.
97. Vilsboll, T., Agerso, H., Krarup, T., and Holst, J.J., Similar elimination rates of glucagon-like peptide-1 in obese type 2 diabetic patients and healthy subjects, *J. Clin. Endocrinol. Metab.,* 88, 220–224, 2003.
98. Drucker, D.J., The biology of incretin hormones, *Cell. Metab.,* 3, 153–165, 2006.
99. Adrian, T.E., Ferri, G.L., Bacarese-Hamilton, A.J., Fuessl, H.S., Polak, J.M., and Bloom, S.R., Human distribution and release of a putative new gut hormone, peptide YY, *Gastroenterology,* 89, 1070–1077, 1985.
100. Feltrin, K.L., Little, T.J., Meyer, J.H., Horowitz, M., Smout, A.J., Wishart, J., Pilichiewicz, A.N., Rades, T., Chapman, I.M., and Feinle-Bisset, C., Effects of intraduodenal fatty acids on appetite, antropyloroduodenal motility, and plasma CCK and GLP-1 in humans vary with their chain length, *Am. J. Physiol. Regul. Integr. Comp. Physiol.,* 287, R524–R533, 2004.
101. Berglund, M.M., Hipskind, P.A., and Gehlert, D.R., Recent developments in our understanding of the physiological role of PP-fold peptide receptor subtypes, *Exp. Biol. Med. (Maywood),* 228, 217–244, 2003.
102. Nonaka, N., Shioda, S., Niehoff, M.L., and Banks, W.A., Characterization of blood-brain barrier permeability to PYY3–36 in the mouse, *J. Pharmacol. Exp. Ther.,* 306, 948–953, 2003.
103. Boggiano, M.M., Chandler, P.C., Oswald, K.D., Rodgers, R.J., Blundell, J.E., Ishii, Y., Beattie, A.H., Holch, P., Allison, D.B., Schindler, M., Arndt, K., Rudolf, K., Mark, M., Schoelch, C., Joost, H.G., Klaus, S., Thone-Reineke, C., Benoit, S.C., Seeley, R.J., Beck-Sickinger, A.G., Koglin, N., Raun, K., Madsen, K., Wulff, B.S., Stidsen, C.E., Birringer, M., Kreuzer, O.J., Deng, X.Y., Whitcomb, D.C., Halem, H., Taylor, J., Dong, J., Datta, R., Culler, M., Ortmann, S., Castaneda, T.R., and Tschop, M., PYY3–36 as an anti-obesity drug target, *Obes. Rev.,* 6, 307–322, 2005.
104. Batterham, R.L., Le Roux, C.W., Cohen, M.A., Park, A.J., Ellis, S.M., Patterson, M., Frost, G.S., Ghatei, M.A., and Bloom, S.R., Pancreatic polypeptide reduces appetite and food intake in humans, *J. Clin. Endo. Metab.,* 88, 3989–3992, 2003.

13 Gastrointestinal Sensorineural Function in the Control of Food Intake

Gary J. Schwartz

CONTENTS

13.1 INTRODUCTION

The upper gastrointestinal tract is a critical site for the negative feedback control of food intake. Its significance is supported by studies in human and nonhuman primates, as well as in rodents, demonstrating that, when nutrients fail to stimulate the proximal duodenum during sham feeding, both meal duration and the amount of food consumed are dramatically increased. Furthermore, infusions of nutrients directly into the duodenum at rates that mimic the physiological time course of gastric emptying have been shown to potently and dose-dependently reduce subsequent food intake. Gastrointestinal nutrients also potently slow gastric emptying, depending on their caloric density, providing a local means by which nutrient absorption and nutrient-stimulated gut hormone release are regulated to modulate energy availability and thereby help determine energy balance. During a typical meal, which is the functional unit of ingestion in humans, nonhuman primates, and rodents, the majority of ingested food accumulates within the stomach, pending its controlled gastric emptying into small intestinal sites that mediate nutrient absorption. Nutrient absorption begins within minutes of the onset of a meal, and, depending on the amount of food consumed, persists for several hours following meal termination. This temporal distribution of nutrients means that upper gastrointestinal sites continue to be stimulated by food during and following the onset of nutrient absorption. Both gastric and upper intestinal sites are richly innervated with intrinsic, enteric neurons, as well as with extrinsic sensory vagal and nonvagal visceral afferent neurons that are responsive to meal-related mechanical, chemical, neuropeptide, and neurotransmitter stimuli. Chemical or surgical interruption of this meal-stimulated sensory neural traffic between the gut and the brain impedes the flow of negative feedback signals that normally contribute to the control of food intake by limiting meal size. The extrinsic neural innervation of the upper gut, in turn, projects to a wide range of interconnected central nervous system targets that can collectively be considered the central distribution of the gut–brain neuraxis. This neuraxis includes the termination sites of incoming gut afferents in the caudal hindbrain, as well as forebrain projection areas in hypothalamic, limbic, and other telencephalic regions involved in the processing of meal-stimulated visceral input. This chapter will review recent advances in our understanding of the sensory capabilities of the gut–brain neuraxis in the reception, transmission, and integration of meal-stimulated signals that contribute to the control of food intake from a basic science perspective in rodent models and, in doing so, suggest sites and modes of action by which altering gastrointestinal sensorineural processing can modulate human feeding.

13.2 GUT–BRAIN NEUROAXIS

The neuroanatomical extent of the afferent distribution of upper gut information to the brain has recently been approached using an H129 strain of herpes simplex virus which undergoes transneuronal transport.[1] Injections into the ventral wall of the rat stomach revealed that the virus was transneuronally transported into a range of spinal, hindbrain, and forebrain sites in neurologically intact rats. Initially, labeling was detected in vagal sensory neurons in the nodose ganglion and spinal viscerosensory neurons in the celiac superior mesenteric ganglion, as well as their respective targets in the brain stem nucleus of the solitary tract and thoracic dorsal horn. At later time points, additional hindbrain and forebrain viscerosensitive regions were labeled, including the caudal brain stem lateral and medial parabrachial nuclei, and in the forebrain, the hypothalamic dorsomedial, paraventricular, supraoptic, arcuate, and lateral subnuclei, the central nucleus of the amygdala, lateral and medial septal nuclei, and agranular insular cortex. Surgical transection of vagal afferent roots as they enter the brain stem attenuated transneuronal transport and infection of neurons within the brain stem nucleus of the solitary tract, demonstrating a critical role for the afferent vagus in the transmission of meal-related gut signals. Vagal afferent innervation of the proximal small intestine may be particularly important in determining the negative feedback effects of nutrients; the paucity of small intestinal vagal afferent terminations in animals deficient in neurotensin-4 results in a feeding phenotype characterized by reduced sensitivity to the satiating effects of gastrointestinal lipids.[2]

This gut vagal afferent pathway, however, is not unique in its ability to convey meal-related signals to the central nervous system sites modulating food intake. Nonvagal, splanchnic afferents have also been implicated in the control of meal size and nutrient detection, and surgical interruption of these visceral afferents by removal of the celiac-superior mesenteric ganglionic plexus in rats blocks the ability of duodenal fat emulsions or carbohydrate solutions to attenuate subsequent feeding.[3] To appreciate the molecular sources of food-stimulated negative feedback, it is essential to characterize the receptor subtypes and signaling mechanisms available to these peripheral sensory paths.

13.3 GUT SIGNALING IN THE ABSORPTIVE PHASE — CANDIDATE MEDIATORS

Gut afferent fibers have been demonstrated to be activated by nutrients as well as by peptides and neurochemicals that are released following gastrointestinal exposure to nutrients. For example, glucose, as a product of the nutrient absorptive process, has been described as a potent modulator of vagal activity in afferents supplying the hepatic portal vein.[4] A novel dimension of gut feedback secondary to intestinal nutrient exposure has been identified by the recent work of Mithieux et al.,[5] demonstrating an intrinsic cycle within the gut wall whereby dietary protein induces intestinal gluconeogenesis, which in turn stimulates hepatic portal glucoreceptors in the afferent vagus. This mechanism has been proposed to contribute to the feeding inhibitory effects of high-protein diets.[5] Insulin has also been shown to modulate activity in gut vagal afferents both in hepatic portal afferents and, more recently, in duodenal afferents in pigs. Hyperinsulinemia increased the basal activity of duodenal vagal mechanoreceptors without altering the magnitude of responses to mechanical distension stimuli.[6] Thus, hepatic and duodenal sites are stimulated during nutrient absorption to help determine gut vagal afferent signaling.

Receptors for multiple meal-stimulated gut–brain peptides have also been localized to vagal sensory neurons. These include, but are not limited to, cholecystokinin A (CCKA) receptors, serotonin-3 (5HT3) receptors, as well as mRNA for ghrelin, leptin, peptide YY (PYY), and glucagon-like peptide-1 (GLP-1) receptors. Peripheral roles for ligands of each of these receptors have been proposed in the feedback control of energy intake. Examples of results from rodent studies of these compounds reveal a variety of ways in which these signaling molecules act alone or in concert to generate feeding modulatory signals at peripheral and brain stem levels of the gut–brain neuraxis.

Intestinal luminal glucose and maltose stimulate a subpopulation of 5HT-sensitive small intestinal vagal afferent nodose neurons, via 5HT3/4R.[7] Intestinal glucose also stimulates local release of 5HT into the mesenteric lumen.[8] Peripheral administration of the 5HT3R antagonist ondansetron has been shown to mediate intestinal lipid- and glucose-induced satiation as well as lipid-induced activation of the brain stem nucleus of the solitary tract (NTS) in regions where gut vagal afferents terminate.[9,10] 5HT3 receptors also are present in gut-recipient areas of the NTS and contribute to the control of meal size.[11] Although it remains unclear whether these brain stem 5HT3 receptors are on vagal afferent terminals ascending from the gut or on NTS neurons themselves, either possibility is consistent with the idea that this receptor subtype plays a critical role in mediating the central processing of nutrient-induced gut negative feedback signals.

Vagal afferents also integrate responses to multiple simultaneously occurring meal-stimulated signals. For example, a subpopulation of duodenal vagal afferents are stimulated by both CCK and 5HT, and combinations of these stimuli are more effective in modulating vagal afferent activity than either stimulus alone.[12] This integrative capacity may play a role in the ability of combinations of CCKA antagonists and ondansetron to completely account for intestinal lipid-induced suppression of food intake.[13] Ondansetron has also been shown to reduce binge frequency in bulimics, suggesting this receptor subtype as a potential therapeutic target as part of a combined strategy to augment the feeding inhibitory effects of orally ingested nutrients.[14] Taken together, these results suggest that translational work could be done using ondansetron (1) to selectively examine the extent to which 5HT3R blockade affects the temporal and spatial patterns of human neural activation produced by a meal using current imaging strategies, and (2) to develop animal models of the 5HT3R-dependent patterns of neuronal activation produced by meals. These data also underscore the potential for conservative functions for gut–brain peptides released during nutrient absorption: (1) nutrient stimulated gastrointestinal factors can act by multiple neurohumoral modes, paracrine as well as endocrine; (2) they can act at multiple sites simultaneously; and (3) their actions at multiple sites along the gut–brain axis may serve a common behavioral outcome — the regulation of energy intake.

Ghrelin is a novel feeding stimulatory gut peptide whose secretion is negatively regulated by food consumption, particularly by delivery of nutrients to the lumen of the small intestine.[15] Ghrelin receptors have been localized to rat and mouse nodose ganglion neurons, the sensory cell bodies of vagal afferent fibers that innervate a range of supra- and subdiaphragmatic targets, including the stomach and small intestine.[16–17] Ghrelin has also been recently demonstrated to inhibit gut afferent mechanosensitivity to circumferential tension in mouse.[17] It would not be surprising if ghrelin receptors were specifically expressed by vagal afferent neurons carrying meal-related signals from the upper gastrointestinal tract to the CNS; however, the role for vagal afferent receptors in mediating ghrelin-induced increases in feeding remains unclear. Initial reports demonstrated that vagotomy blocked feeding stimulation caused by ghrelin, and, consistent with a role for the afferent vagus in transmitting negative feedback signals that limit food intake, that ghrelin itself attenuated the neurophysiological multiunit activity of gut vagal afferents.[18] Additionally, humans undergoing vagotomy in the course of gastric or esophageal surgery fail to increase feeding in response to ghrelin.[19] More recent experiments designed to refine this analysis in rodents have instead revealed that selective gut deafferentation fails to alter the increase in food intake that is induced by peripheral ghrelin, and that local ghrelin infusion is not an adequate stimulus to affect neurophysiological activity in single-unit studies of gastric and duodenal vagal afferents.[20] Although there are additional neuronal ghrelin receptor message-expressing sites distributed across brain stem and hypothalamic levels of the gut–brain axis,[21] it is not yet known how, or whether, these sites modify the processing of meal-related signals, or how such actions may be related to the control of food intake during a meal.

The adiposity hormone leptin provides an additional important focus for peri- and postabsorptive neurohumoral signals in the control of food intake. Circulating leptin levels are proportional to body adiposity, reflecting the consequences of effective nutrient absorption and storage. Leptin is also present in the rodent and human stomach,[22–23] where, upon insulin stimulation, it is released to contact either neural or duodenal luminal absorptive sites. The functional long-form leptin receptor is expressed at these loci in rodents and humans,[24–25] and intestinal leptin can modulate the absorptive flux of nutrients across the gut epithelium and into the bloodstream.[26] Long-form leptin receptors are also distributed across several nodes of the gut–brain neuraxis, including primary gut vagal afferents,[27] nodose ganglion neurons receiving gut input,[28–29] brain stem neurons receiving gut input,[30–33] and hypothalamic neuronal populations activated by meals and implicated in the control of food intake, such as the arcuate and ventromedial nuclei.[32–33] This distribution raises the possibility that leptin can act at multiple sites along the gut–brain axis simultaneously to modulate food intake, and new evidence strongly supports this view. Local celiac arterial but not jugular vein infusion of leptin reduces feeding, and this reduction is blocked by vagotomy or by capsaicin, a neurotoxin that selectively destroys a subpopulation of vagal afferents. These data support a role for vagal afferent leptinergic signals in its local feeding inhibitory actions. Peripheral leptin has also been shown to modulate neurophysiological activity in primary gut vagal afferents[34] as well as nodose ganglion neurons receiving input from gastric and intestinal primary vagal sensors.[35] In the forebrain, leptin modulates the neurophysiological activity of multiple feeding-related hypothalamic neuronal subpopulations, including the arcuate, lateral, and ventromedial nuclei.[36]

Leptin exposure also modifies the peripheral and central nervous system responses to meal-related stimuli in a manner that is consistent with a role in the control of feeding. Reductions in food intake produced by celiac artery leptin infusions are augmented by coinfusion of the gut satiety peptide CCK.[37] Combinations of central leptin and peripheral CCK or gastric nutrient loads reduce meal size and increase the number of neurons expressing c-fos, a marker of cellular activation, in gut-recipient regions of the NTS.[38–39] Furthermore, combinations of gastric distention and central leptin produce a greater degree of activation in gut-recipient NTS neurons than either stimulus alone.[40–41] Taken together, these data support a role for integration in gut-recipient nodose and brain stem neurons in the early neural processing of food-related signals during meal consumption and absorption. In this regard, both hindbrain and forebrain sites along the gut–brain axis share another potentially critical morphological feature — the presence of a relatively leaky blood–brain barrier with a specialized circulatory network that has the potential for a greater degree of neuronal exposure to nutrient and neurohumoral meal-related signals. In the hindbrain this role is served by the area postrema adjacent to the NTS,[42–43] while the median eminence adjacent to the hypothalamic arcuate nucleus provides preferred bloodborne access.[44]

As leptin receptors have been localized to peripheral and central levels of the human gut–brain axis, including the neocortex,[33] functional imaging studies following a meal under different systemic leptin conditions could provide important clues as to (1) the neuroanatomical targets of putative leptinergic modulation of the neural processing of a meal in humans, (2) the degree to which the metabolic context modulates the meal-induced patterns of activation, and (3) any correlations among leptin levels, meal-stimulated neural activation, and meal size and duration.

Glucagon-like peptide-1 (GLP-1), secreted by ileal L-cells in response to intestinal nutrient exposure, is a significant candidate mediator of food-stimulated negative feedback signaling during the digestive process. In addition to its central inhibitory effects on feeding, peripheral systemic administration of the GLP-1 receptor agonist exendin 4 potently reduces food intake and gastric emptying in rodents and in both human and nonhuman primates.[45–46] GLP-1 receptors are present at multiple sites along the rodent and human gut–brain neuraxis, in nodose ganglion cells supplying vagal afferents, brain stem gut recipient neurons, and hypothalamic neuronal populations that have been implicated in the control of food intake.[47–50] In rats, GLP-1 stimulates hepatic portal vagal afferents, nodose ganglion neurons, and hypothalamic proopiomelanocortin (POMC) neurons,[51–53] while recent human studies using fluorodeoxyglucose demonstrate that GLP-1 significantly reduces cerebral glucose metabolism in both the hypothalamus and brain stem.[50] A functional role for this pathway is also supported by recent work in rats demonstrating that surgical interruption of the gut–brain axis at either the peripheral vagal or the brain stem-hypothalamic linkages attenuates GLP-1-induced reductions in food intake.[54]

GLP-1 elicits a coordinated set of responses that limit nutrient distribution, including increasing insulin secretion, reducing gastric emptying to limit the rate of nutrient absorption, and modulating feeding behavior directly. Neuroimaging across multiple targets during plasma GLP-1 excursions can, therefore, provide a window on the pattern of neural activation associated with each of these coordinated effects. In progress toward this end, peak postprandial levels of GLP-1 have been positively correlated with increased levels of brain activation in hypothalamic and dorsal prefrontal cortical regions associated with human satiation.[55] Parallel studies in rodents and nonhuman primates have not been performed, but would permit more extensive and hypothesis-driven investigations of the importance of these areas in the neural processing of GLP-1 signals that modify feeding. In addition, there is behavioral evidence that intraluminal intestinal protein infusions increase the inhibitory effect of GLP-1 on food intake in humans;[56] here again, imaging studies could be useful in identifying neuroanatomical sites of convergent activation or integration that are important in this effect. Furthermore, complimentary data evaluating GLP-1 interactions with other gastrointestinal negative feedback stimuli in rodent models would significantly increase the strength of the translational approach to understanding the role of meal-stimulated gut–brain peptides in the control of food intake.

The above types of peripheral and central signal interactions reflect three critical features of the neural processing of nutrient stimulation in the control of food intake:

1. There is neuroanatomical convergence of multiple meal-stimulated peri- and postabsorptive signals throughout the gut–brain axis.
2. The nervous system response to meal-related signals that occurs during and after nutrient absorption depends on the metabolic context in which they are delivered, and, in some cases, on secretions related to stored nutrients.
3. Individual elements along the gut–brain axis have the capacity to integrate signals arising from multiple meal-related stimuli to modify neural activity and feeding.

13.4 CHEMICAL SENSING IN THE GUT

As a future direction, there is a growing body of literature demonstrating that nutrient transporters, gustatory, and even olfactory transducer elements are present within the gastrointestinal tract and may play an important role in nutrient detection and/or absorption. These include the intestinal assessment of fat transporters, such as CD36, ApoIV, as well as gustducin-like proteins and taste receptors for chemical compounds that are psychophysically reported as sweet and bitter substances. Recent examples reveal the ways in which such intestinal molecules may mediate the control of food intake through multiple simultaneous transduction and absorption events. The fatty acid transporter CD36 is localized to the small intestinal mucosa and has been linked to fat absorption and plasma cholesterol levels.[57] The jejuno-ileal satiety factor ApoIV mediates chylomicron formation, stimulates duodenal vagal afferents, is involved in the intestinal detection of intestinal lipid, and acts peripherally, as well as in the arcuate hypothalamus, to inhibit feeding.[58–60] Enteroendocrine cells of the brush border of the small intestine express the taste receptor protein alpha gustducin and coexpress either 5HT or GLP-1, as well as olfactory receptors linked to 5HT release upon odorant stimulation.[61–65] These data suggest a linkage between nutrient detection and release of neurohumoral factors that may directly (via vagal or brain stem signaling) or indirectly (via their ability to inhibit gastric emptying) affect food intake and absorption during a meal. More recently, sweet taste receptors have been localized to, and characterized in, the rat and mouse small intestine, where they have the ability to mediate glucose transport.[66] Such findings begin to blur the line between detection and transport in the sequence of events leading to propagation of negative feedback signals during absorption that limit food intake. The biochemical linkages between the functions of these transducer cells, transporters, and extrinsic neural elements that carry meal-related signals to the brain remain an open avenue of investigation.

13.5 ELECTRICAL GUT STIMULATION

Given the multiplicity of gut vagal afferent meal-related signals demonstrated to inhibit food intake, it is not unreasonable to suggest that vagal stimulation *per se* may be effective in modulating energy balance. Gastric electrical stimulation, which typically activates gut vagal afferents, has been reported to induce chronic reductions in body weight gain and food intake in rabbits,[67] dogs,[68] and more recently, in pigs,[69] an animal model that more closely approximates human gut vagal neuroanatomy. Gastric distension-sensitive neurons in the rat ventromedial hypothalamic nucleus also respond to gastric electrical stimulation.[70] Chronic vagal stimulation in the context of therapy for severe, treatment-resistant depression has been reported to reduce body weight in the absence of reduced food intake[71] and alters reporting of craving for sweet foods in response to food images.[72] Gastric pacing in morbidly obese patients has been associated with significant weight loss, reduced basal levels of leptin and GLP-1, and reduced prandial excursions of CCK and somatostatin,[73–74] and a single report demonstrates acute reductions in food intake during stimulation.[75] Human vagal stimulation is amenable to analysis by fMRI,[76] and as vagal trunk and gastric pacing stimulation becomes more refined and specific, their roles in modulating food intake and the relationships between any feeding modulatory actions and differential activation of the human gut–brain axis may be more coherently assessed.

13.6 FOREBRAIN NEURAL REPRESENTATION OF A MEAL

Work in nonhuman primates has demonstrated a significant role for anterior cortical sites, particularly the orbitofrontal cortex, in the processing of meal-related stimuli.[77] More recent studies by Pritchard and colleagues have revealed a novel taste-responsive area in the medial orbitofrontal cortex that integrates taste with postoral nutrient stimulation,[78] where feeding a caloric beverage to satiety modulates single-unit gustatory neurophysiological responses.[79] There is some preliminary concordance between human and nonhuman primate study results, in that both appetitive and consummatory aspects of food stimuli affect orbitofrontal cortex activity in humans; the orbitofrontal cortex is more metabolically active during presentation of either pictures of food or food itself.[80–82] Glucose ingestion also alters human hypothalamic function, and both energy content and sweet taste may be required for these effects, as ingestion of glucose, but not other nonsweet, caloric solutions results in a significant and persistent reduction in hypothalamic activation.[83] Sweet and nonsweet equicaloric glucose and maltodextrin solutions did not differ in their ability to elevate plasma insulin and glucose. Thus, the hypothalamic response does not depend on these postabsorptive measures. Oral glucose at doses that produce plasma levels lower than those produced by intravenous infusions of glucose that are effective for MRI changes, produces a more profound and longer lasting suppression of BOLD fMRI than intravenous glucose and a concomitant prolonged elevation in plasma insulin.[84] These data suggest that the neurohumoral factors driven by oral rather than intravenous glucose availability play an important role in modulating the hypothalamic response to glucose. In rats, orally consumed glucose has been shown to differentially modulate hypothalamic activity as assessed by micro-PET as a function of time relative to the glucose meal.[85] Better temporal and spatial resolution applied to these studies and more rational stimulus presentation designed to mimic the postabsorptive availability of nutrients will increase the interpretability of new data.

A major concern from a translational perspective is that, while human studies have begun to evaluate the pattern of neural responses to both appetitive and consummatory aspects of food intake, this has not been systematically approached in animal models. Overall, results from both human and animal studies are difficult to interpret coherently because of the variety of stimuli used, including appetitive aspects of meal taking such as the sight, taste, and smell of food, which will maximally stimulate the orosensory and olfactory apparatus while minimally engaging sites involved in nutrient absorption, versus studies in which imaging is performed after more substantial caloric intake, where the absorptive consequences of nutrient ingestion of a meal may influence the pattern of activation. In addition, the brain stem is not commonly assessed in these studies, and given the extent and concentration of meal-related neurohumoral signals available to this area, refinement of human neuroimaging technology to permit assessment of this area (1) is likely to reveal significant changes in distinct metabolic conditions and (2) has the potential to identify therapeutic neurochemical and neuroanatomical targets in the diagnosis or treatment for eating and metabolic disorders.

13.7 A TRANSLATIONAL APPROACH TO GUT–BRAIN COMMUNICATION IN THE CONTROL OF FOOD INTAKE

Finally, from a technical perspective, there are early reports that may provide a translational approach to bridging the gaps in understanding the biological basis of human food-stimulated imaging and that found in animal models. Recent work of Lazovic and colleagues has fruitfully compared measures of c-fos activation following colorectal distension to fMRI performed in anesthetized rats,[86] and gastric distension can be used as a potent stimulus in functional human neuroimaging.[87] Paired studies of c-fos activation and fMRI in rats following 5HT2C stimulation or antagonists, implicated both in anxiety and feeding, engaged many telencephalic structures implicated in gut–brain axis activation, including the paraventricular and dorsomedial hypothalamus and cingulate and orbitofrontal cortices.[88] These data demonstrate that parallels in the pattern of activation can be identified and quantified and suggest that c-fos and fMRI may provide distinct, but complimentary spatial information and temporal resolution, respectively. Furthermore, the overlap of c-fos and fMRI activation provides the opportunity to characterize the neurochemical phenotypes and interconnectivity of activated neurons, helping to both more clearly establish the neural representation and processing of a meal and target neurochemical and/or neuropeptide factors acting in particular central locations relevant for the control of feeding.

ACKNOWLEDGMENTS

Supported by NIH DK047208 and the Skirball Institute.

REFERENCES

1. Rinaman, L. and Schwartz, G., Anterograde transneuronal viral tracing of central viscerosensory pathways in rats, *J. Neurosci.*, 24, 2782, 2004.
2. Chi, M.M. and Powley, T.L., NT-4-deficient mice lack sensitivity to meal-associated preabsorptive feedback from lipids, *Am. J. Physiol. Regul. Integr. Comp. Physiol.*, 292, R2124, 2007.
3. Sclafani, A., Ackroff, K., and Schwartz, G.J., Selective effects of vagal deafferentation and celiac-superior mesenteric ganglionectomy on the reinforcing and satiating action of intestinal nutrients, *Physiol. Behav.*, 78, 285, 2003.
4. Nagase, H. et al., Hepatic glucose-sensitive unit regulation of glucose-induced insulin secretion in rats, *Physiol. Behav.*, 53, 139, 1993.
5. Mithieux, G. et al., Portal sensing of intestinal gluconeogenesis is a mechanistic link in the diminution of food intake induced by diet protein, *Cell Metab.*, 2, 321, 2005.
6. Blat, S. and Malbert, C.H., Insulin modulates duodenal vagal afferent basal activity, *Auton. Neurosci.*, 122, 29, 2005.

7. Zhu, J. et al., Intestinal serotonin acts as a paracrine substance to mediate vagal signal transmission evoked by luminal factors in the rat, *J. Physiol.,* 530, 431, 2001.
8. Freeman, S.L. et al., Luminal glucose sensing in the rat intestine has characteristics of a sodium-glucose cotransporter, *Am. J. Physiol. Gastrointest. Liver Physiol.,* 291, G439, 2006.
9. Savastano, D.M., Hayes, M.R., and Covasa, M., Serotonin-type 3 receptors mediate intestinal lipid-induced satiation and Fos-like immunoreactivity in the dorsal hindbrain, *Am. J. Physiol. Regul. Integr. Comp. Physiol.,* 292, R1063, 2007.
10. Savastano, D.M., Carelle, M., and Covasa, M., Serotonin-type 3 receptors mediate intestinal Polycose- and glucose-induced suppression of intake, *Am. J. Physiol. Regul. Integr. Comp. Physiol.,* 288, R1499, 2005.
11. Hayes, M.R. and Covasa, M., Dorsal hindbrain 5-HT3 receptors participate in control of meal size and mediate CCK-induced satiation, *Brain Res.,* 1103, 99, 2006.
12. Li, Y., Wu, X.Y., and Owyang, C., Serotonin and cholecystokinin synergistically stimulate rat vagal primary afferent neurones, *J. Physiol.,* 559, 651, 2004.
13. Savastano, D.M. and Covasa, M., Intestinal nutrients elicit satiation through concomitant activation of CCK(1) and 5-HT(3) receptors, *Physiol. Behav.,* 292, R1061–R1062, 2007.
14. Faris, P.L. et al., Effect of decreasing afferent vagal activity with ondansetron on symptoms of bulimia nervosa: a randomised, double-blind trial, *Lancet,* 355, 792, 2000.
15. Overduin, J. et al., Role of the duodenum and macronutrient type in ghrelin regulation, *Endocrinology,* 146, 845, 2005.
16. Burdyga, G. et al., Ghrelin receptors in rat and human nodose ganglia: putative role in regulating CB-1 and MCH receptor abundance, *Am. J. Physiol. Gastrointest. Liver Physiol.,* 290, G1289, 2006.
17. Page, A.J. et al., Ghrelin selectively reduces mechanosensitivity of upper gastrointestinal vagal afferents, *Am. J. Physiol. Gastrointest. Liver Physiol.,* 292, G1376, 2007.
18. Date, Y. et al., The role of the gastric afferent vagal nerve in ghrelin-induced feeding and growth hormone secretion in rats, *Gastroenterology,* 123, 1120, 2002.
19. le Roux, C.W. et al., Ghrelin does not stimulate food intake in patients with surgical procedures involving vagotomy, *J. Clin. Endocrinol. Metab.,* 90, 4521, 2005.
20. Arnold, M. et al., Gut vagal afferents are not necessary for the eating-stimulatory effect of intraperitoneally injected ghrelin in the rat, *J. Neurosci.,* 26, 11052, 2006.
21. Zigman, J.M. et al., Expression of ghrelin receptor mRNA in the rat and the mouse brain, *J. Comp. Neurol.,* 494, 528, 2006; erratum in *J. Comp. Neurol.,* 499, 69, 2006.
22. Bado, A. et al., The stomach is a source of leptin, *Nature,* 394, 790, 1998.
23. Sobhani, I. et al., Vagal stimulation rapidly increases leptin secretion in human stomach, *Gastroenterology,* 122, 259, 2002.
24. Aparicio, T. et al., Leptin and Ob-Rb receptor isoform in the human digestive tract during fetal development, *J. Clin. Endocrinol. Metab.,* 90, 6177, 2005.
25. Barrenetxe, J. et al., Distribution of the long leptin receptor isoform in brush border, basolateral membrane, and cytoplasm of enterocytes, *Gut,* 50, 797, 2002.
26. Ducroc, R. et al., Luminal leptin induces rapid inhibition of active intestinal absorption of glucose mediated by sodium-glucose cotransporter 1, *Diabetes,* 54, 348, 2005.
27. Buyse, M. et al., Expression and regulation of leptin receptor proteins in afferent and efferent neurons of the vagus nerve, *Eur. J. Neurosci.,* 14, 64, 2001.
28. Peiser, C. et al., Leptin receptor expression in nodose ganglion cells projecting to the rat gastric fundus, *Neurosci. Lett.,* 320, 41, 2002.
29. Burdyga, G. et al., Expression of the leptin receptor in rat and human nodose ganglion neurones, *Neuroscience,* 109, 339, 2002.
30. Williams, K.W., Zsombok, A., and Smith, B.N., Rapid inhibition of neurons in the dorsal motor nucleus of the vagus by leptin, *Endocrinology,* 148, 1868, 2007.

31. Williams, K.W. and Smith, B.N., Rapid inhibition of neural excitability in the nucleus tractus solitarii by leptin: implications for ingestive behaviour, *J. Physiol.*, 573, 395, 2006.
32. Elmquist, J.K. et al., Distributions of leptin receptor mRNA isoforms in the rat brain, *J. Comp. Neurol.*, 395, 535, 1998.
33. Burguera, B. et al., The long form of the leptin receptor (OB-Rb) is widely expressed in the human brain, *Neuroendocrinology*, 71, 187, 2000.
34. Gaige, S., Abysique, A., and Bouvier, M., Effects of leptin on cat intestinal vagal mechanoreceptors, *J. Physiol.*, 543, 679, 2002.
35. Peters, J.H., Ritter, R.C., and Simasko, S.M., Leptin and CCK selectively activate vagal afferent neurons innervating the stomach and duodenum, *Am. J. Physiol. Regul. Integr. Comp. Physiol.*, 290, R1544, 2006.
36. Dhillon, H. et al., Leptin directly activates SF1 neurons in the VMH, and this action by leptin is required for normal body-weight homeostasis, *Neuron*, 49, 191, 2006.
37. Peters, J.H. et al., Leptin-induced satiation mediated by abdominal vagal afferents, *Am. J. Physiol. Regul. Integr. Comp. Physiol.*, 288, R879, 2005.
38. Emond, M. et al., Leptin amplifies the feeding inhibition and neural activation arising from a gastric nutrient preload, *Physiol. Behav.*, 72, 123, 2001.
39. Emond, M. et al., Central leptin modulates behavioral and neural responsivity to CCK, *Am. J. Physiol.*, 276, R1545, 1999.
40. Schwartz, G.J. and Moran, T.H., Leptin and neuropeptide y have opposing modulatory effects on nucleus of the solitary tract neurophysiological responses to gastric loads: implications for the control of food intake, *Endocrinology*, 143, 3779, 2002.
41. Huo, L. et al., Leptin and the control of food intake: neurons in the nucleus of the solitary tract are activated by both gastric distension and leptin, *Endocrinology*, 148, 2189, 2007.
42. Gross, P.M. et al., Metabolic activation of efferent pathways from the rat area postrema. *Am. J. Physiol.*, 258, R788, 1990.
43. Gross, P.M. et al., Subregional topography of capillaries in the dorsal vagal complex of rats: II. Physiological properties, *J. Comp. Neurol.*, 306, 83, 1991.
44. Cheunsuang, O., Stewart, A.L., Morris, R., Differential uptake of molecules from the circulation and CSF reveals regional and cellular specialisation in CNS detection of homeostatic signals, *Cell Tissue Res.*, 325, 397, 2006.
45. Scott, K.A. and Moran, T.H., The GLP-1 agonist exendin-4 reduces food intake in nonhuman primates through changes in meal size, *Am. J. Physiol. Regul. Integr. Comp. Physiol.*, 2007 [Epub ahead of print].
46. Chelikani, P.K., Haver, A.C., and Reidelberger, R.D., Intravenous infusion of glucagon-like peptide-1 potently inhibits food intake, sham feeding, and gastric emptying in rats, *Am. J. Physiol. Regul. Integr. Comp. Physiol.*, 288, R1695, 2005.
47. Merchenthaler, I., Lane, M., and Shughrue, P., Distribution of pre-pro-glucagon and glucagon-like peptide-1 receptor messenger RNAs in the rat central nervous system, *J. Comp. Neurol.*, 403, 261, 1999.
48. Nakagawa, A. et al., Receptor gene expression of glucagon-like peptide-1, but not glucose-dependent insulinotropic polypeptide, in rat nodose ganglion cells, *Auton. Neurosci.*, 110, 36, 2004.
49. Vahl, T.P. et al., GLP-1 receptors expressed on nerve terminals in the portal vein mediate the effects of endogenous GLP-1 on glucose tolerance in rats, *Endocrinology*, 2007 [Epub ahead of print].
50. Alvarez, E. et al., The expression of GLP-1 receptor mRNA and protein allows the effect of GLP-1 on glucose metabolism in the human hypothalamus and brainstem, *J. Neurochem.*, 92, 798, 2005.
51. Nishizawa, M. et al., The hepatic vagal reception of intraportal GLP-1 is via receptor different from the pancreatic GLP-1 receptor, *J. Auton. Nerv. Sys.*, 80, 14, 2000.

52. Kakei, M. et al., Glucagon-like peptide-1 evokes action potentials and increases cytosolic Ca2+ in rat nodose ganglion neurons, *Auton. Neurosci.*, 102, 39, 2002.
53. Ma, X., Bruning, J., and Ashcroft, F.M., Glucagon-like peptide 1 stimulates hypothalamic proopiomelanocortin neurons, *J. Neurosci.*, 27, 7125, 2007.
54. Abbott, C.R. et al., The inhibitory effects of peripheral administration of peptide YY(3-36) and glucagon-like peptide-1 on food intake are attenuated by ablation of the vagal-brainstem-hypothalamic pathway, *Brain Res.*, 1044, 127, 2005.
55. Pannacciulli, N. et al., Postprandial glucagon-like peptide-1 (GLP-1) response is positively associated with changes in neuronal activity of brain areas implicated in satiety and food intake regulation in humans, *Neuroimage*, 35, 511, 2007.
56. Degen, L. et al., Effects of a preload on reduction of food intake by GLP-1 in healthy subjects, *Digestion*, 74, 78, 2006.
57. Nassir, F. et al., CD36 is important for fatty acid and cholesterol uptake by the proximal but not distal intestine, *J. Biol. Chem.*, 282, 19493, 2007.
58. Glatzle, J. et al., Apolipoprotein A-IV stimulates duodenal vagal afferent activity to inhibit gastric motility via a CCK1 pathway, *Am. J. Physiol. Regul. Integr. Comp. Physiol.*, 287, R354, 2004.
59. Whited, K.L. et al., Apolipoprotein A-IV is involved in detection of lipid in the rat intestine, *J. Physiol.*, 569, 949, 2005.
60. Shen, L. et al., Hypothalamic apolipoprotein A-IV is regulated by leptin, *Endocrinology*, 148, 2681, 2007.
61. Rozengurt, E., Taste receptors in the gastrointestinal tract. I. Bitter taste receptors and alpha-gustducin in the mammalian gut, *Am. J. Physiol. Gastrointest. Liver Physiol.*, 291, G171, 2006.
62. Sutherland, K. et al., Phenotypic characterization of taste cells of the mouse small intestine, *Am. J. Physiol. Gastrointest. Liver Physiol.*, 292, G1420, 2007.
63. Dyer, J. et al., Expression of sweet taste receptors of the T1R family in the intestinal tract and enteroendocrine cells, *Biochem. Soc. Trans.*, 33, 302, 2005.
64. Bezencon, C., le Coutre, J., and Damak, S., Taste-signaling proteins are coexpressed in solitary intestinal epithelial cells, *Chem. Senses*, 32, 41, 2007.
65. Braun, T. et al., Enterochromaffin cells of the human gut: sensors for spices and odorants, *Gastroenterology*, 132, 1890, 2007.
66. Mace, O.J. et al., Sweet taste receptors in rat small intestine stimulate glucose absorption through apical GLUT2, *J. Physiol.*, 582, 379, 2007.
67. Sobocki, J. et al., The cybergut. An experimental study on permanent microchip neuromodulation for control of gut function, *Acta Chir. Belg.*, 102, 68, 2002.
68. Chen, J.Z. et al., Reverse gastric pacing reduces food intake without inducing symptoms in dogs, *Scand. J. Gastroenterol.*, 41, 30, 2006.
69. Matyja, A. et al., Effects of vagal pacing on food intake and body mass in pigs, *Folia Med. Cracov.*, 45, 55, 2004.
70. Sun, X. et al., Excitatory effects of gastric electrical stimulation on gastric distension responsive neurons in ventromedial hypothalamus (VMH) in rats, *Neurosci. Res.*, 55, 451, 2006.
71. Pardo, J.V. et al., Weight loss during chronic, cervical vagus nerve stimulation in depressed patients with obesity: an observation, *Int. J. Obes.*, 2007, Jun 12 [Epub ahead of print].
72. Bodenlos, J.S. et al., Vagus nerve stimulation acutely alters food craving in adults with depression, *Appetite*, 48, 145, 2007.
73. Bonatti, H. et al., Laparoscopically implanted gastric pacemaker after kidney-pancreas transplantation: treatment of morbid obesity and diabetic gastroparesis, *Obes. Surg.*, 17, 100, 2007.

74. Cigaina, V. and Hirschberg, A.L., Gastric pacing for morbid obesity: plasma levels of gastrointestinal peptides and leptin, *Obes. Res.*, 11, 1456, 2003.
75. Yao, S. et al., Retrograde gastric pacing reduces food intake and delays gastric emptying in humans: a potential therapy for obesity? *Dig. Dis. Sci.*, 50, 1569, 2005.
76. Nahas, Z. et al., Serial vagus nerve stimulation functional MRI in treatment-resistant depression, *Neuropsychopharmacology*, 32, 1649, 2007.
77. Rolls, E.T., Sensory processing in the brain related to the control of food intake, *Proc. Nutr. Soc.*, 66, 96, 2007.
78. Pritchard, T.C. et al., Gustatory neural responses in the medial orbitofrontal cortex of the old world monkey, *J. Neurosci.*, 25, 6047, 2005.
79. Pritchard, T.C., Schwartz, G.J., and Scott, T.R., Taste in the medial orbitofrontal cortex of the macaque, *Ann. N.Y. Acad. Sci.*, in press.
80. DelParigi, A. et al., Sensory experience of food and obesity: a positron emission tomography study of the brain regions affected by tasting a liquid meal after a prolonged fast, *Neuroimage*, 24, 436, 2005.
81. Porubská, K. et al., Subjective feeling of appetite modulates brain activity: an fMRI study, *Neuroimage*, 32, 1273, 2006.
82. Rothemund, Y. et al., Differential activation of the dorsal striatum by high-calorie visual food stimuli in obese individuals, *Neuroimage*, 37, 410, 2007.
83. Smeets, P.A. et al., Functional magnetic resonance imaging of human hypothalamic responses to sweet taste and calories, *Am. J. Clin. Nutr.*, 82, 1011, 2005.
84. Smeets, P.A. et al., Oral glucose intake inhibits hypothalamic neuronal activity more effectively than glucose infusion. *Am. J. Physiol. Endocrinol. Metab.*, 293, E754–E758, 2007.
85. Tabuchi, E. et al., Spatio-temporal dynamics of brain activated regions during drinking behavior in rats, *Brain Res.*, 951, 270, 2002.
86. Lazovic, J. et al., Regional activation in the rat brain during visceral stimulation detected by c-fos expression and fMRI, *Neurogastroenterol. Motil.*, 17, 548, 2005.
87. Stephan, E. et al., Functional neuroimaging of gastric distention, *J. Gastrointest. Surg.*, 7, 740, 2003.
88. Stark, J.A. et al., Functional magnetic resonance imaging and c-Fos mapping in rats following an anorectic dose of m-chlorophenylpiperazine, *Neuroimage*, 31, 1228, 2006.

14 Conscious and Unconscious Regulation of Feeding Behaviors in Humans: Lessons from Neuroimaging Studies in Normal Weight and Obese Subjects

P. Antonio Tataranni and Nicola Pannacciulli

CONTENTS

14.1 INTRODUCTION

The prevalence of overweight and obesity is reaching epidemic proportions in many industrialized countries, especially the United States.[1] Weight gain results from a chronic disruption of energy balance, such that energy intake persistently exceeds energy expenditure. Although the pathogenesis of obesity is not completely understood, in most cases excessive accumulation of fat is probably due to the interaction between genetic factors and environmental conditions, such that changes in the environment operate on a predisposing genetic milieu to cause weight gain by creating an energy imbalance between intake and expenditure.[2]

Studies of twins reared apart, as well as adoptee and kin, indicate that approximately two thirds of the variability in body size is attributable to genetic factors.[3–7] From prospective studies in Pima Indians, it is possible to ascribe 12% of the variability in body mass index (BMI) to metabolic rate, 5% to fat oxidation, and another probable 10% to the level of spontaneous physical activity.[8] Hence, familial traits, such as energy expenditure and nutrient partitioning, explain only a minor portion of the genetic variability of body size, indicating that a major portion is related to genetic factors involved in the regulation of food intake.

Therefore, central to the pathogenesis of obesity is the feedback system involving peripheral hormones, such as leptin and insulin, and metabolites, such as glucose and free fatty acids (FFA), as well as neurochemicals in the brain, and the neural and endocrine messages that respond to the intake of food.[9] In this context, several different areas of the brain receive information from the environment (external stimuli), as well as peripheral tissues (internal stimuli), which is processed to generate meaningful responses affecting food intake and body weight control. External stimuli include visual, olfactory, taste, auditory, and tactile stimuli. Internal stimuli include preabsorptive stimuli (osmolality, gastric distension, etc.) and postabsorptive stimuli (such as changes in the activity of autonomic fibers), as well as metabolites, hormones, and other factors originating from various tissues, circulating in the blood, and activating corresponding sensors directly in the brain (glucose, amino acids, insulin, leptin, etc.).

14.2 UNCONSCIOUS (HOMEOSTATIC) REGULATION OF FOOD INTAKE

Adiposity signals, such as the hormones insulin and leptin, whose circulating concentrations are proportional to body fat mass, and metabolic signals, such as FFA and glucose, whose plasma concentrations are dependent on the metabolism of circulating nutrients, convey information about the body energy stores to the brain.[10] Neuronal systems sense these inputs and set out responses affecting feeding behavior, autonomic outflow, and substrate metabolism to promote homeostasis of both energy stores and fuel metabolism, such that energy intake is inhibited, while simultaneously increasing energy expenditure, in times of plenty, whereas energy intake is stimulated, while simultaneously decreasing energy expenditure, when deficiency of stored energy occurs.[10–12]

14.2.1 The Role of the Hypothalamus

The hypothalamus plays a crucial role in the homeostatic regulation of food intake and energy balance, as pointed out mainly by animal studies.[13] This organ is, in fact, strategically located in the midst of the mammalian neuraxis and receives relevant information about the status of body energy stores, as well as their changes, via internal state signals that have access to various hypothalamic nuclei through multiple routes, including hormone receptors, metabolite sensors, and afferent neural pathways.[14] This information is processed within the hypothalamus, thanks to rich intrahypothalamic connections facilitating redistribution and processing of incoming inputs, and then drives pituitary–endocrine and neuronal–autonomic effectors through output pathways.[15] In fact, the hypothalamus has widespread neural projections to most endocrine systems and both sympathetic and parasympathetic centers involved in the flux, storage, mobilization, and utilization of fuels.[14]

The role of the hypothalamus in monitoring energy intake has also been confirmed by human studies. In fact, administration of a 75-g glucose load after an overnight fast led to a decrease in hypothalamic activity, as measured by functional magnetic resonance imaging (fMRI), which was localized in the medial hypothalamus, previously implicated in controlling feeding behavior and regulating plasma glucose concentrations.[16] This decrease in hypothalamic neuronal activity in response to the glucose load was significantly correlated with the fasting plasma insulin concentrations, indicating a dynamic interaction between neuronal and biochemical signals.[16] Similarly, glucose administration in lean subjects was associated with a prolonged decrease in the hypothalamic fMRI signal,[17] possibly related to decreases in neuronal activity in the lateral hypothalamic area (LHA), which is known to contain glucose-sensitive neurons.[18] The time course and dose dependency of this response indicated a possible association with changes in the plasma insulin concentrations.[17] Finally, a decrease in regional cerebral blood flow ([rCBF], a marker of neuronal activity), as measured by ^{15}O-water positron emission tomography (PET), was observed also following the administration of a satiating amount of a liquid formula meal after a 36-hour fast in both lean and obese men.[19,20]

The exact meaning of such reduction in hypothalamic activity after nutrient intake, as well as its neurophysiological underpinnings is not clear. It may be that the condition of hunger elicited by a 12- or 36-hour fast was associated with a high basal activity of the hypothalamus, which was reduced by the energy intake. Alternatively, nutrient intake may directly activate inhibitory pathways to the hypothalamus, causing a decrease in hypothalamic activity. However, human studies on the role of the hypothalamus in the regulation of energy intake suffer from important limitations related to the small size and deep location of this organ, which lines the lateral walls of the third ventricle and is surrounded by a very rich vascular network, thus making it difficult and technically demanding to image the effects of food stimuli in this part of the brain.

14.3 CONSCIOUS (HEDONIC/COGNITIVE) REGULATION OF FEEDING BEHAVIORS

There is much more to the neural regulation of food intake than just processing physiologic signals aimed at achieving the homeostasis of energy balance. Ingestive behavior is made up of several phases.[15] The initiation phase is prompted by internal state signals, such as the replenishment of body energy stores, coupled with the incentive value of food, which produce the stimulus to eat. The procurement phase provides the subject with the means to satisfy this drive to eat, via search or preparation of the desired food. The consummation phase starts when the food is present and provides sensory associations (for example, between taste and postabsorptive changes) that are stored as memory representations. The termination phase occurs when satiation signals reach a certain level, stored information is recalled (learned satiety), or another behavior becomes more important. Remarkably, all these phases making up ingestive behavior are affected not only by the internal state, but also by the incentive value of goal object, as well as reward expectancy and learning and memory systems.

14.3.1 The Role of Reward in the Regulation of Food Intake

A pivotal feature of the regulation of food intake, especially in humans, is that such processed and modulated internal state information interfaces with external, hedonic, and cognitive information in telencephalic structures. The hypothalamus, in fact, has widespread neural projections to several brain regions, including cortical areas, from which it also receives inputs.

The remarkable expansion of the cerebral cortex represents one of the most relevant breakthroughs of human evolution, allowing for higher neural functions, such as cognition, language, planning, consciousness, and emotions. This has provided human beings with new ways to guarantee and satisfy nutritional needs, as well as a higher level of control over energy intake. In fact, a very complex representation of nutrients and nutrient-related environment is afforded by the flexible and multifaceted computational capability of the cerebral cortex, in which countless pieces of sensory information pertaining to the physical attributes of potential nutrients, their relationship to the environment, and their psychochemical and neural interaction with the organism are collected through all senses and systematically processed within specialized subcortical and cortical areas.

14.3.1.1 Reward Circuitries

Food reward is a primary drive for feeding and attributes affective value to eating behaviors. Food reward is embedded in the brain as a distributed neural system, stretching all the way from the hindbrain nucleus of the solitary tract and parabrachial nucleus through the limbic (hypothalamus, amygdala) and cortical (insula, operculum) gustatory pathways.[21] Food reward hinges on the taste, smell, sight, and feeling of food and of the act of eating, as well as their integration. The neuroanatomical correlates of taste and olfaction, which are known to be primary reinforcers of food intake, have been well described.

14.3.1.2 Taste

Taste perception is mediated by a multisynaptic neuronal pathway involving peripheral taste nerves (facial, glossopharyngeal, and vagus nerves), as well as central neurons arising in the hindbrain nucleus of the solitary tract, ventral posteriomedial nucleus of the thalamus, primary gustatory cortex (frontal opercular and anterior insular cortices), secondary gustatory cortex (orbitofrontal cortex), and amygdala.[22] The orbitofrontal cortex and amygdala have, in turn, reciprocal connections with the lateral hypothalamus.[22] Human studies have provided additional information about brain regions that participate in the sensation of taste. Surgical excision of the anterior temporal lobe in epileptic patients was associated with defects in taste quality recognition.[23] Discrimination of 0.18% saline from pure water was associated with significantly higher neuronal activity in the thalamus, insular cortex, anterior cingulate gyrus, parahippocampal gyrus, lingual gyrus, caudate nucleus, and temporal gyrus.[24] Aversive gustatory stimulation activated limbic circuits, including the amygdala and orbitofrontal cortex, in humans, confirming results from animal studies that implicate the amygdala and its connections in the recognition of aversive stimuli.[25] Similarly, ^{15}O-water PET measurements of rCBF, a marker of local neuronal activity, of paralimbic and limbic areas and the temporal lobe of the human brain in response to taste perception of a liquid meal in the context of extreme hunger confirmed that the temporal cortex, thalamus, cingulate cortex, caudate, and hippocampal formation are preferentially affected by taste stimulation also in this setting.[26]

14.3.1.3 Olfaction

Olfactory inputs from the olfactory bulb reach the insula, and from there, connections reach the piriform and medial orbitofrontal cortices.[27,28] Neuroimaging studies of taste and smell have shown a high degree of overlapping between areas activated by the two stimulations and demonstrated that independent presentation of a tastant or an odorant produces overlapping activation in regions of the insula, amygdala, and orbitofrontal cortex.[29,30] In addition, the insula, orbitofrontal cortex, and anterior cingulate are key components of the network underlying taste–smell integration, from which flavor arises.[31,32] In synthesis, the cortical representations of the chemical senses (taste and smell) are in the limbic and paralimbic cortices, regions of the brain that are thought to be important for processing the internal and motivational states, as well as the affective significance of external objects, thus confirming that a higher level of neural control than the hypothalamus-mediated homeostatic regulation is deeply involved in eating behavior.

14.3.1.4 Pleasure and Aversion

An fMRI study on healthy volunteers showed that the level of reward drive was strongly correlated with activation to pictures of appetizing foods in a neural network including ventral striatal, amygdala, midbrain, orbitofrontal, and ventral pallidal regions, areas involved in food reward.[33] Since levels of reward drive and related constructs predict relative body weight, food cravings, and hyperphagia,[34] a heightened responsivity of this network to food cues may increase reward drive, thus promoting compulsive-eating disorders and, possibly, weight gain.

Different brain regions are recruited in relation to changes in the affective significance associated with feeding (as the reward value of a certain food changes from pleasant to aversive). In fact, differential activation of brain regions was reported in a PET study of volunteers eating chocolate (a food with high reward value) to beyond satiety, depending on whether subjects ate chocolate when they were highly motivated to eat and rated the chocolate as pleasant (primary gustatory cortex, striatum, midbrain, subcallosal region, and caudomedial orbitofrontal cortex) or whether they were highly motivated not to eat and rated the chocolate as unpleasant (parahippocampal gyrus, caudolateral orbitofrontal and prefrontal cortices).[35] This indicates that different neural substrates underlie two motivation systems related to the affective salience of feeding, the former dealing with positive/appetitive stimuli and the latter with negative/aversive stimuli.

Similarly, a significant correlation between the activation of the human orbitofrontal cortex, as measured by fMRI, and the decrease in subjective pleasantness of a liquid food, when eaten to satiety, was reported.[36] Consistently, the activation of the orbitofrontal cortex was greater in response to the administration of a satiating liquid meal (that is, a meal proportional to each subject's body size) than in response to a fixed, smaller amount of the same liquid meal in lean and obese men.[37] These results are consistent with an important role for the orbitofrontal cortex in human emotion and motivation associated with eating.

14.3.1.5 The Role of Dopaminergic Circuits

These findings lend support to the central role of dopaminergic circuits in the regulation of food intake also in humans. Several animal studies have implicated dopamine in feeding behavior. Rats with lesions of the dopamine system are aphagic and die from starvation.[38] Feeding increases dopamine turnover in the ventral striatum, namely the nucleus accumbens.[39] Conversely, dopamine antagonists block the reward quality of food.[40,41] By using [^{11}C]raclopride PET scanning before and after feeding in healthy humans, eating a favorite meal was associated with dopamine release, which was proportional to the perceived pleasantness of the meal, in the dorsal striatum, including caudate and putamen, but not the ventral striatum, namely nucleus accumbens.[42] These findings may be at variance with animal studies involving the ventral striatum as a major player in the representation of rewards, such as drug reward. On the other hand, evidence from animal studies also indicates that it is the dorsal, rather than ventral, striatum that plays the key role in feeding and food reward. In fact, lesions of the nucleus accumbens did not reduce food consumption in rats,[43] whereas microinjections of a dopamine antagonist into the caudate-putamen, but not the nucleus accumbens, reduced food-rewarded lever pressing in rats.[44] In synthesis, striatal dopamine participates in food intake regulation by modulating motivational and reward processing.

14.3.2 Integration of Hedonic and Cognitive Control of Eating Behavior

Human studies using functional neuroimaging techniques have shown that areas involved in the unconscious and conscious regulation of food intake are connected in a network integrating homeostatic, hedonic, and even cognitive stimuli to provide a full-fledged control system linking physiologic stimuli with affective motivation and decision making. In particular, hunger, as elicited by a 36-hour fast in lean men, was associated with increased neuronal activity in the hypothalamus, insular, orbitofrontal and anterior cingulate cortices, striatum, hippocampal and parahippocampal formations, precuneus, thalamus, and cerebellum; whereas, satiety, as induced by the administration of a liquid meal providing 50% of the daily resting metabolic rate, was associated with increased neuronal activity in the dorsolateral and ventromedial prefrontal cortices.[20]

By using a different paradigm, in which subjects were scanned before and after imagining themselves in a restaurant and considering a number of items on a menu, the participation of the above brain areas in a network underlying feeding behavior has been further confirmed.[45] In such an experimental setting, increased activation in response to a hungry state was shown in the hypothalamus, amygdala, striatum, insula, and anterior cingulate cortex. Satiety, in contrast, was associated with increased activation in the lateral orbitofrontal and temporal cortices.[45]

In summary, these functional neuroimaging studies have demonstrated that the neural substrates of the motivation to eat in humans are represented in a network of midbrain, diencephalic, and cortical areas integrating intrinsic and extrinsic factors, with each area playing a possibly distinct but integrated role in the process: physiological responses mainly represented in the brain stem and hypothalamus, more complex motivational and affective responses represented in the amygdala, striatum, and insula, and higher cognitive control represented in the prefrontal cortex.

The hypothalamus, with its widespread connections, including those directed toward the midbrain, may provide a route by which food-related cues generate autonomic and hormonal/metabolic responses to feeding. The amygdala is involved in the activation of the cephalic-phase insulin response[46] and responds to the sight of foodstuffs. The striatum may integrate information from different components of the limbic system and provide a route for learned stimuli to influence behavioral responses. The cortical areas, such as orbitofrontal, prefrontal, frontal, and temporal cortices, may provide a higher level of regulation of eating, pertaining motivational and inhibitory control.

The implications of understanding this network are far-reaching both in terms of increasing the knowledge on the normal regulation of the motivation to eat and for understanding disorders in which this system is dysfunctional, such as obesity and eating disorders.

14.4 NEURAL ABNORMALITIES IN HUMAN OBESITY

Atypical neuronal responses to food-related stimuli of some brain areas involved in the regulation of eating behavior have been reported in functional neuroimaging studies of obese versus lean people. Exposure to food was associated with an increase in rCBF, as measured by ^{99m}Tc-ethyl-cysteine-dimer single photon emission computed tomography (SPECT), in obese, but not lean, women in the right temporal and parietal cortices, and the right parietal cortex activation was associated with an enhanced feeling of hunger with exposure to food.[47] This increased neuronal response to food exposure in the above cortical areas of obese women may be due either to food-elicited hyperactivity of the temporal and parietal cortices or to an initially lower activity of these areas.

Obese subjects had significantly higher basal metabolic activity, as measured by 2-deoxy-2[^{18}F]fluoro-d-glucose (FDG) PET, in the bilateral parietal somatosensory cortex in the regions where sensation to the mouth, lips, and tongue are located.[48] The enhanced activity in regions involved with sensory processing of food might make obese subjects more sensitive to the rewarding properties of food and contribute to their overeating.

14.4.1 Differences in Taste Processing between Lean and Obese Subjects

Sensory experience of food, as evaluated by tasting 2 ml of an artificially flavored liquid formula meal, was associated with greater increases in rCBF, as measured by ^{15}O-water PET, in the middle-dorsal insula and midbrain, and greater decreases in the posterior cingulate, temporal, and orbitofrontal cortices in obese compared to lean individuals.[49] In particular, the greater insular response in obese versus lean subjects may be an expression of greater central sensitivity to the fat content and/or texture of the liquid meal, as the insular cortex has been shown to be activated by oral fat and food texture.[50] These results may help understand the neuroanatomical correlates of abnormal eating behavior and their relationship with human obesity. In fact, sensory perception of food in the mouth represents the driving force behind the motivation to eat for many individuals,[22] and the preference for highly palatable food may contribute to weight gain, thus possibly underlying the current epidemic of obesity.[51,52]

14.4.2 Differences in Satiety Processing between Lean and Obese Subjects

In our studies of neurofunctional correlates of hunger, as elicited by a 36-h fast, and satiety, as induced by the administration of a liquid formula meal providing 50% of the subject's measured resting metabolic rate,[53,54] a significant effect of body size was found in the left dorsolateral prefrontal cortex, such that, when compared with lean men, obese men had significantly less activation in the left dorsolateral prefrontal cortex in response to the meal.[37] In addition, percentage of body fat was negatively correlated with the change in rCBF in the left dorsolateral prefrontal cortex after the meal.[37]

14.4.2.1 The Role of the Prefrontal Cortex

The prefrontal cortex has a central role in the inhibition of inappropriate behaviors. In particular, it is important in the suppression of a course of action that is no longer appropriate and for the ability to monitor ongoing actions[55] and may contain a general mechanism for integrating perceptual evidence for decision making.[56,57] Hence, it may well be that an impairment of neuronal activity in the dorsolateral prefrontal cortex in response to a meal in obese men affects satiation, satiety, or both. This would result in hyperphagia, which would, in turn, either lead to obesity, if it represents a primary event, or make weight loss difficult, if it represents an acquired feature of obesity.

In a ^{15}O-water PET study of the brain response to satiety in successful dieters (subjects who had achieved, by diet and physical exercise, the weight loss necessary to reduce their BMI from ≥35 to ≤25 kg/m^2 and had successfully kept their weight stable for at least 3 months) versus nondieters, successful dieters had a greater activation in the right dorsal prefrontal cortex in response to meal consumption compared to nondieters, and this prefrontal activation was associated with the level of dietary restraint.[58] Therefore, it may be speculated that a higher activation of the prefrontal cortex may have provided successful dieters with the high level of dietary restraint needed to successfully pursue weight loss, thus reinforcing the important role of this cortical area in inhibitory control, also with regard to food intake.

This hypothesis of a central role of the prefrontal cortex in the cognitive control of eating behaviors and, possibly, in inducing/perpetuating overeating is confirmed by the results of some, though not all functional neuroimaging studies in subjects with eating disorders. In fact, lateral prefrontal activity, as measured by fMRI, in response to food stimuli was decreased in women with bulimia nervosa compared to subjects with anorexia nervosa and controls.[59] The diminished activity in this region may account for the loss of control on the eating behavior in bulimic patients.

14.4.3 Dopaminergic Abnormalities in Human Obesity

Dopaminergic circuits play a pivotal role in the regulation of food intake also in humans.[60] There is evidence that this neural pathway is impaired in the brains of obese subjects. Striatal dopamine D_2 receptor availability, as measured by [^{11}C]raclopride PET, was significantly reduced in obese compared to lean individuals, and this deficiency was correlated with BMI.[61] This reduction may represent either a down-regulation, to compensate for dopamine increases caused by chronic overstimulation from feeding, or a marker of propensity to addictive behaviors, therefore perpetuating overeating as a means to compensate for the decreased function of reward circuits.

14.4.4 Structural Brain Abnormalities in Obesity

Obesity is also associated with morphological abnormalities of the brain, as demonstrated by animal studies. Overeating may have adverse effects on the nervous system of rodents by increasing susceptibility of neural cells to dysfunction and degeneration.[62] There is also mounting evidence from animal models that dietary restriction has striking neuroprotective effects.[63] The lack of leptin in the genetically obese *ob/ob* mouse is associated with structural abnormalities of the brain, including reduced brain weight and cortical brain volume, delayed maturation of neurons and glial cells, and increased susceptibility to neurodegeneration.[64,65] Also human obesity seems to negatively affect brain morphology. Prospective studies have demonstrated that overweight is a risk factor for Alzheimer's disease,[66] and a high BMI is associated with cerebral atrophy of the temporal region.[67]

By using voxel-based morphometry (VBM), an MRI-based whole-brain technique detecting region-wise differences in brain tissue composition of stereologically normalized brains, gray matter density was found to be reduced in the frontal operculum (belonging to the primary gustatory cortex), postcentral gyrus (indicated as putative secondary gustatory area), middle frontal gyrus (belonging to the prefrontal cortex), cerebellum (bidirectionally connected with the hypothalamus), and putamen (central relay in the reward circuitry) of obese subjects compared to lean individuals.[68] Theoretically, these changes in brain tissue composition in areas directly involved in the regulation of eating at different levels, may explain individual vulnerability to addictive behaviors including overeating, promoting obesity, or the difficulty overweight individuals have in losing weight, perpetuating obesity. Additionally, these structural abnormalities in the brains of obese people may represent the morphological substrate of the functional abnormalities previously reported in the dorsal striatum[61] and the prefrontal cortex[68] of obese individuals.

14.5 CONCLUSIONS

It is well established that the neural regulation of eating behavior spans the range of nonconscious (homeostatic) and conscious (hedonic and cognitive) events. Hence, functional neuroimaging represents an increasingly important tool for investigating how different regions of the brain work together to coordinate normal eating behaviors and how they conspire to produce or perpetuate obesity and other eating disorders. Nonetheless, methodological challenges associated with this technologically advancing field still remain. Therefore, it is pivotal for successful progress in the field to capitalize on methodological approaches that complement the role of imaging in the study of the normal and abnormal regulation of food intake.

14.5.1 Future Directions

Applying to human studies research techniques successfully developed in animal models certainly represents an important step forward and may be a winning approach to determine the extent to which neurofunctional and neurostructural correlates of normal and abnormal responses to specific stimuli identified by neuroimaging techniques are necessary for the behavior of interest. These strategies include:

1. Lesion, stimulation, and neural tract tracing studies.
2. Reversible "lesion" studies, such as transcranial magnetic stimulation.
3. Electrophysiological recording techniques (e.g., event-related potentials and magnetoencephalography), which have the temporal resolution needed

to help determine the time course of the activation/deactivation responses of different brain regions.

4. Transcriptomic and proteomic studies, using postmortem brain tissue from the brain regions implicated in imaging studies to assess the molecular processes involved in the normal and abnormal regulation of food intake.
5. *In vivo* hybridization techniques, using antisense DNA probes with high specific radioactivity for SPECT or PET, also combined with adenoviral vector-mediated expression.

14.5.2 Gaps

In particular, it is important to pursue also in human studies areas which have recently been demonstrated to have a pivotal role in the regulation of food intake in animals. One of these areas is represented by the role of gastrointestinal vagal afferents in the control of food intake. The vagus nerve is the primary neuroanatomic substrate in the gut–brain axis, transmitting meal-related signals elicited by nutrient contact with the gastrointestinal tract to sites in the central nervous system that mediate ingestive behavior.[69–72] Its role in the regulation of human eating behavior and, especially, the integration with the higher, conscious central control of food intake is still poorly understood in humans.

Another important area, related to the central control of food intake and still unaddressed in humans, is the nutrient sensing in the brain. Over the past 50 years, there has been extensive debate about what these brain circuits actually monitor to maintain energy balance, the main hypotheses being that the hypothalamus monitors either the storage and use of carbohydrate (glucostatic theory) or the storage and metabolism of fat (lipostatic theory). The glucostatic theory maintains that, as neurons use glucose as their primary fuel, fluctuations in glucose availability or usage are monitored and linked to the control of eating behaviors, such that food intake is elicited when the glucose supply to tissues becomes insufficient and is terminated when glucose concentrations are restored to their physiological levels.[73] Prospective studies in humans, showing that a higher carbohydrate balance[74] and a greater postload glucose response[75] are both protective against body weight gain, have provided indirect support to the role of glucose sensing in the long-term regulation of body weight in humans, possibly via its effects on food intake. The lipostatic theory posits that the energy homeostasis system is set to regulate total body fat in response to feedback signals from fat depots to the brain, including fatty acids, leptin, and insulin.[10,12] There is also growing evidence that fatty acid metabolism within discrete hypothalamic regions can function as a sensor for nutrient availability, integrating multiple nutritional and hormonal signals.[11,12,76] These findings have provided novel insights into how neurons monitor fuels and their oxidation, indicating that fuel sensing spans beyond an exclusive focus on glucose. These observations underscore the centrality of brain fuel-sensing mechanisms in the organism's overall regulation of energy homeostasis. These findings, however, have largely been obtained from *in vitro* and animal studies. The capacity to transfer them to human tests of the regulation of energy balance is urgently needed and will provide a better understanding of the integration of homeostatic needs with conscious control in the regulation of food intake and energy balance.

REFERENCES

1. Hedley, A.A., Ogden, C.L., Johnson, C.L., Carroll, M.D., Curtin, L.R., and Flegal, K.M., Prevalence of overweight and obesity among US children, adolescents, and adults, 1999–2002, *JAMA,* 2004, 291(23), 2847–2850.
2. Tremblay, A., Perusse, L., and Bouchard, C., Energy balance and body-weight stability: impact of gene-environment interactions, *Br. J. Nutr.,* 2004, 92 (Suppl. 1), S63–S66.
3. Allison, D.B., Kaprio, J., Korkeila, M., Koskenvuo, M., Neale, M.C., and Hayakawa, K., The heritability of body mass index among an international sample of monozygotic twins reared apart, *Int. J. Obes. Relat. Metab. Disord.,* 1996, 20(6), 501–506.
4. Bouchard, C., Perusse, L., Leblanc, C., Tremblay, A., and Theriault, G., Inheritance of the amount and distribution of human body fat, *Int. J. Obes.,* 1988, 12(3), 205–215.
5. Bouchard, C. and Perusse, L., Heredity and body fat, *Annu. Rev. Nutr.,* 1988, 8, 259–277.
6. Sakul, H., Pratley, R., Cardon, L., Ravussin, E., Mott, D., and Bogardus, C., Familiality of physical and metabolic characteristics that predict the development of non-insulin-dependent diabetes mellitus in Pima Indians, *Am. J. Hum. Genet.,* 1997, 60(3), 651–656.
7. Tataranni, P.A., Mechanisms of weight gain in humans, *Eur. Rev. Med. Pharmacol. Sci.,* 2000, 4(1–2), 1–7.
8. Ravussin, E. and Bogardus, C., Energy balance and weight regulation: genetics versus environment, *Br. J. Nutr.,* 2000, 83 (Suppl. 1), S17–S20.
9. Bray, G.A., Obesity is a chronic, relapsing neurochemical disease, *Int. J. Obes. Relat. Metab. Disord.,* 2004, 28(1), 34–38.
10. Schwartz, M.W. and Porte, D., Jr., Diabetes, obesity, and the brain, *Science,* 2005, 307(5708), 375–379.
11. Obici, S., Zhang, B.B., Karkanias, G., and Rossetti, L., Hypothalamic insulin signaling is required for inhibition of glucose production, *Nat. Med.,* 2002, 8(12), 1376–1382.
12. Seeley, R.J. and Woods, S.C., Monitoring of stored and available fuel by the CNS: implications for obesity, *Nat. Rev. Neurosci.,* 2003, 4(11), 901–909.
13. Barsh, G.S. and Schwartz, M.W., Genetic approaches to studying energy balance: perception and integration, *Nat. Rev. Genet.,* 2002, 3(8), 589–600.
14. Simerly, R.B., Anatomical substrates of hypothalamic integration, in *The Rat Nervous System,* Paxinos, G., Ed., Academic Press, San Diego, CA, 1995, pp. 353–376.
15. Berthoud, H.R., Multiple neural systems controlling food intake and body weight, *Neurosci. Biobehav. Rev.,* 2002, 26(4), 393–428.
16. Liu, Y., Gao, J.H., Liu, H.L., and Fox, P.T., The temporal response of the brain after eating revealed by functional MRI, *Nature,* 2000, 405(6790), 1058–1062.
17. Smeets, P.A., de Graaf, C., Stafleu, A., van Osch, M.J., and van der, G.J., Functional MRI of human hypothalamic responses following glucose ingestion, *Neuroimage,* 2005, 24(2), 363–368.
18. Oomura, Y., Input-output organization in the hypothalamus relating to food intake behavior, in *Physiology of the Hypothalamus,* Morgane, P.J. and Panksepp, J., Eds., Marcel Dekker, New York, NY, 1980, pp. 557–620.
19. Gautier, J.F., Chen, K., Salbe, A.D. et al., Differential brain responses to satiation in obese and lean men, *Diabetes,* 2000, 49(5), 838–846.
20. Tataranni, P.A., Gautier, J.F., Chen, K., et al., Neuroanatomical correlates of hunger and satiation in humans using positron emission tomography, *Proc. Natl. Acad. Sci. U.S.A.,* 1999, 96(8), 4569–4574.
21. Berridge, K.C., Food reward: brain substrates of wanting and liking, *Neurosci. Biobehav. Rev.,* 1996, 20(1), 1–25.
22. Drewnowski, A., Taste preferences and food intake, *Annu. Rev. Nutr.,* 1997, 17, 237–253.

23. Small, D.M., Jones-Gotman, M., Zatorre, R.J., Petrides, M., and Evans, A.C., A role for the right anterior temporal lobe in taste quality recognition, *J. Neurosci.,* 1997, 17(13), 5136–5142.
24. Kinomura, S., Kawashima, R., Yamada, K., et al., Functional anatomy of taste perception in the human brain studied with positron emission tomography, *Brain Res.,* 1994, 659(1–2), 263–266.
25. Zald, D.H., Lee, J.T., Fluegel, K.W., and Pardo, J.V., Aversive gustatory stimulation activates limbic circuits in humans, *Brain,* 1998, 121 (Pt 6), 1143–1154.
26. Gautier, J.F., Chen, K., Uecker, A., et al., Regions of the human brain affected during a liquid-meal taste perception in the fasting state: a positron emission tomography study, *Am. J. Clin. Nutr.,* 1999, 70(5), 806–810.
27. Carmichael, S.T., Clugnet, M.C., and Price, J.L., Central olfactory connections in the macaque monkey, *J. Comp. Neurol.,* 1994, 346(3), 403–434.
28. Carmichael, S.T. and Price, J.L., Architectonic subdivision of the orbital and medial prefrontal cortex in the macaque monkey, *J. Comp. Neurol.,* 1994, 346(3), 366–402.
29. Gottfried, J.A., Deichmann, R., Winston, J.S., and Dolan, R.J., Functional heterogeneity in human olfactory cortex: an event-related functional magnetic resonance imaging study, *J. Neurosci.,* 2002, 22(24), 10819–10828.
30. Small, D.M., Gregory, M.D., Mak, Y.E., Gitelman, D., Mesulam, M.M., and Parrish, T., Dissociation of neural representation of intensity and affective valuation in human gustation, *Neuron,* 2003, 39(4), 701–711.
31. Small, D.M., Jones-Gotman, M., Zatorre, R.J., Petrides, M., and Evans, A.C., Flavor processing: more than the sum of its parts, *Neuroreport,* 1997, 8(18), 3913–3917.
32. Small, D.M., Voss, J., Mak, Y.E., Simmons, K.B., Parrish, T., and Gitelman, D., Experience-dependent neural integration of taste and smell in the human brain, *J. Neurophysiol.,* 2004, 92(3), 1892–1903.
33. Beaver, J.D., Lawrence, A.D., van Ditzhuijzen, J., Davis, M.H., Woods, A., and Calder, A.J., Individual differences in reward drive predict neural responses to images of food, *J. Neurosci.,* 2006, 26(19), 5160–5166.
34. Davis, C., Strachan, S., and Berkson, M., Sensitivity to reward: implications for overeating and overweight, *Appetite,* 2004, 42(2), 131–138.
35. Small, D.M., Zatorre, R.J., Dagher, A., Evans, A.C., and Jones-Gotman, M., Changes in brain activity related to eating chocolate: from pleasure to aversion, *Brain,* 2001, 124(9), 1720–1733.
36. Kringelbach, M.L., O'Doherty, J., Rolls, E.T., and Andrews, C., Activation of the human orbitofrontal cortex to a liquid food stimulus is correlated with its subjective pleasantness, *Cereb. Cortex,* 2003, 13(10), 1064–1071.
37. Le, D.S., Pannacciulli, N., Chen, K., et al., Less activation of the left dorsolateral prefrontal cortex in response to a meal: a feature of obesity, *Am. J. Clin. Nutr.,* 2006, 84(4), 725–731.
38. Ungerstedt, U., Adipsia and aphagia after 6-hydroxydopamine induced degeneration of the nigro-striatal dopamine system, *Acta Physiol. Scand. Suppl.,* 1971, 367, 95–122.
39. Hernandez, L. and Hoebel, B.G., Feeding and hypothalamic stimulation increase dopamine turnover in the accumbens, *Physiol. Behav.,* 1988, 44(4–5), 599–606.
40. Hsiao, S. and Smith, G.P., Raclopride reduces sucrose preference in rats, *Pharmacol. Biochem. Behav.,* 1995, 50(1), 121–125.
41. Wise, R.A., Spindler, J., deWit, H., and Gerberg, G.J., Neuroleptic-induced "anhedonia" in rats: pimozide blocks reward quality of food, *Science,* 1978, 201(4352), 262–264.
42. Small, D.M., Jones-Gotman, M., and Dagher, A., Feeding-induced dopamine release in dorsal striatum correlates with meal pleasantness ratings in healthy human volunteers, *Neuroimage,* 2003, 19(4), 1709–1715.

43. Salamone, J.D., Mahan, K., and Rogers, S., Ventrolateral striatal dopamine depletions impair feeding and food handling in rats, *Pharmacol. Biochem. Behav.*, 1993, 44(3), 605–610.
44. Beninger, R.J. and Ranaldi, R., Microinjections of flupenthixol into the caudate-putamen but not the nucleus accumbens, amygdala or frontal cortex of rats produce intra-session declines in food-rewarded operant responding, *Behav. Brain Res.*, 1993, 55(2), 203–212.
45. Hinton, E.C., Parkinson, J.A., Holland, A.J., Arana, F.S., Roberts, A.C., and Owen, A.M., Neural contributions to the motivational control of appetite in humans, *Eur. J. Neurosci.*, 2004, 20(5), 1411–1418.
46. Roozendaal, B., Oldenburger, W.P., Strubbe, J.H., Koolhaas, J.M., and Bohus, B., The central amygdala is involved in the conditioned but not in the meal-induced cephalic insulin response in the rat, *Neurosci. Lett.*, 1990, 116(1–2), 210–215.
47. Karhunen, L.J., Lappalainen, R.I., Vanninen, E.J., Kuikka, J.T., and Uusitupa, M.I., Regional cerebral blood flow during food exposure in obese and normal-weight women, *Brain*, 1997, 120 (Pt 9), 1675–1684.
48. Wang, G.J., Volkow, N.D., Felder, C., et al., Enhanced resting activity of the oral somatosensory cortex in obese subjects, *Neuroreport*, 2002, 13(9), 1151–1155.
49. DelParigi, A., Chen, K., Salbe, A.D., Reiman, E.M., and Tataranni, P.A., Sensory experience of food and obesity: a positron emission tomography study of the brain regions affected by tasting a liquid meal after a prolonged fast, *Neuroimage*, 2005, 24(2), 436–443.
50. de Araujo, I.E. and Rolls, E.T., Representation in the human brain of food texture and oral fat, *J. Neurosci.*, 2004, 24(12), 3086–3093.
51. Blundell, J.E. and King, N.A., Overconsumption as a cause of weight gain: behavioural-physiological interactions in the control of food intake (appetite), *Ciba Found. Symp.*, 1996, 201, 138–154.
52. Salbe, A.D., DelParigi, A., Pratley, R.E., Drewnowski, A., and Tataranni, P.A., Taste preferences and body weight changes in an obesity-prone population, *Am. J. Clin. Nutr.*, 2004, 79(3), 372–378.
53. Del Parigi, A., Gautier, J.F., Chen, K., et al., Neuroimaging and obesity: mapping the brain responses to hunger and satiation in humans using positron emission tomography, *Ann. N.Y. Acad. Sci.*, 2002, 967, 389–397.
54. Tataranni, P.A. and DelParigi, A., Functional neuroimaging: a new generation of human brain studies in obesity research, *Obes. Rev.*, 2003, 4(4), 229–238.
55. Shallice, T., *From Neuropsychology to Mental Structure*, Cambridge University Press, Cambridge, UK, 1998.
56. Heekeren, H.R., Marrett, S., Bandettini, P.A., and Ungerleider, L.G., A general mechanism for perceptual decision-making in the human brain, *Nature*, 2004, 431(7010), 859–862.
57. Heekeren, H.R., Marrett, S., Ruff, D.A., Bandettini, P.A., and Ungerleider, L.G., Involvement of human left dorsolateral prefrontal cortex in perceptual decision making is independent of response modality, *Proc. Natl. Acad. Sci. U.S.A.*, 2006, 103(26), 10023–10028.
58. DelParigi, A., Chen, K., Salbe, A.D., et al., Successful dieters have increased neural activity in cortical areas involved in the control of behavior, *Int. J. Obes.*, 2006, 31, 440–448.
59. Uher, R., Murphy, T., Brammer, M.J., et al., Medial prefrontal cortex activity associated with symptom provocation in eating disorders, *Am. J. Psychiatry*, 2004, 161(7), 1238–1246.
60. Wang, G.J., Volkow, N.D., and Fowler, J.S., The role of dopamine in motivation for food in humans: implications for obesity, *Expert Opin. Ther. Targets*, 2002, 6(5), 601–609.

61. Wang, G.J., Volkow, N.D., Logan, J., et al., Brain dopamine and obesity, *Lancet,* 2001, 357(9253), 354–357.
62. Mattson, M.P., Duan, W., and Guo, Z., Meal size and frequency affect neuronal plasticity and vulnerability to disease: cellular and molecular mechanisms, *J. Neurochem.,* 2003, 84(3), 417–431.
63. Mattson, M.P., Duan, W., Lee, J., and Guo, Z., Suppression of brain aging and neurodegenerative disorders by dietary restriction and environmental enrichment: molecular mechanisms, *Mech. Ageing Dev.,* 2001, 122(7), 757–778.
64. Bereiter, D.A. and Jeanrenaud, B., Altered neuroanatomical organization in the central nervous system of the genetically obese (ob/ob) mouse, *Brain Res.,* 1979, 165(2), 249–260.
65. Sriram, K., Benkovic, S.A., Miller, D.B., and O'Callaghan, J.P., Obesity exacerbates chemically induced neurodegeneration, *Neuroscience,* 2002, 115(4), 1335–1346.
66. Gustafson, D., Rothenberg, E., Blennow, K., Steen, B., and Skoog, I., An 18-year follow-up of overweight and risk of Alzheimer disease, *Arch. Intern. Med.,* 2003, 163(13), 1524–1528.
67. Gustafson, D., Lissner, L., Bengtsson, C., Bjorkelund, C., and Skoog, I., A 24-year follow-up of body mass index and cerebral atrophy, *Neurology,* 2004, 63(10), 1876–1881.
68. Pannacciulli, N., Del Parigi, A., Chen, K., Le, D.S., Reiman, E.M., and Tataranni, P.A., Brain abnormalities in human obesity: a voxel-based morphometric study, *Neuroimage,* 2006, 31(4), 1419–1425.
69. Moran, T.H., Ladenheim, E.E., and Schwartz, G.J., Within-meal gut feedback signaling, *Int. J. Obes. Relat. Metab. Disord.,* 2001, 25 (Suppl. 5), S39–S41.
70. Schwartz, G.J., The role of gastrointestinal vagal afferents in the control of food intake: current prospects, *Nutrition,* 2000, 16(10), 866–873.
71. Schwartz, G.J. and Azzara, A.V., Sensory neurobiological analysis of neuropeptide modulation of meal size, *Physiol. Behav.,* 2004, 82(1), 81–87.
72. Schwartz, G.J., Biology of eating behavior in obesity, *Obes. Res.,* 2004, 12 (Suppl. 2), 102S–106S.
73. Mayer, J., Regulation of energy intake and the body weight: the glucostatic theory and the lipostatic hypothesis, *Ann. N.Y. Acad. Sci.,* 1955, 63(1), 15–43.
74. Eckel, R.H., Hernandez, T.L., Bell, M.L., et al., Carbohydrate balance predicts weight and fat gain in adults, *Am. J. Clin. Nutr.,* 2006, 83(4), 803–808.
75. Pannacciulli, N., Ortega, E., Koska, J., Salbe, A.D., Bunt, J.C., and Krakoff, J., Glucose response to an oral glucose tolerance test predicts weight change in non-diabetic subjects, *Obesity,* 2006, 15, 632–639.
76. Lam, T.K., Schwartz, G.J., and Rossetti, L., Hypothalamic sensing of fatty acids, *Nat. Neurosci.,* 2005, 8(5), 579–584.

15 Macronutrients: Complexity of Intake Control

Pawel K. Olszewski and Allen S. Levine

CONTENTS

15.1 INTRODUCTION

Food is defined as a substance which consists of nutrients and can be ingested and assimilated as a source of energy by the organism. Thus, energy derived from food is the primary reason for consummatory behavior to occur, as hunger serves as a driving force and a key signal for the animal to seek nutritive ingestants and replenish the lacking calories. However, feeding is a complex behavior since it is controlled by many other crucial factors, such as reward, stress, and social interactions. Also, the intricate characteristics of food further modify consummatory activity; ingestants differ in their caloric content, nutrient composition, texture, and flavor, to name a few. These properties play a decisive role in acceptability and preference toward diets as well as physiological outcome resulting from consumption of a given tastant.

Carbohydrate, fat, and protein are the three major classes of macronutrients. They allow animals to sustain all essential biochemical processes, enabling the proper functioning of the organism. In real life, macronutrients are rarely available in their pure forms, but rather they are part of chemically complex foods; hence they concurrently affect various physiological parameters and preference toward a given diet.[1,2] In laboratory conditions, it is possible to create ingestants whose content is strictly controlled, which gives a possibility of offering diets that contain only one macronutrient or a known combination of two or three of them. It is important to note that, regardless of the multiform composition of tastant, not only are animals capable of discriminating between individual macronutrient components of tastants, but they have innate preferences toward specific macronutrients, and these preferences can be shifted through a change in energy status, peptidergic activity, or genetic manipulations.[1–4]

In this chapter we will focus on two major aspects of consumption of macronutrients: how these compounds are sensed by animals and how macronutrient intake is affected by peptidergic systems.

15.2 APPETITE FOR MACRONUTRIENTS: A GUSTATORY COMPONENT

The peripheral gustatory system plays an extremely important function in the regulation of consummatory behavior; in the absence of olfactory cues or along with the olfactory system, it acts as the first "barrier" whose role is to detect and distinguish the beneficial and nutritive ingestants from those that can jeopardize homeostasis of the organism.[5,6] As a result, taste receptors in mammals have evolved to recognize a wide variety of chemical agents. Therefore, the liking and preference of some foods and avoidance of other ones is based, to a large extent, on the integration of orosensory stimulation.[3]

Initially, the gustatory system was thought to respond to only several basic tastes including sweet, sour, salty, and bitter. This classification was based on the perception described by human subjects and was later enriched with the recognition of the monosodium glutamate taste termed umami. Animal species, similarly to humans, are capable of discerning between the five tastes, although they may differ in their perception of particular chemicals. Recent evidence suggests that specific macronutrients, some of which had been considered earlier to act almost exclusively via nongustatory mechanisms,[7] can also be detected by taste receptors.[3]

Attraction to high-fat diets was long recognized to depend on their smell and texture.[7] However, the intake of fat-rich foods is associated with the exposure of the oral cavity to fatty acids, and some of the taste receptors appear to be capable of detecting these chemicals. In 1997, Fukuwatari et al. found that the putative membrane fatty acid transporter (FAT) protein and its mRNA are present in the epithelial layer of circumvallate papillae. Immunohistochemical analysis revealed that FAT immunoreactivity is localized primarily in the apical part of taste bud cells, possibly gustatory cells, in the circumvallate papillae.[8] Gilbertson et al. performed patch-clamp recordings of isolated taste receptors of the rat and found that fatty acids prolong stimulus-induced depolarization of these cells by acting on potassium channels.[9] Importantly, the lipolytic activity of lingual lipase supports an adequate stimulation of fatty acid receptors when food is rich in triacylglycerides. In fact, administration of a potent lipase inhibitor, orlistat, in rats diminishes their preference for triacylglycerides as assessed in a very short-lasting two-bottle test, which further suggests that the gustatory aspect of fat intake plays a crucial role in the attractiveness of fat as an ingestant.[10] This notion is supported by the findings that sated rats exhibit a similar preference toward nutritive and nonnutritive oils, which suggests that flavor cues play an essential role in the development of an animal's preference to fatty foods.[11] This preference can be shifted toward nutritive ingestants through deprivation, signifying the importance of postoral stimulation and the capability to sense both flavor and energy density. Importantly, the ability to perceive the flavor of fatty acids appears to be independent from age and can be observed even in infant rats.[11] Finally, it should be noted that receptors tend to be particularly sensitive to *cis*-polyunsaturated fatty acids, which further supports the concept that the role of the taste system is to aid in the process of recognizing essential nutrients.

The fact that nutritive elements belong to a given class of macronutrients does not mean that they exhibit a similar flavor profile. This is particularly true considering carbohydrates, which induce a wide array of responses of the taste system. The sweet flavor associated with sucrose, glucose, or fructose is extremely appealing to numerous animal species and it is readily chosen over other flavors. On the other hand, starch is perceived as "unattractive."[2] Stimulation of taste receptors with natural substances perceived as sweet causes an elevation of cAMP levels in depolarized cells.[12] This stimulation leads to a robust consummatory response, and the mechanism seems to be innate, as the increase in feeding has been observed even in preweanling rats offered a sucrose solution through sublingual catheters.[13]

Studies on transgenic animals revealed that the presence of two proteins, T1R2 and T1R3, is crucial for the proper functioning of the sweet taste detection system; T1R2 and T1R3 form a complex needed for the receptor responsiveness to molecules perceived as sweet, though T1R3 protein alone may serve as a receptor as well.[14] Molecular deletion of either T1R2- or T1R3-encoding genes only partially affected an animal's ability to recognize sucrose; it was necessary to construct double-knockout mice to completely impair the ability to detect sweet-tasting sugars.[15,16]

Interestingly, the ability of humans to perceive flavor of carbohydrates is subpar in comparison to the gustatory system of rats. Extensive evidence suggests that rats may have a different receptor or a set of receptors for carbohydrates. Ramirez used a conditioned taste aversion paradigm followed by a two-bottle test to show that these animals can distinguish starch-containing suspensions from nonstarch tastants similar in texture.[17]

Although starch itself is not a particularly preferred nutrient by rodents, rats are attracted to the taste of polysaccharides derived from starch. Polycose, a starch-derived maltodextrin preparation, is perceived as bland by humans. Yet rats find it palatable, and they can easily detect its appealing flavor rather than rely only on this substance's rewarding postingestive effects, as evidenced by the studies in which Polycose was offered for a brief period of time or in sham-feeding experiments.[18] Sako and coworkers conducted an important study in which they found that aversive conditioning to Polycose did not generalize to sugars, such as sucrose, maltose, glucose, and fructose, and vice versa.[19] Gurmarin, a sweet taste-suppressing polypeptide, strongly inhibited chorda tympani nerve responses to those carbohydrates, but had practically no effect on Polycose-induced neural activity.[19] It is noteworthy that rats are not the only rodents that have been proposed to express distinct receptors for carbohydrate subclasses: Golden Syrian hamsters, Mongolian gerbils, and Egyptian spiny mice also distinguish Polycose from sugars.[20] To date, it has not been clarified whether T1R2 and T1R3 proteins participate in the process of Polycose detection. However, T1R3 is essential for the recognition and response to the disaccharide trehalose.[21]

The chemical nature of sweet-tasting nutrients is very diverse and is not restricted to the wide class of carbohydrates. Certain amino acids also produce a sensation perceived as a sweet taste. In fact, amino acids are often assigned to a category of either sweet or bitter, where many l-isomers are frequently reported as sweet, whereas d-isoforms typically taste bitter. Interestingly, the umami flavor — the appearance of which signals protein content of an ingestant — conveyed by the l-glutamate molecule can be recognized by a receptor system somewhat similar to that necessary for detection of sweet carbohydrates. It has been found that T1R1 and T1R3, as well as a truncated form of the type 4 metabotropic glutamate receptor, participate in this process.[16] A characteristic quality of umami is its potentiation by inosine- or guanosine 5′-monophosphates, which broadens receptor sensitivity to amino acids other than glutamate.[22]

The fact that certain macronutrient taste recognition-related mechanisms appear to have a common core may reflect the complexity of foods and the necessity for macronutrient flavors to be readily and concurrently detected for the purpose of supplying an organism with adequate energy. In line with that, in rats the majority of fungiform and palate papillae respond to multiple tastes[9]; this also seems to make the process of flavor integration more efficient. Hence, the organization of oral macronutrient detection systems appears to employ numerous mechanisms and pathways to discern between specific compounds. Yet at the same time, it shows a certain level of overlap to enable fast and simultaneous recognition of multiple nutritive agents present in composite diets.

15.3 APPETITE FOR MACRONUTRIENTS: IT IS NOT ONLY ABOUT TASTE

The flavor of foods, including the flavor of specific macronutrients, is typically not the sole reason for liking or avoiding particular ingestants. Energy density and metabolic consequences related to macronutrient intake — thus the postoral aspects of consumption — contribute to the preference exhibited towards fat, carbohydrates, and protein. An extensive body of evidence supports the notion that postingestive processes modify acceptance of macronutrients.[3] At least some of these mechanisms may rely on the presence of cells in the gastrointestinal tract that share structural and biochemical features of taste receptor cells found in the tongue,[23,24] although a plethora of pre- and postabsorptive events presumably play a crucial role as well.[3]

The involvement of postingestive effects in long-term preference toward fat in mice was shown by Suzuki et al.[25] These investigators found by the means of a short-term (30-minutes long) two-bottle test that palatability of the sorbitol fatty acid esters, nondigestible fat substitutes with low energy density, was similar to that of corn oil. Thus, the intake of both ingestant types resulted in a somewhat similar stimulation of taste receptors in the oral cavity, presumably leading to similar taste perception, in these animals. However, in the long-term two-bottle choice test, where both gustatory and postprandial feedback mechanisms were triggered, mice did not continue to eat the fat substitute, but their preference shifted toward corn oil. Furthermore, the reinforcing properties of sorbitol fatty acid ester versus corn oil were examined in a conditioned place preference test. Mice infused intragastrically with corn oil just prior to conditioning showed reinforcing effects of the calorie-dense fat on the consumption of sorbitol fatty acid ester. Importantly, placing corn oil in the stomach without subsequent orosensory stimulation did not show any such reinforcing effects against corn oil.[25] Those experiments provided evidence that both orosensory and postoral mechanisms are crucial in the development of macronutrient preference and associated reinforcement.

Lucas et al. determined that intragastric fat, although less potent than carbohydrates, is a powerful reinforcement stimulus, which further supports the concept that postoral events propel a drive to seek this macronutrient.[26] Ackroff et al. performed a study in which various sources of fat, including corn oil, safflower oil, vegetable shortening, and beef tallow, were tested as intragastric reinforcing agents.[27] They determined that fat sources differing in fatty acid composition with respect to chain length and saturation, are capable of conditioning flavor preferences. Fats with high polyunsaturated content or with low saturated fat content are most effective.

In an elegant study, Suzuki et al.[28] confirmed that a postingestive energy signal serves as a crucial factor in the reinforcing effects and palatability of fat. They injected mice with a beta-oxidation blocker, mercaptoacetate, or saline. Reinforcing effects and palatability response were examined with conditioned place preference and one-bottle tests, respectively. In conditioned place preference tests, the mercaptoacetate-treated animals exhibited reinforcement-related effects when offered a 40% sucrose solution, which is not metabolized via the beta-oxidation pathway, but not when given 100% corn oil. The saline group exhibited reinforcing effects when offered sucrose solution as well as when presented with corn oil. In addition, a one-bottle test revealed that the mercaptoacetate group lacked preference toward the corn oil.[28]

A different approach aimed at discerning whether macronutrients are sensed postorally was utilized by Tracy et al.[29] These investigators employed a taste aversion paradigm which relies on pairing exposure to a novel tastant with an unpleasant gastrointestinal sensation induced by a toxic agent, such as lithium chloride. As a result, tastant avoidance, which can differ in magnitude, develops. The authors demonstrated that when corn oil, that had never been tasted by the animals, was delivered via a catheter into the stomach or into the duodenum and a peripheral injection of aversion-inducing lithium chloride was administered right after the fat infusion, preference for that nutrient was subsequently reduced at the first period of contact by mouth. In fact this ability to detect, recognize, and integrate intragastric macronutrient-derived stimulation appeared as a phenomenon that could be generalized to other macronutrient classes as well; a similar outcome was noted when a carbohydrate, maltodextrin, was used.[29] In line with these findings, the results of another study suggested that nutrient-derived stimulation of the gastrointestinal tract may potentiate learning about nonnutritive flavors.[30]

The phenomenon of a gastrointestinal macronutrient sensing system, which seems to act in a direct and an indirect manner, also governs carbohydrate consumption. When isocaloric glucose and fructose solutions are presented concurrently, rats acquire preference toward glucose during even a short course of exposure, regardless of their initial preference profile.[31,32] Hence, it seems that animals develop glucose preference based on the different postingestive actions related to each carbohydrate. Thus, it is not surprising that glucose acts as a more effective reinforcing agent than fructose. A stronger preference toward a nonnutritive flavored ingestant can be induced by providing it along with an intragastric infusion of glucose rather than fructose.[33] Other studies confirmed that fructose was capable of acting as an intragastric reinforcing agent, primarily in energy-deficient rats, by employing lengthy exposure training sessions, or by pairing fructose infusions with sweetened solution exposure.[34,35]

Furthermore, a greater propensity to acquire glucose compared to fructose can be generalized to more complex carbohydrates: rats develop a preference toward the disaccharides Polycose and maltose, which are glucose-based, over another disaccharide, sucrose, which is broken down into fructose and glucose.[32] In reinforcement studies utilizing macronutrient infusions, Azzara and Sclafani found that intragastric loading of sucrose or maltose powerfully conditioned flavor preferences relative to control infusions of water. In line with other experiments, the flavor paired with maltose stomach loading was significantly preferred to the flavor paired with intragastrically delivered sucrose.[36] Apparently, specific caloric value and energy density of fructose- versus glucose-rich carbohydrates does not account for the differences in the preference profile toward these nutrients. In fact, energy density of the infused macronutrient seems to play a key role regardless of the carbohydrate content of the solution, since a high concentration of macronutrient tends to counteract the reinforcing action driven by the compound, probably as a result of the satiating effect of energy-dense food.[37] This may be due to the fact that the processes of macronutrient calorie detection versus reinforcement appear to utilize distinct integration mechanisms. Sclafani et al. found that gut vagal afferents and splanchnic nerves are not essential for flavor–nutrient preference conditioning, whereas both vagal afferents and splanchnic nerves are implicated in macronutrient-induced satiation.[38]

Taking into account the aforementioned data on carbohydrates and fat, it should not be surprising that postoral consequences of protein intake affect preference toward this macronutrient as well as associative behaviors. When an oral delay regimen was used, in which different short-term cue flavors were followed, after a 10-minute delay, by presentation of one nutrient solution, including one that contained protein, or a nonnutritive solution, the animals displayed similar preferences for nutrient-paired flavors.[39] In an interesting study, Baker et al. subjected rats to 4-hour food deprivation. After this relatively brief period of having no access to food, animals were infused intragastrically with casein; at the time of infusion, animals drank a distinctively flavored nonnutritive fluid. On the experimental day, when the same food-deprivation and solution presentation protocol was applied, the rats showed conditioned preference for the flavor.[40] Perez et al. confirmed that rats develop preference toward flavors paired with intragastric infusion of protein.[39] In macronutrient self-selection studies, these investigators also found that gastric infusion of protein diminished subsequent oral intake of this macronutrient, which suggests that the presence of protein may be sensed in the gut, and hence, protein appetite may be temporarily reduced. One should note, however, that the combination of oral and intragastric stimulation serves as the most effective method of signaling the nutritional status of the organism.[39]

Finally, there is another aspect of macronutrient intake: sensory-dependent satiety. This issue was initially raised in human studies[41]; however, it was later examined in advanced animal models in relation to gastrointestinal macronutrient sensing abilities. Investigations primarily utilized infusions of macronutrients into the stomach and duodenum. Burggraf et al. found that an intragastric load of glucose or lipid in rats significantly reduced total intake of a high-carbohydrate and a high-fat diet presented concurrently. At the same time, glucose was more effective than lipid at decreasing carbohydrate intake. Interestingly, this satiating action of macronutrients was greater upon their intragastric rather than intravenous delivery, which signifies the importance of gastrointestinal macronutrient sensory effects.[42] Conversely, an infusion of fat via a duodenal cannula suppressed oral intake of the fat solution faster and for a longer time period, than did an infusion of an isocaloric sucrose solution.[43] In another experiment, rats received gastric preloads of either carbohydrate, fat, or protein, and they were allowed to self-select their diet from the three pure macronutrients. Carbohydrate load generated a decrease in the intake of carbohydrate only, whereas fat and protein affected consumption of all nutrients, although each evoked a more profound and lengthy reduction in the intake of the corresponding nutrient.[44]

Data described above are consistent with the notion that there is a clear relationship between oral and gastrointestinal detection of macronutrients. Under natural conditions, these two sensory system levels appear to supply intertwined signals which allow for a proper selection of quality and amount of ingestants in relation to their macronutrient composition.

15.4 NEURAL AGENTS AND MACRONUTRIENT INTAKE CONTROL

Foods available in the environment differ in their composition, flavor, and texture. Animals display individual preferences toward certain ingestants. These preferences can fluctuate, reflecting energy needs and physiological, psychological, and health status of an animal. Macronutrients provide the energy necessary to maintain the functioning of the organism, and they are also a source of a positive reinforcement. It should not be surprising, therefore, that ingestion of macronutrients is influenced by neuropeptides involved in the regulation of energy homeostasis and those associated with reward.[2] In the brain, these substances are organized into a complex network, and activity of components of this circuitry plays a decisive role in the regulation of food intake. Central networks "communicate" with the periphery by utilizing reciprocal neuronal connections or via hormonal feedback. Gustatory and postoral stimuli related to macronutrient intake affect the activity of these neuropeptidergic systems, and in turn, they may lead to changes in meal patterns, preferences, reinforcement, and other direct and indirect consequences of macronutrient consumption.[1,2]

Following the initial reports showing that neuropeptides could alter food intake in general, investigators started examining whether these substances could also influence the intake of individual macronutrients. The outcome of those experimental trials indeed indicated that specific peptides may control intake of particular macronutrients; however, the relationship appears to be very complex and dependent on a number of circumstances. This complexity is apparent regardless of a hunger- or reward-related nature of action of a given peptide.

For example, it has been found that central injections of neuropeptide Y (NPY), which serves as a potent inducer of hunger- or energy-driven consummatory behavior, cause a more robust feeding response toward high-carbohydrate foods than toward fat or protein in male rats.[45] However, the same group of investigators found that female animals repeatedly injected with NPY in the hypothalamic paraventricular nucleus (PVN) ate more carbohydrate (additional 26.4 kcal per day) and fat (additional 48.5 kcal per day), whereas their protein intake remained unchanged when the three compounds were presented concurrently.[45] Glass et al. treated rats with NPY and offered them a choice between the following diet combinations: (1) high-fat diet versus high-cornstarch, (2) high-fat diet versus high-sucrose, and (3) high-fat versus high-Polycose. As a result of NPY administration, animals ate more of both the high-fat and high-carbohydrate diets when Polycose or corn starch served as sources of carbohydrate. When the high-sucrose and high-fat diets were offered concurrently, rats significantly increased the intake of the sucrose diet only. Thus the source of carbohydrate has a marked effect on the ability of NPY to affect macronutrient consumption.[46] To add to the confusion, energy density of a macronutrient mitigates the orexigenic action of NPY: this neuropeptide has a very weak effect on dilute 10% sucrose solution intake when calorically dense chow is presented at the same time.[47] On the other hand, Primeaux et al. found that intra-amygdalar infusions of NPY did not affect calorie intake in rats, but induced a shift in preference from a high-fat/low-carbohydrate diet to a low-fat/high-carbohydrate one.[48] Furthermore, in reinforcement studies, Altizer and Davidson showed that NPY injections paired with a conditioned stimulus of either high-sucrose or high-fat food did not augment the capacity of a cue associated with sucrose to promote conditioned appetitive behavior.[49] Finally, there is an unresolved issue of the presence of NPY in taste receptor cells and its possible role in conveying taste-related signals. Also, the NPY Y1 receptors are expressed by some taste bud cells where NPY appears to enhance an inwardly rectifying potassium current. Interestingly, it has been suggested that NPY may have, in this case, a more pronounced role in the perception of bitter flavors than in detecting specific macronutrient-associated flavors.[50]

The relationship between macronutrient intake and orexigenic peptides involved in reward mechanisms seems as complex as with hunger-related NPY described above. Opioids have been one of the most extensively studied groups of such substances. In basic feeding experiments, opioid receptor agonists belonging to all subclasses of the opioid family, namely endorphins, dynorphins, and enkephalins, have been found to increase consumption of palatable tastants more potently than of less attractive tastants. Antagonists induce an opposite effect.[1] Initial macronutrient studies revealed that opioid agonists increased intake of fat to a greater extent than intake of carbohydrate or protein. Conversely, consumption of a high-fat diet increased gene expression and peptide levels of enkephalins and dynorphins in the hypothalamus.[51]

Subsequently it was suggested that opioids may simply be involved in the control of reward-related feeding rather than affect a specific macronutrient intake. For example, it was shown that naloxone was much more effective in decreasing intake of a high-sucrose diet than a high-cornstarch or high-Polycose diet in food-restricted rats, and in that paradigm, sucrose was the most attractive tastant.[52] In an interesting study, Gosnell and coworkers classified rats into carbohydrate, fat, or intermediate preferers based on daily food intakes of high-fat and high-carbohydrate diets presented concurrently. Animals were injected with morphine or saline and offered both diets. Morphine increased intake of a preferred diet rather than selectively increasing intake of only a high-fat diet.[53] With a similar base preference classification protocol, opioid-like neuropeptide nociceptin/orphanin FQ increased intake of both high-carbohydrate and high-fat diet offered concurrently only in fat-preferring animals.[54] These observations suggest that innate preferences toward foods may influence what macronutrient animals select in response to a given peptidergic stimulation.

Moreover, reinforcement studies utilizing two-bottle tests revealed that the endogenous opioid system did not seem to play a major role in either the acquisition or expression of flavor preference learning in paradigms where carbohydrates were used as conditioned stimuli.[55,56] On the other hand, studies showed that it is possible that opioid receptor blockade alters perception of the taste of sweet carbohydrates and, thus, decreases their rewarding value. At the same time, it was important to learn that the taste of nutrients remains discriminable following administration of opioid antagonists. For example, naloxone did not affect sucrose discrimination in rats taught to discern 10% sucrose from water in a two-lever operant chamber. In that study animals continued to press the appropriate sucrose lever following naltrexone injection, which suggests that these tastants are still discriminable and that, perhaps, the rewarding value of sucrose decreases as a result of the treatment.[57]

The aforementioned data clearly indicate that, due to a plethora of variables inherently present in studies where food and feeding behavior are the focus of interest, experimental procedures would rarely yield a straightforward answer regarding neuropeptidergic control of macronutrient intake. Environment, social cues, innate preference toward macronutrients, food content, flavor, and texture, to name a few, modify a consummatory response. Neuropeptides that control feeding in general also affect intake of macronutrients; however these peptides — regardless of being indisputably a driving force in macronutrient preference and consumption — should be also viewed as part of a dynamic mechanism which actively responds to multiple aspects and circumstances of feeding behavior.

15.5 QUEST FOR ANSWERS: ANIMAL VERSUS HUMAN STUDIES

The majority of studies on the processes governing macronutrient intake have been performed using laboratory animals, primarily rats and mice, as model organisms. A crucial question has been raised whether data derived from animal experiments should be viewed as translatable to the terms of human physiology. Clearly, as with virtually any physiological system, mechanisms related to macronutrient selection in various species share both similarities and differences. For example, as mentioned before, even though rodents recognize sweet, bitter, salty, sour, and umami flavors, they may also be — contrary to humans — endowed with the ability to distinguish between mono-, di-, and polysaccharides.[19] However, using laboratory animals instead of humans in basic research offers several advantages, including relative genetic uniformity of a population studied, strict control of overall consumption profile, and ability to determine physiological variables or behavioral responses not attainable in human subjects due to technical or ethical issues. Finally, animal experiments provide a chance to examine macronutrient preference without the influence of the subjects' bias towards tastants due to, for example, social or societal types of pressure commonly experienced by humans. Conversely, it is important to remember that those advantages of studies involving animals may serve as a drawback, for example, for epidemiologists wishing to describe macronutrient preferences in human populations whose members do not typically live in social isolation or present extremely high levels of genetic similarity to other individuals in the cohort. Therefore, it seems that for quite a while animal and human research will go hand in hand and offer complementary answers.

15.6 CONCLUSIONS

Complexity of the mechanisms responsible for the regulation of food intake reflects the complexity of foods. Macronutrients, which are essential for the proper functioning of the organism, constitute merely an element of chemically heterogenous ingestants. Thus, the role of the feeding regulation system is to propel consummatory behavior that promotes sufficient intake of macronutrients. This system incorporates fast and accurate detection of these compounds in the oral cavity and in the gastrointestinal tract, recognition of postoral processes related to consumption, and reinforcement of consummatory behavior that leads to acquisition of appropriate amounts of macronutrients. Certain neuropeptides aid in integration of feeding-related information and, hence, affect intake and preference toward macronutrients.

REFERENCES

1. Levine, A.S. and Billington, C.J., Opioids as agents of reward-related feeding: A consideration of the evidence, *Physiol. Behav.,* 82, 57, 2004.
2. Levine, A.S. and Billington, C.J., Why do we eat? A neural systems approach, *Annu. Rev. Nutr.,* 17, 597 1997.
3. Sclafani, A., Psychobiology of food preferences, *Int. J. Obes. Relat. Metab. Disord.,* 25 (Suppl. 5), S13, 2001.
4. Alexander, J. et al., Distinct phenotypes of obesity-prone AKR/J, DBA2J and C57BL/6J mice compared to control strains, *Int. J. Obes. (Lond.),* 30, 50 2006.
5. Takeda, M. et al., Preference for corn oil in olfactory-blocked mice in the conditioned place preference test and the two-bottle choice test, *Life Sci.,* 69, 847, 2001.
6. Ramirez, I., Role of olfaction in starch and oil preference, *Am. J. Physiol.,* 265, R1404, 1993.
7. Kinney, N.E. and Antill, R.W., Role of olfaction in the formation of preference for high-fat foods in mice, *Physiol. Behav.,* 59, 475, 1996.
8. Fukuwatari, T. et al., Expression of the putative membrane fatty acid transporter (FAT) in taste buds of the circumvallate papillae in rats, *FEBS Lett.,* 414, 461, 1997.
9. Gilbertson, T.A. et al., Fatty acid modulation of K+ channels in taste receptor cells: Gustatory cues for dietary fat, *Am. J. Physiol.,* 272, C1203, 1997.
10. Kawai, T. and Fushiki, T., Importance of lipolysis in oral cavity for orosensory detection of fat, *Am. J. Physiol. Regul. Integr. Comp. Physiol.,* 285, R447, 2003.
11. Ackroff, K., Vigorito, M., and Sclafani, A., Fat appetite in rats: The response of infant and adult rats to nutritive and non-nutritive oil emulsions, *Appetite,* 15, 171, 1990.
12. Cummings, T.A., Powell, J., and Kinnamon, S.C., Sweet taste transduction in hamster taste cells: Evidence for the role of cyclic nucleotides, *J. Neurophysiol.,* 70, 2326, 1993.
13. Ackerman, S.H. et al., Intake of different concentrations of sucrose and corn oil in preweanling rats, *Am. J. Physiol.,* 262, R624, 1992.

14. Montmayeur, J.P. and Matsunami, H., Receptors for bitter and sweet taste, *Curr. Opin. Neurobiol.,* 12, 366, 2002.
15. Damak, S. et al., Detection of sweet and umami taste in the absence of taste receptor T1r3, *Science,* 301, 850, 2003.
16. Zhao, G.Q. et al., The receptors for mammalian sweet and umami taste, *Cell,* 115, 255, 2003.
17. Ramirez, I., Rats discriminate between starch and other substances having a similar texture, *Physiol. Behav.,* 53, 373, 1993.
18. Sclafani, A. and Mann, S., Carbohydrate taste preferences in rats: Glucose, sucrose, maltose, fructose and polycose compared, *Physiol. Behav.,* 40, 563, 1987.
19. Sako, N. et al., Differences in taste responses to Polycose and common sugars in the rat as revealed by behavioral and electrophysiological studies, *Physiol. Behav.,* 56, 741, 1994.
20. Feigin, M.B., Sclafani, A., and Sunday, S.R., Species differences in polysaccharide and sugar taste preferences, *Neurosci. Biobehav. Rev.,* 11, 231, 1987.
21. Ariyasu, T. et al., Taste receptor T1R3 is an essential molecule for the cellular recognition of the disaccharide trehalose, *In Vitro Cell. Dev. Biol. Anim.,* 39, 80, 2003.
22. Conigrave, A.D. and Hampson, D.R., Broad-spectrum L-amino acid sensing by class 3 G-protein-coupled receptors, *Trends Endocrinol. Metab.,* 17, 398, 2006.
23. Hofer, D., Puschel, B., and Drenckhahn, D., Taste receptor-like cells in the rat gut identified by expression of alpha-gustducin, *Proc. Natl. Acad. Sci. U.S.A.,* 93, 6631, 1996.
24. Newson, B. et al., Ultrastructural observations in the rat ileal mucosa of possible epithelial "taste cells" and submucosal sensory neurons, *Acta Physiol. Scand.,* 114, 161, 1982.
25. Suzuki, A. et al., Integration of orosensory and postingestive stimuli for the control of excessive fat intake in mice, *Nutrition,* 19, 36, 2003.
26. Lucas, F., Ackroff, K., and Sclafani, A., High-fat diet preference and overeating mediated by postingestive factors in rats, *Am. J. Physiol.,* 275, R1511, 1998.
27. Ackroff, K., Lucas, F., and Sclafani, A., Flavor preference conditioning as a function of fat source, *Physiol. Behav.,* 85, 448, 2005.
28. Suzuki, A., Yamane, T., and Fushiki, T., Inhibition of fatty acid beta-oxidation attenuates the reinforcing effects and palatability to fat, *Nutrition,* 22, 401, 2006.
29. Tracy, A.L. et al., The gastrointestinal tract "tastes" nutrients: evidence from the intestinal taste aversion paradigm, *Am. J. Physiol. Regul. Integr. Comp. Physiol.,* 287, R1086, 2004.
30. Tracy, A.L. and Davidson, T.L., Comparison of nutritive and nonnutritive stimuli in intestinal and oral conditioned taste aversion paradigms, *Behav. Neurosci.,* 120, 1268, 2006.
31. Ackroff, K. and Sclafani, A., Flavor preferences conditioned by sugars: rats learn to prefer glucose over fructose, *Physiol. Behav.,* 50, 815, 1991.
32. Ackroff, K. and Sclafani, A., Sucrose to Polycose preference shifts in rats: the role of taste, osmolality and the fructose moiety, *Physiol. Behav.,* 49, 1047, 1991.
33. Ackroff, K., Sclafani, A., and Axen, K.V., Diabetic rats prefer glucose-paired flavors over fructose-paired flavors, *Appetite,* 28, 73, 1997.
34. Ackroff, K. and Sclafani, A., Fructose-conditioned flavor preferences in male and female rats: Effects of sweet taste and sugar concentration, *Appetite,* 42, 287, 2004.
35. Ackroff, K. et al., Flavor preferences conditioned by intragastric fructose and glucose: Differences in reinforcement potency, *Physiol. Behav.,* 72, 691, 2001.
36. Azzara, A.V. and Sclafani, A., Flavor preferences conditioned by intragastric sugar infusions in rats: Maltose is more reinforcing than sucrose, *Physiol. Behav.,* 64, 535, 1998.
37. Sclafani, A., Flavor preferences conditioned by sucrose depend upon training and testing methods: Two-bottle tests revisited, *Physiol. Behav.,* 76, 633, 2002.
38. Sclafani, A., Ackroff, K., and Schwartz, G.J., Selective effects of vagal deafferentation and celiac-superior mesenteric ganglionectomy on the reinforcing and satiating action of intestinal nutrients, *Physiol. Behav.,* 78, 285, 2003.

39. Perez, C., Lucas, F., and Sclafani, A., Carbohydrate, fat, and protein condition similar flavor preferences in rats using an oral-delay procedure, *Physiol. Behav.,* 57, 549, 1995.
40. Baker, B.J. et al., Protein appetite demonstrated: Learned specificity of protein-cue preference to protein need in adult rats, *Nutr. Res.,* 7, 481, 1987.
41. Johnson, J. and Vickers, Z., Factors influencing sensory-specific satiety, *Appetite,* 19, 15, 1992.
42. Burggraf, K.K., Willing, A.E., and Koopmans, H.S., The effects of glucose or lipid infused intravenously or intragastrically on voluntary food intake in the rat, *Physiol. Behav.,* 61, 787, 1997.
43. Foster, L.A., Boeshore, K., and Norgren, R., Intestinal fat suppressed intake of fat longer than intestinal sucrose, *Physiol. Behav.,* 64, 451, 1998.
44. Bartness, T.J. and Rowland, N., Dietary self-selection in normal and diabetic rats after gastric loads of pure macronutrients, *Physiol. Behav.,* 31, 546, 1983.
45. Stanley, B.G. et al., Paraventricular nucleus injections of peptide YY and neuropeptide Y preferentially enhance carbohydrate ingestion, *Peptides,* 6, 1205, 1985.
46. Glass, M.J. et al., Role of carbohydrate type on diet selection in neuropeptide Y-stimulated rats, *Am. J. Physiol.,* 273, R2040, 1997.
47. Giraudo, S.Q. et al., Differential effects of neuropeptide Y and the mu-agonist DAMGO on "palatability" versus "energy," *Brain Res.,* 834, 160, 1999.
48. Primeaux, S.D., York, D.A., and Bray, G.A., Neuropeptide Y administration into the amygdala alters high fat food intake, *Peptides,* 27, 1644, 2006.
49. Altizer, A.M. and Davidson, T.L., The effects of NPY and 5-TG on responding to cues for fats and carbohydrates, *Physiol. Behav.,* 65, 685, 1999.
50. Zhao, F.L. et al., Expression, physiological action, and coexpression patterns of neuropeptide Y in rat taste-bud cells, *Proc. Natl. Acad. Sci. U.S.A.,* 102, 11100, 2005.
51. Chang, G.Q. et al., Dietary fat stimulates endogenous enkephalin and dynorphin in the paraventricular nucleus: role of circulating triglycerides, *Am. J. Physiol. Endocrinol. Metab.,* 292, E561, 2007.
52. Weldon, D.T. et al., Effect of naloxone on intake of cornstarch, sucrose, and polycose diets in restricted and nonrestricted rats, *Am. J. Physiol.,* 270, R1183, 1996.
53. Gosnell, B.A., Krahn, D.D., and Majchrzak, M.J., The effects of morphine on diet selection are dependent upon baseline diet preferences, *Pharmacol. Biochem. Behav.,* 37, 207, 1990.
54. Olszewski, P.K. et al., Effect of nociceptin/orphanin FQ on food intake in rats that differ in diet preference, *Pharmacol. Biochem. Behav.,* 73, 529, 2002.
55. Azzara, A.V. et al., Naltrexone fails to block the acquisition or expression of a flavor preference conditioned by intragastric carbohydrate infusions, *Pharmacol. Biochem. Behav.,* 67, 545, 2000.
56. Baker, R.W. et al., Naltrexone does not prevent acquisition or expression of flavor preferences conditioned by fructose in rats, *Pharmacol. Biochem. Behav.,* 78, 239, 2004.
57. O'Hare, E.O. et al., Naloxone administration following operant training of sucrose/water discrimination in the rat, *Psychopharmacology (Berl.),* 129, 289, 1997.

16 Macronutrients, Feeding Behavior, and Weight Control in Humans

James Stubbs, Stephen Whybrow, and Nik Mazlan Mamat

CONTENTS

16.1 INTRODUCTION: THE STUDY OF HUMAN FOOD INTAKE

We live in a society obsessed with the influence of diet composition and food on health, energy intake (EI), and body weight control. While much of life in preindustrial societies has been concerned with locating, obtaining, or cultivating adequate quantities of appropriate foods, many people living in industrialized societies spend considerable time and effort attempting to avoid excess food intake. For many individuals this has become an active process. The food industry in any Western society is worth billions of dollars per annum. In addition, consumers spend several billion dollars on products they hope will help them avoid excess food intake or remedy the consequences of overconsumption. The composition of the diet we eat is now considered a primary cause of morbidity and mortality (e.g., obesity, coronary heart disease[1]). Our growing knowledge of the effects of the diet on health offers a potential means of preventing certain illnesses or alleviating the effects of others through nutritional support. The market economy has recognized the potential in this area, and now "functional foods," "nutraceuticals," and diets of specific compositions are available with the promise of increased consumer longevity, health, and well-being. Despite at least two decades of intensive research on the role of macronutrients in the control of feeding behavior, there are relatively few commonly agreed facts or a strong consensus on the way macronutrients influence feeding and weight control in humans.

16.2 FACTS ABOUT HUMAN FEEDING BEHAVIOR

It appears difficult to pinpoint the major facts that scientists have discovered about food intake. This is largely because we are dealing with a form of *behavior,* which operates according to probabilistic rather than deterministic principles. This also has implications for those seeking to unravel the specific molecular mechanisms thought to be important in controlling feeding behavior. If clear facts about feeding are rather elusive, then mechanistic explorations of the molecular basis of feeding must be more difficult to describe in concrete terms.

Reliable quantitative and qualitative facts about food intake are also difficult to obtain because the act of measurement may influence what is being measured. This is exemplified by current concerns over the nature and extent of misreporting of dietary intakes.[2] Even more frustrating to both the scientist and the general public is the problem of communicating the results of research to a population eager to understand how to regulate their own body weight and improve health and fitness. Once research findings have been reduced by the media to easily digested "sound bites" deemed fit for public consumption, the information being relayed has become distorted. This is often so in science. However, the field of ingestive behavior, energy balance, and obesity is constantly the subject of media interest, and so this problem of media misrepresentation of our results is more acute. Thus we have cycled from a ubiquitous emphasis on increasing carbohydrate (CHO) intake during the 1980s to 1990s to a renewed interest in low CHO diets as a means of successful weight control in the first years of the new millennium. The consequences for consumer confidence in scientific research in this area has been catastrophic.

While food intake may be under voluntary behavioral control, macronutrient intake may not, since people cannot usually recognize the amount of protein, fat, or CHO they have ingested on a day-to-day basis. The study of food intake should concentrate on the way in which environmental, cognitive, or biological factors impinge on behavior. Not-eating (one aspect of which is satiety) is also a form of behavior. Consequently, events that prevent eating are also important. Understanding how energy balance is maintained requires an understanding of the forms of behavior that promote weight stability. Avoiding obesity development and developing strategies for its treatment require an appreciation of the mechanisms that influence the behaviors leading to weight gain and those that can bring about a sustained weight loss, respectively.

One of the most important mechanisms that influence feeding is learning. In many laboratory studies where manipulations of the macronutrient content and energy density (ED) of the diet are made, the manipulation itself is covert. Thus subjects are naive to the manipulation and do not have the opportunity to learn to modify their behavior as they would do in real life. This implies that many laboratory studies should yield larger effects than are seen in real life. In the case of dietary macronutrients and ED at least (see sections that follow) this appears to be so.

16.2.1 Definitions

For the purposes of this chapter, diet is defined as water (g·day^{-1}), protein (MJ·day^{-1}), carbohydrate (MJ·day^{-1}), fat (MJ·day^{-1}), energy (MJ·day^{-1}), energy density (MJ·kg^{-1}), and amount of food eaten (kg·day^{-1}). Energy density is defined as the energy per kg of wet weight of ready-to-eat food.

16.2.2 Human Feeding Behavior in Our Current Environment

With regard to the development of obesity, the evidence from the human literature suggests the following:

1. In the short-term, it is remarkably easy to perturb energy balance in either a positive or a negative direction. Changing the composition or ED of the diet can generate considerable energy imbalances.[3–5]
2. In the medium- to longer-term, the evidence suggests that humans defend against induced energy deficits, regardless of body weight at the outset of the induced deficit.[6,7] Over the same time window, we are remarkably tolerant of moderate increases in energy balance. Thus American adults, on average, gain 0.2 to 2.0 kg per year.[8]
3. While tolerant of positive energy balances, we do not eat anywhere near the maximum levels of EI that is readily obtainable by selecting commonly available foods. This behavior is apparent only in certain pathological states such as genetically determined leptin deficiency or binge eating, where intakes of 30 MJ a day have been reported.[3]
4. It seems, therefore, that there is a tonic control on EI, which limits a very rapid weight gain in most people. There is little evidence that such tonic control operates through negative feedback loops, as for tightly regulated

physiological systems, such as breathing. In other words, there is little evidence that, as fat mass accumulates, physiological signals become stronger and limit further gain in fat mass.[9] The exact nature and strength of the mechanisms that restrain excess EI in humans is currently unclear.

5. There is greater evidence that energy deficits do induce signals that elevate appetite and EI. As weight loss proceeds, these signals appear to become stronger, until they become the primarily motivational forces governing an individual's behavior.[10] There are a number of signaling systems in the periphery that interlink with the peptide messenger systems of the brain to increase intake when energy deficits significantly deplete tissue stores.[11] The extent to which these systems are involved in the control of day-to-day feeding behavior in humans is currently less clear.
6. As regards depletion of body tissues during periods of energy deficit, research has focused almost exclusively on fat.[11] This is despite the fact that in the clinical setting a negative nitrogen balance and loss of lean tissue are known to compromise physiological function. Loss of lean tissue during therapeutic weight loss may be a major factor signaling to the brain that physiological integrity is being eroded. The signals are as yet unknown.

Given these "facts" about food intake in the current environment, it is valuable to consider how the food environment has changed in recent decades.

16.2.3 Changes in the Food Environment

The diet we eat has changed considerably since the World War II. Fat contributes more to the diet now than in the 1930s, although recently it appears to be decreasing slightly.[12,13] Consumption of sugars added to the diet has increased steadily.[14] The way we eat has also changed, with restaurant meals, processed foods, and soft drinks being a bigger part of the diet than previously.[15,16] These changes have contributed to a food environment containing a wider range of relatively inexpensive, highly palatable, and energy-dense foods than ever before. It is frequently considered axiomatic that the ready availability of these foods contributes to current secular trends in increasing prevalence of obesity. In the last two decades a large amount of work has been conducted examining the role of diet composition in appetite and energy balance control.[17] We now have a clearer idea of the nutritional attributes of the diet that tend to elevate or limit excess EI. To understand this better, it is important to consider how the macronutrient composition of foods relates to dietary ED and EI.

16.3 THE RELATIONSHIP BETWEEN DIETARY MACRONUTRIENTS AND THE ENERGY DENSITY OF FOODS

As macronutrients come in the diet, fat is more energy dense (37 $kJ \cdot g^{-1}$) than either carbohydrate (16 $kJ \cdot g^{-1}$) or protein (17 $kJ \cdot g^{-1}$), while alcohol is 29 $kJ \cdot g^{-1}$.[18]

An analysis of 1032 ready-to-eat foods from the British food composition tables shows that the primary determinants of ED are water and fat (Figure 16.1).

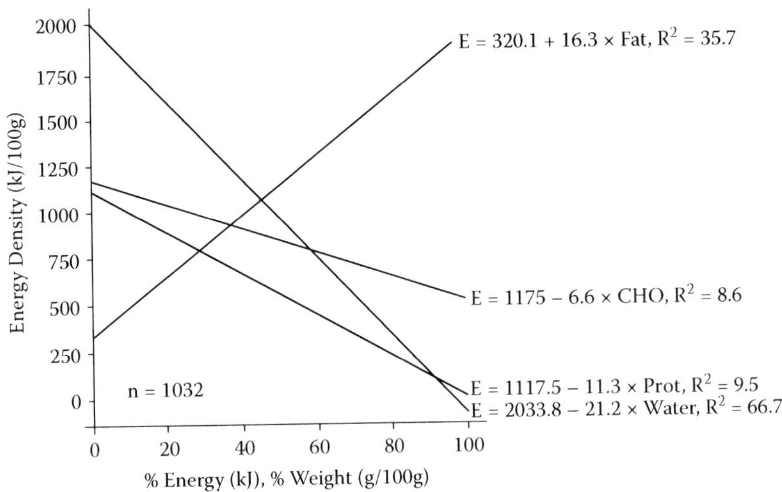

FIGURE 16.1 Analysis of the determinants of energy density in 1032 ready-to-eat foods from the British food tables.

Fat elevates ED, and water decreases ED. Protein and CHOs contribute very little to dietary ED *per se*.[3] Thus, the ED of foods is mainly determined by a fat–water seesaw. If high-protein, high-CHO, and high-fat foods are selected so that the two remaining macronutrients are equally represented (in MJ), then high-protein foods are less energy-dense than high-CHO foods, which are less energy-dense than high-fat foods (Figure 16.2). There is about 50% overlap in ED between each category.[19]

Although CHO and protein have relatively small and variable effects on energy density, there appears to be consistent evidence, whether foods or the overall diets of individuals are considered, that water and fat content are the main determinants of energy density.[3,20–25]

Many "lower-fat" alternatives of foods are of a similar ED to their more traditional counterparts,[22] because in these products fats are largely replaced by readily assimilated starches and disaccharides (Figure 16.3). This has been suggested as an explanation for the failure of the introduction of lower-fat alternative foods to significantly reduce EIs.[26] Having considered the relationship between macronutrients and ED, it is valuable to consider how both ED and the macronutrient content of foods influence satiety and EI.

16.4 ENERGY DENSITY, MACRONUTRIENTS, AND SATIETY

16.4.1 Energy Density

Many laboratory studies have shown that when the ED of foods is covertly increased, subjects tend to eat a similar amount of food and increase EI.[19] Conversely, when the ED of foods is covertly decreased, subjects show a similar lack of change in behavior and so consume less energy. These observations have led some authors to suggest that ED is the primary factor influencing human EI and that dietary macronutrients have

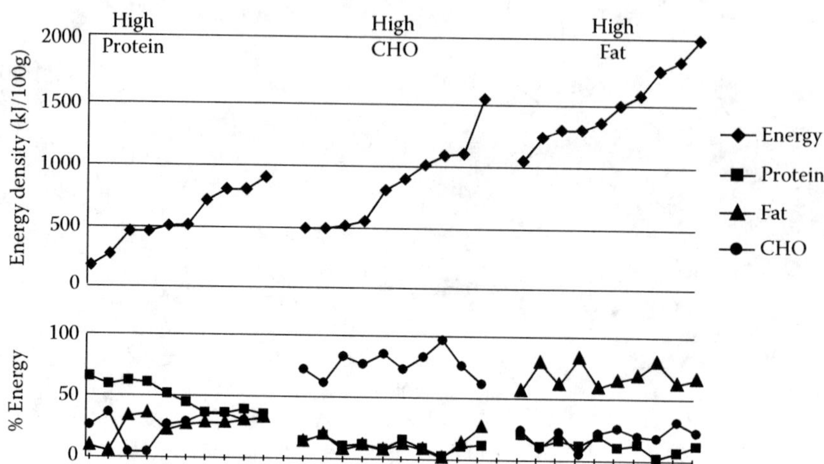

FIGURE 16.2 The macronutrient composition and energy density of selected high-protein, high-carbohydrate, and high-fat foods. The foods were chosen to be high in one macronutrient and to have (as close as possible) an equal energy content derived from the other two macronutrients.

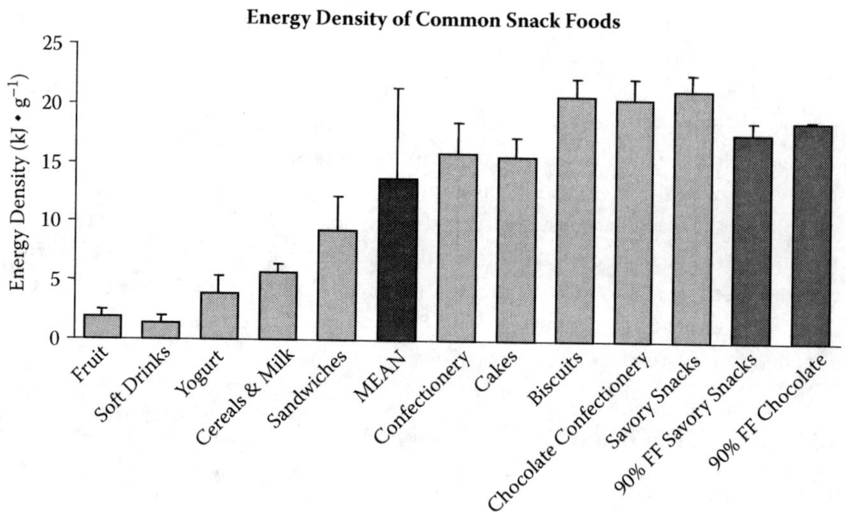

FIGURE 16.3 The energy density of a range of ready-to-eat snack foods taken from the British food tables. (FF = fat-free.)

little or no effect on satiety.[27,28] However, in most of these studies subjects are naive to the manipulation and do not have the time to learn the postingestive consequences of these relatively novel foods. When subjected to familiar foods, compensation is greater. Thus when Mazlan et al.[29] gave subjects 0, 1.5, and 3.0 MJ of covertly manipulated snack foods a day, which were either high in fat or high in sugar, subjects did not compensate EI over 7 days. In contrast the same energy intakes from familiar, commercial snack foods that were 2 to 3 times more energy dense resulted in around 50% EI compensation in free-living consumers.[30] Furthermore, compensation was a direct function of habitual consumption of commercial snack foods, illustrating the importance of learning as a mechanism of caloric compensation.

Yeomans et al.[31] showed that subjects learn to compensate more accurately when high- and low-energy density versions of the same food are paired to distinct flavors than when the foods remained covertly manipulated. Thus EI is not a simple function of the ED of the diet, although, especially in the short-to-medium term, changes in the ED of foods can have an effect on EI, due to the lack of precision with which food intake is regulated.[32] The simplest means of altering the ED of a food is to add or remove water from it. However, in free-living subjects, large variations in water intake do not have much discernable impact on EI.[25] Thus, there must be additional components to the diet that differ between high- and low-energy density foods, which lead to their tendency to elevate or constrain EI. These constituents are the macronutrients protein, CHO, fat, and alcohol, water, and structural components such as dietary fiber.

16.5 PROTEIN

Protein appears to be the macronutrient that elevates satiety and suppresses EI to a greater extent than any of the other macronutrients. Careful retrospective analysis of food records[19,33] indicates that protein exerts a postingestive action over and above the contribution from energy *per se*. Protein also exerts a large influence on satiety in the laboratory. Some studies using pure macronutrient loads delivered to the stomach, or solutions quickly swallowed by subjects wearing nose clips,[34,35] have found that all macronutrients have equal satiating power. It is intriguing in this regard that sensory cues (especially taste) may be important in clearly identifying the effects of nutrient ingestion. Miller and Teates[36] found that rats were able to select from nutritionally different diets to stabilize the protein energy ratio at 0.14. However, when subjected to impairment of oral somatosensory input, they were unable to maintain a stable selection pattern. The authors hypothesized that selection between protein and CHO (or energy) at least "involves an associative learning process in which somatosensory inputs effect feeding activity and/or the properties of the food link dietary choice behavior to later metabolic consequences."

It also appears that there is a critical threshold in the amount of protein required to suppress subsequent EI, because studies that have found little effect of protein relative to other macronutrient preloads have only used small amounts of energy as protein in the preload.[34,37] Hill and Blundell[38] found that a high-protein (HP) meal (31% of 2.1 MJ) produced a greater sensation of fullness and a decreased desire to eat, relative to a high-carbohydrate (H-CHO) meal (52%) of the same energy content.

They also found that both obese and normal-weight subjects reduced their subsequent meal intakes by 19 and 22%, respectively, after a HP (54% of 2 MJ) meal compared to a H-CHO meal (63% of 2 MJ) with weight of food held constant.[39] Barkeling et al.[40] gave 20 normal-weight women a high-protein (43% of 2.6 MJ) or a high-CHO (69% of 2.6 MJ) lunch. EI at a subsequent evening meal was depressed by 12% more after consumption of the HP than the high-CHO meal. Booth et al.[41] also found that a HP meal reduced the intake of a subsequent test meal by 26% relative to a virtually protein-free meal in normal-weight individuals. Thus, protein appears to be particularly satiating when given at moderate and large amounts.

This apparent appetite-restraining effect of protein has not yet been given a strong theoretical basis. Essential amino acids when ingested in excess of requirements form a physiological stress that must be disposed of by oxidation. It is known that animals will alter feeding behavior in order to alleviate a physiological stress.[42] Pigs, in particular, appear capable of learning to select a protein:energy ratio in the diet that is optimal for growth,[43,44] as can rats.[36] The protein:energy ratio of foods may be important in influencing feeding. Malnourished children find it difficult to tolerate nutritional supplements whose protein:energy ratio is too high. Millward has hypothesized that lean tissue deposition may be an important factor driving appetite during catch-up growth in children.[45]

16.5.1 Protein and the Prevention of Weight Regain

Stubbs and Elia have suggested that lean tissue depletion during weight loss may be at least as important as adipose tissue depletion in increasing appetite and driving intake upward.[46] This concept has been long neglected. One seminal study has enabled the relationship between tissue loss and subsequent feeding behavior to be determined.[47] The results were quite remarkable and have been revisited by Dulloo.[48,49] During the Minnesota semistarvation study a group of lean men were chronically underfed for 24 weeks, consuming ~40% of their normal EI throughout this period. During this time they lost ~70% of their fat mass and ~18 to 20% of their lean body mass. For the next 12 weeks, they were incrementally refed in a mandatory manner. By the end of this period, they were still in a deficit of ~25% for fat mass and 12 to 15% for lean body mass. During the final 8 weeks subjects had *ad libitum* access to a range of foods. During this period EI initially increased to 160% of requirements and gradually subsided to preweight-loss levels. However, by this time fat mass had reached 170% of preweight-loss values, while lean body mass had returned to preweight-loss levels.[48,49] These relationships are depicted in Figure 16.4. Thus, the cessation of postweight-loss hyperphagia coincided with a massive overshoot of fat mass, but precise repletion of lean body mass. There are very few data sets of this extremity or quality available, which highlights the importance of conducting more detailed longitudinal studies with this degree of precision and accuracy. If depletion of lean tissue during weight loss stimulates hunger, then increased protein intake, subsequent to significant weight loss, may replete lean tissue faster and help stabilize body weight at a new, lower level. While there is evidence to support this hypothesis in growing children,[45] there is little evidence that this mechanism operates at the levels of weight loss adult humans usually achieve (~10% of original body weight).[50,51]

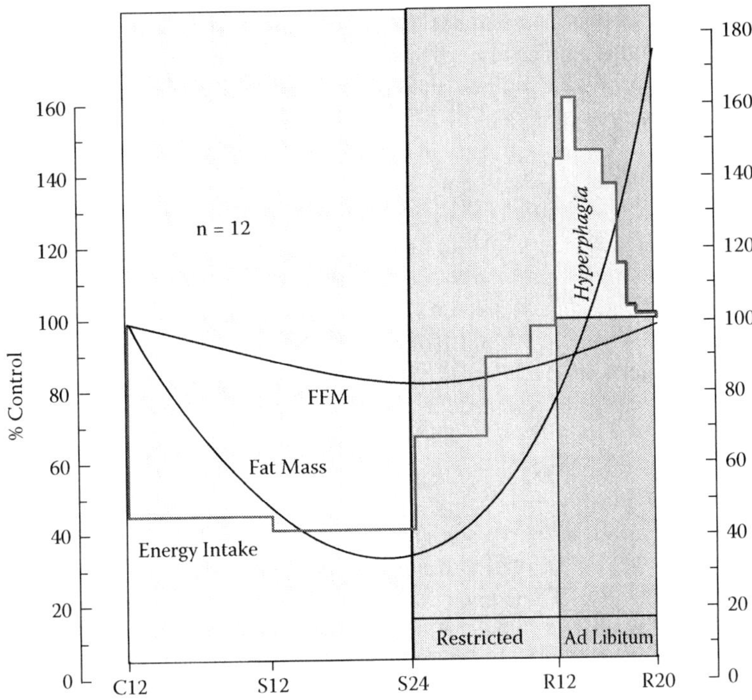

FIGURE 16.4 Relationship between energy intake and tissue change during 6 months severe undernutrition, 3 months rehabilitation, and 2 months *ad libitum* feeding in 12 of the subjects who took part in the Minnesota study. Of particular note is the fact that *ad libitum* energy intake returned to pre-underfeeding levels at approximately the time lean tissue returned to baseline values. By this time fat mass had overshot baseline, and reached ~170% of original levels.

It can be seen from the arguments outlined in this discussion that the physiological regulation of lean tissue may be a critical factor exerting feedback on subsequent EI. When subjects are in energy balance, excess protein intake does not increase the size of lean body mass.[52] Instead it is disposed of by transamination, deamination, and urea production. This regulation of protein balance by obligatory oxidative disposal predicts a suppression of subsequent EI.[5] During undernutrition, lean body mass becomes depleted.[47,52,53] The Keys data from the Minnesota semistarvation study suggest that, when food is available *ad libitum,* subjects do not stop eating when fat mass is repleted, but when lean body mass is repleted. Thus, there is evidence that the regulation of lean tissue (which helps maintain normal physiological function), through oxidation of excess and repletion of deficits in protein intake, may exert some negative feedback effect on longer-term EI.[46] The role of lean tissue in this respect has been largely ignored. It is important to understand how both lean and adipose tissue changes relate to longer-term energy balance.[46–49] This is again important in the clinical setting, since loss of lean tissue in disease compromises physiological function and can complicate further the effects of disease. Understanding how loss of fat and lean tissue relate to other aspects of function, health, and well-being will be critical in improving sustained weight loss.

16.5.2 Protein and Weight Loss

The last few years has seen a frenzy of interest in the role of high-protein diets in promoting weight loss. A well conducted study by Skov et al. showed that a low-fat diet which was high in protein was more effective at reducing weight than a low-fat diet that was high in CHO.[54] This finding in combination the high satiety value of protein and with current concerns about the role of some CHOs in weight control has led to a renaissance of interest in the role of high-protein diets in weight control. As is often the case in this area of research, these concepts have overshot their logical conclusion, leading to renewed interest in low-CHO, high-protein diets. Four major studies have now been conducted to examine the effect of high-protein, low-fat, weight-reducing diets on body weight over 6 to 12 months.[55–58]

On average high-protein, low-CHO, weight-reducing diets produced around 4 kg greater weight loss within 6 months relative to normal-protein, high-CHO diets. However, these differences were not apparent at 12 months, demonstrating no clear long-term advantage of such diets to lose weight. A diet that is very high in protein and very low in CHO tends to be extremely monotonous, and there are limits to the palatability of such diets, making adherence difficult. Furthermore, it appears that the initial success of such diets is due to the high satiety value of protein, and there seems little need to drastically reduce CHO intake to achieve this effect, as demonstrated by the Skov study.[54] This notion has recently found experimental support in a study by Weigle et al., who kept the CHO content of the diet constant and altered the amount of protein and fat for 2 weeks per dietary treatment.[59] Nineteen subjects spent 2 weeks consuming a diet comprising 15% protein, 35% fat, and 50% CHO. They then spent 2 weeks on an isoenegetic diet comprising 30% protein, 20% fat, and 50% CHO. Following this they consumed *ad libitum* a diet composed of 30% protein, 20% fat, and 50% CHO. During the fixed-intake phase subjects experienced greater satiety on the high-protein diet. When they fed *ad libitum* on this diet they lost 5 kg over the 12 weeks. Thus, the apparent effect of so-called low-CHO diets appears to be due to the fact that they are high in protein and there is no apparent need to minimize CHO intake.

It is worth mentioning one caveat in relation to high- and low-protein diets. People rarely discuss what exactly a high- or low-protein diet means. On average, Western adults consume around 10 to 20% of their EI from protein when they are in approximate energy balance. As Westerterp-Plantenga et al. note, when considering weight-reducing diets the absolute amount of protein as well as the percentage of EI from protein should be taken into account.[50] This is because a very-low-energy diet containing, for example, 40% protein may still only contain moderate amounts relative to requirements.

16.6 CARBOHYDRATES

The public perception of CHOs has oscillated in recent decades. Throughout the 1970s there was a tendency to view CHOs (especially refined forms) as conducive to weight gain. This reached its logical extreme with perceptions of sugars as "pure, white, and deadly" by Yudkin.[60] Since then, and until recently, the nutritional perception of CHOs has improved dramatically. By the mid-1990s, dietary fat had developed a reputation of near demonic proportions as the dietary villain of the late twentieth century and was squarely blamed as the major dietary constituent promoting excess EI. Dietary CHO was generally viewed in generic terms as a beneficial nutrient whose ingestion could promote all manner of positive outcomes with reference to weight control.[61] The positive effects of carbohydrates on energy balance were enshrined in the predictions of JP Flatt's glycogenostatic model of energy balance control.[62] The general perceptions about CHOs and energy balance at this time were as follows:

1. It was generally accepted that CHOs are absorbed, metabolized, and stored with less bioenergetic efficiency than dietary fat. Indeed, a general perception was developing that, because *de novo* lipogenesis appears limited when humans feed on Western diets, CHO ingestion does not promote fat storage.[63,64]
2. At the same time there was a renaissance of interest in CHO-specific models of feeding. The notion that CHO metabolism or stores exert powerful negative feedback on EI became quite firmly established in the field of energy and nutrient balance.[9,17]
3. The simultaneous focus of researchers and health professionals on dietary fat as the pivotal nutrient promoting high levels of EI reinforced CHO-specific models of feeding. HF hyperphagia was seen as due to the tendency for subjects to eat to CHO balance rather than energy balance.[9,17]
4. By the same reasoning, diets high in CHOs were deemed to be more satiating, specifically because they were high in CHOs.
5. The extension of this logic led to the notion amongst some that it was difficult if not virtually impossible to overeat on a high-CHO diet.[63,64]
6. Finally, epidemiological observations have shown that, in subjects self-recording their food intakes, the percentage of EI from fat and CHOs are reciprocally related to each other. One form of this relationship has been termed the fat–sugar seesaw. It has been noted in one seminal study that high-sugar consumers also tend to be thinner than HF consumers are.[65] This led to the suggestion that sugar displaces fat energy from the diet, and since fat is conducive to weight gain, high-sugar intakes may well protect against obesity.[66]

Carbohydrates had never had it so good. Fat reduction became the order of the day, and the low-fat (LF) food market rapidly expanded.[67,68] The fat reduction message is now so strong that consumers appear to focus on fat avoidance as a primary nutritional objective while foraging for food in local supermarkets. The food industry has gone to great lengths to diversify products in the direction of LF, lower fat, and high-CHO foods that have sufficient sensory appeal that consumers will continue to select them. A major sensory attribute of high-CHO foods, which is almost ubiquitously appealing, is sweetness.

In recent years, there have been some doubts about the paramount role of CHOs as the central nutrient around which energy balance is regulated and body weight controlled.[9,17]

1. While excess CHO is stored with less efficiency than fat, the relevance of these effects to free-living Western consumers has been questioned.
2. Several rigorous tests of CHO-specific models of feeding have suggested that CHO oxidation, or stores, *per se* do not exert powerful unconditioned negative feedback on EI.[9,17,19,69] Rather, as macronutrients come in the diet (where fat is disproportionately energy dense), there appears to be a hierarchy in the satiating efficiency of the macronutrients. Per MJ of energy ingested, protein, CHO, and fat produce supercaloric, approximately isocaloric, and subcaloric compensation, respectively. Furthermore, statistical modeling shows that models including all three macronutrients explain far more of the variance in EI, either in the laboratory, or in free-living subjects.[19] When ED is controlled, protein is still far more satiating than CHOs or fats, and the differences in the satiating efficiency of CHOs and fats become more subtle (see below).[3,17,19]
3. HF hyperphagia can be explained by the high palatability and ED of HF foods (which facilitate greater levels of intake) and the low postabsorptive satiety value of fat (which prevents subsequent compensatory decreases in EI). While CHO is more satiating than fat, excess fat intake is not necessarily driven by a need to eat to maintain CHO balance.
4. There appear to be several reasons why many high-CHO foods are more satiating than HF foods. First, they are usually (but not always) less energy dense than HF foods. Many high-CHO foods contain dietary fiber, which limits rates of ingestion and digestion, both of which can have a limiting effect on EI. High-CHO foods that are dry will tend to exert a higher osmotic load in the gut than will HF foods of similar moisture content. When the energy content and ED of high-CHO and HF foods are compared, readily assimilated CHO is more satiating than fat. This difference in the satiating capacity of fat and CHO can be deemed to be independent of ED or palatability. However, this effect is much weaker than when HF, ED foods are compared to lower-fat less ED foods that are high in CHO.[61] Thus the nutrient-specific differences in the satiating effects of fats and CHOs need to be considered in relation to the structure and composition of the foods in which those nutrients abound.[61]
5. Frequently, it has been stated that there is no evidence that foods high in CHOs promote overconsumption. This may be due to the fact that the majority of studies examining the effects of high-CHO and HF foods on feeding behavior compared HF, more energy-dense foods to high-CHO (LF), less energy-dense foods. The majority of studies that demonstrate the effects of fat in promoting excess EI examined how adding fat to the diet influences feeding. Recently a few studies have examined how adding CHOs to food affects feeding behavior or EI.[61] In one study at least, increasing the ED of the diet by dramatically increasing the maltodextrin content led to marked elevations of EI over 14 days, as shown in Figure 16.5.[70]
6. While the fat–sugar seesaw has become a well-recognized phenomenon, the phenomenon itself has been harder to pin down. The fact that fat and sugar, or even fat and CHO, are reciprocally related to each other in the diet

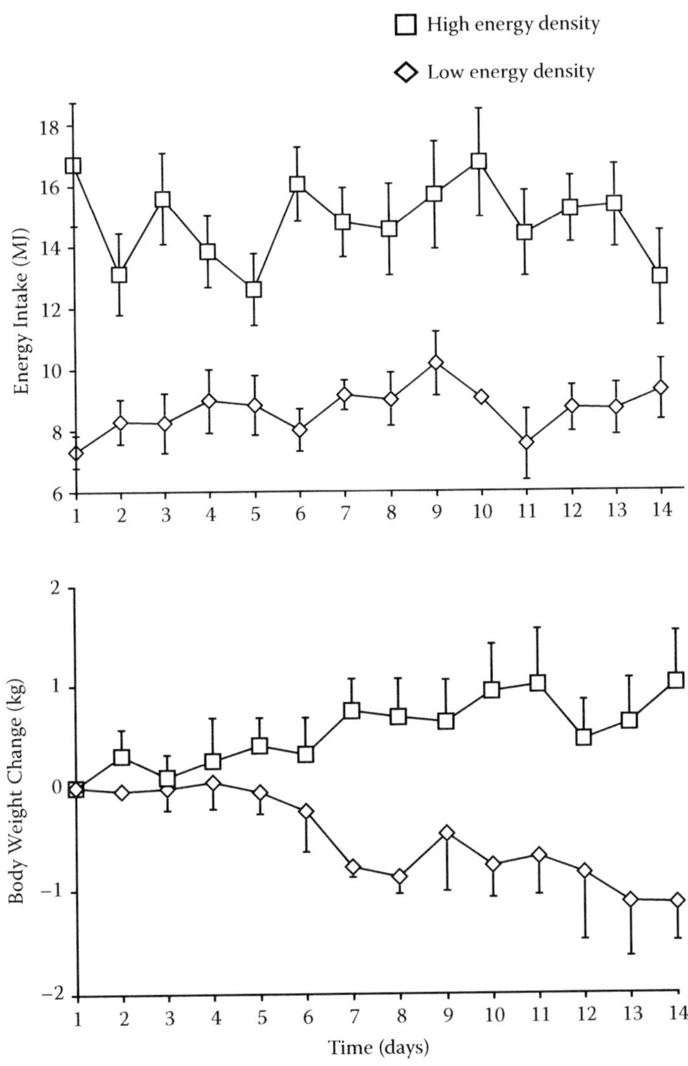

FIGURE 16.5 Energy intake and change in body weight of six men who fed *ad libitum* on low- and high-energy density diets that were both high in percent energy from carbohydrate (> 60%) for 2 weeks per treatment.

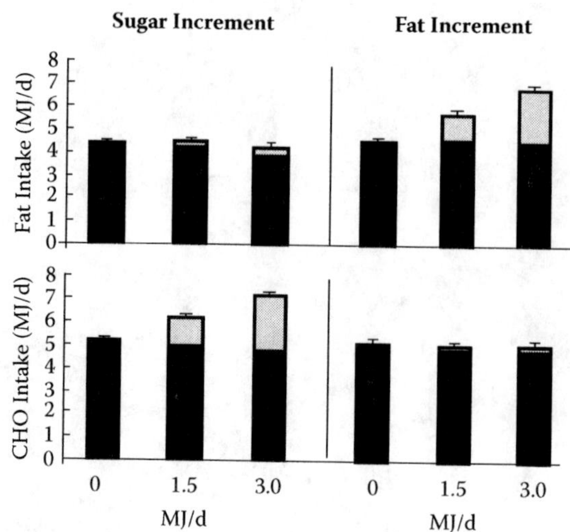

FIGURE 16.6 The impact of 0, 1.5, and 3.0 MJ/day of high-fat or high-sugar mandatory snacks on the intake of fat and carbohydrate, when subjects had *ad libitum* access to a counterbalanced selection of high-protein, high-carbohydrate, and high-fat foods, over the course of 7 days.

is almost inevitable, given that they are the main energy-providing macronutrients.[71] Adding fats and sugars into the diet in an incremental manner does not produce a fat:sugar seesaw effect.[29,30] The energy from fat- or sugar-rich snacks is largely added to voluntary EI with no macronutrient specific compensation (Figure 16.6).

16.6.1 Types of Carbohydrate and Appetite Control

Carbohydrates can be simple (short-chain sugars), complex (starches and nonstarch polysaccharides), or the intermediate-chain-length oligosaccharides. Very little is known about the vast range of different starches and their various structures in relation to appetite and energy balance.[61] These are still uncharted landscapes on the research horizon.

High-CHO foods most capable of limiting EI (both voluntary and metabolizable) are those rich in unavailable complex carbohydrates (UCCs). However, there is a catch, because in general, humans are not too fond of these foods, and as typified by the average Western diet, when given the choice they tend to select a diet comprising 37 to 42% fat, 10 to 20% sugar, and a variable amount of high-glycemic-index starches. The average Western adult's fiber intake is spectacularly low.[72,73] It is likely that dietary fiber exerts a secondary indirect effect on satiety and EI. Many high-CHO foods of a low ED (such as fruits and vegetables) have a lot of intracellular water bound into their food matrix by structural CHOs. When water is ingested in addition to food, it empties from the stomach more quickly than the solid phase and so has little effect on delaying gastric emptying or in activating associated satiety signals. However, when water is bound into the food matrix by structural CHOs a greater time is required to digest them and empty the stomach, and this may account for why the low ED of such foods is associated with slower nutrient release and delayed postabsorptive signals associated with their ingestion.

16.6.2 Glycemic Index of Foods, Satiety, and Energy Intake

In the light of the recent doubts aired about the central role that CHOs may play in limiting weight gain, attention has again focused on the impact of the glycemic index or load of CHOs on satiety and EI. The glycemic index of a CHO is its capacity (relative to a white bread standard) to increase plasma glucose and insulin. The evidence relating to the glycemic index of CHOs currently cannot be interpreted due to the heterogeneity of study designs, vehicles, and treatments used and, indeed, doubts as to whether the glycemic index of a food is a physiological constant. In a recent review of this area Raben examined 31 short-term studies and found that, relative to high glycemic index foods, 15 studies found reduced hunger when subjects consumed low-GI foods, but 16 studies showed no difference. Seven studies showed a reduced food intake when subjects consumed low-GI foods, but 16 studies showed no difference. Of 20 longer-term studies (up to 6 months) 4 showed greater weight loss with low-GI diets, while 15 showed no difference. A major problem with many of these studies is that, while GI is the main focus of the dietary manipulation, several other attributes of the diet are often altered to achieve the change in GI. These include the starch, fiber, and sugar content of foods, their physical state and degree of preparation (raw foods have a lower GI than cooked), and the orosensory and physical properties of the foods. Thus in many cases it is not GI *per se* that is being altered. While there appears to be something associated with the GI of foods that sometimes affects satiety and feeding behavior, exactly what this is has not become clearly apparent. This should be an area of future research.

It is also worth bearing in mind that there are a number of CHOs with a relatively low GI that are implicated in the development of weight gain. The fructose-based corn syrups which are used as a main CHO sweetener in soft drinks and other foods are a case in point. This raises the question "when do high-CHO foods promote over-consumption?"

16.6.3 How Easy Is It to Overeat on a High-Carbohydrate Diet?

Clearly this depends on the ED, palatability, and the type of CHO in the diets concerned. It has been demonstrated that excess EIs are possible when normal-weight men feed *ad libitum* on HC diets over 14 days.[69] The sensory attribute primarily associated with short-chain CHOs (sweetness) is known to stimulate EI, especially when combined as mixtures with fats.[74] Do the sensory attributes of some sweet foods elevate palatability and hence intake of those foods? Dissolving short-chain CHOs in solution appears to be an effective means of supplementing EI. The majority of snack foods produced (rather than sold) tend to be high in CHO and ED. These considerations suggest that there is considerable scope for HC foods to promote high levels of EI and in some cases energy balanced (EB). The exact conditions under which this occurs, and in whom, are presently unclear. In a recent series of studies Mazlan et al. have shown that the addition of mandatory snacks (ED = 550 kJ/100 g) which were rich in sugar, fat, or starch led to elevated EIs over 7 days in men, women, and lean and overweight subjects.[75] While short-term studies show that low-energy density preloads that are high in sugar induce caloric compensation, a longer-term study has shown that a less energy-dense, high-sugar diet consumed *ad libitum* led to similar EIs in women as a higher-fat, more energy-dense diet. This was because subjects ate more food on the high-sugar diet.[76] It appears that the high-sugar diet stimulated the greatest food intake — presumably due to its high level of sweetness. It also appears that sugar can stimulate appetite and leads to excess EI (and obesity) in rats. Several data from studies in rats have shown that overeating of simple sugars such as glucose and sucrose, has led to obesity, especially if those sugars are in solution.[77–79] There is recent evidence that this is also the case in humans. Raben et al. investigated the effect of medium-term (10 weeks) supplementation with either sucrose or artificial sweeteners (primarily as drinks) on *ad libitum* food intake and body weight in overweight subjects.[80] Two groups of overweight subjects (36 women, 6 men) consumed dietary supplements containing sucrose or artificial sweeteners for 10 weeks in a parallel design. On average, the sucrose intervention supplemented 3.4 MJ/day and 152 g/day sucrose, and the sweetener intervention added 1.0 MJ/day and 0 g/day sucrose per day. After 10 weeks sucrose supplementation, EI increased (2.6 MJ/day), as did ED, and the percentage of energy from sucrose (to 28 E%) and CHO E%. The percentage of energy from fat and protein decreased. On the sweetener-supplemented diet the only change was a small decrease in sucrose intake (by 4% of EI). Taken together these studies suggest that excess EI can readily occur when subjects consume sweet short-chain CHOs in foods that are rich in readily assimilated energy. It appears we may have to revise our assessments of the capacity of certain CHOs to elevate EI.

16.6.4 Which Carbohydrates (CHOs) Stimulate and Which Protect against Excess Energy Intake (EI)?

The current controversy regarding which CHOs promote and which protect against excess EI is due to a number of factors. First, it seems likely that, as more foods rich in readily assimilated CHOs become available, the ED of high-CHO foods is, on average, increasing. Second, CHO is a term used to describe a range of structures from monosaccharides and disaccharides at one end of the spectrum to a range of unavailable complex CHOs at the other. It is reasonable to state that shorter-chain CHOs are likely to have more of an intake-promoting effect, and unavailable complex CHOs will have more of an intake-restraining effect. There is a broad range of starches and shorter-chain CHOs in between these extremes. Their sensory and physiological effects cannot be predicted from chain length alone, since other factors such as the ratio of alpha to beta links and branching of chains are critically important. There is a vast range of specific CHO subtypes, and their effects on appetite and energy balance are almost virtually unknown at this level. It is also important to recognize that some CHOs may constrain intake because they limit the digestibility of foods. They may not elevate satiety though, and this will add further to the heterogeneity of feeding and motivational responses. As has been discussed throughout this chapter, there are numerous confounding effects which need to be controlled when comparing the effects of different CHOs on appetite, feeding behavior, and energy balance. These include the ED of foods, the presence of other nutrients in foods, the moisture content of foods being compared, the sensory attributes of foods, and the psychological, physiological, and genetic predisposition of the subjects being studied. Indeed, given the number of confounding issues, it is not surprising that, at the present time, it is difficult to give anything more than a preliminary assessment of which CHOs promote and which protect against weight gain.

Given the range of CHO structures available to the food market and the different physicochemical properties they possess, it is particularly important to identify how these potentially beneficial effects of CHO structure can be used to enhance preabsorptive and absorptive-phase satiety signals.

16.6.5 Dietary Fiber

Most work on the effects of different CHOs on EI has been done with UCCs or fiber. The time-energy displacement concept has been invoked to suggest that the addition of UCCs to the diet enhances satiation and limits meal size. This effect is apparent in some of the studies discussed above, and the phenomenon has been used to limit weight gain in farm animals on single feeds.

Over 50 studies have examined the effects of dietary fiber on food intake and body weight, and these have been extensively covered in four reviews,[81–84] to which the reader is referred. In summary, various loads of UCC or fiber at one meal have been shown to decrease both hunger and EI at the next meal, but the effects are relatively modest. Levine and Billington[81] note that 26 of 38 long-term studies have examined the effects of increased UCC ingestion on body weight. The results of this seemingly large number of trials are equivocal because of the different forms of fiber used, the different vehicles chosen (ranging from real foods to tablet formulations), different subject populations, and the varying degrees of experimental control ranging from overt to double-blind manipulations. The conclusion seems to be that supplementing the diet with tolerable levels of extracted UCC appears to have, at best, modest effects in decreasing body weight over several months or more. However, fiber-rich bulky diets of low ED may have different effects, and the reader should consider the methodological issues detailed in a number of references[81–84] before drawing firm conclusions. A major problem with the notion of using dietary fiber to limit intake is that people do not enjoy very fibrous foods. They tend, therefore, not to select them.

16.6.6 Wet versus Dry Carbohydrates

Mattes has conducted a meta-analysis of feeding responses to either liquid or solid manipulations of the nutrient and energy content of the diet.[85] The analysis suggests that the physical state of ingested CHO intake is important in influencing subsequent caloric compensation. The reasons for this are at present unclear, but may relate to the rate, timing, and density at which the energy is ingested. There may be a threshold in these parameters, below which energy is poorly detected. In 1955 Fryer supplemented the diet of college students with a high-CHO drink containing 1.8 MJ/day for 2 months. Compensation was incomplete (~50%) after 8 weeks.[86] The recent study by Raben et al. also confirms that supplementing the diet with wet CHOs can lead to elevations of both EI and body weight in the medium-term.[87]

There is a large range of CHO subtypes whose specific structures, either alone or in combination with other nutrients, are likely to influence appetite and energy balance. At the present time very little is known about which aspects of CHO structure are most likely to influence motivation to eat and feeding behavior. Here lies an expanse of virgin territory for research into the development of functional foods.

16.7 FAT

Numerous laboratory studies have now shown that when humans or animals are allowed to feed *ad libitum* on high-fat energy-dense diets, they consume similar amounts (weight) of food but more energy (which is usually accompanied by weight gain) than when they feed *ad libitum* on lower-fat, less energy-dense diets, as depicted in Figure 16.7.[5,88,89] The ingestion of systematically manipulated HF, energy-dense diets does not appear to elicit compensatory feeding responses. Interestingly, if single midday meals are covertly manipulated, by increasing or decreasing their ED using fat or CHO, under conditions where subjects feed on a range of familiar food items, compensation appears to be more precise.[90,91] When experiments are conducted over similar time frames but the diet is systematically manipulated (subjects cannot select food items of differing composition), compensation for the fat content of the diet is again poor.[92] These observations further suggest that both learning and preabsorptive and absorptive-phase factors play a major role in meal-to-meal compensation. Furthermore, a number of prospective observational epidemiological studies show that fat consumption is a risk factor for subsequent weight gain.[93] However, it is

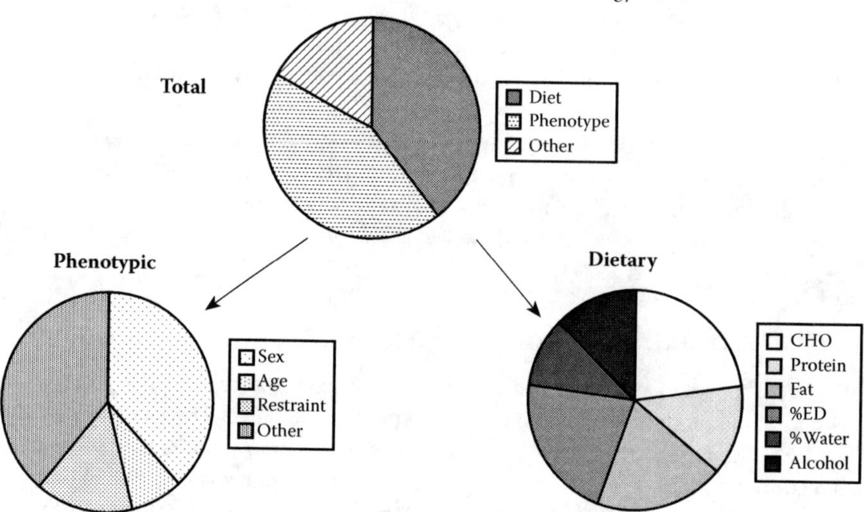

FIGURE 16.7 Pie charts illustrating the percentage of the variability in energy intake ascribable to different sources in 102 subjects self-recording their food intake for 7 consecutive days. Approximately 39% of the variability was due to diet, and ~40% was due to intersubject variability. These two major sources of variation are subdivided further. These charts clearly illustrate that the determinants of energy intake in human adults is multifactorial.

unlikely to be the only risk factor, and few analyses take account of how fat interacts with types of CHOs. For instance, in the short term, sweet high-fat foods have potent effect at stimulating EI.[94]

We are beginning to gain insights into the effects of types of fat on appetite control, due to the search for forms of fat that do not predispose to weight gain. Fat structure varies in terms of (1) chain length, (2) degree of saturation, (3) degree of esterification, and (4) by combining (1–3), through the development of novel structured lipids. Information is scarce and fragmentary in this area, but some provisional patterns are beginning to emerge. Substitution of long-chain triglyceride (LCT) by medium-chain triglyceride (MCT) limits the high levels of EI usually seen with high-fat, energy-dense diets.[95] Although very large doses of MCT are usually required in order to achieve these effects, a recent study has shown that a much lower dose of structured MCT and LCT (14 g/day of medium-long-chain triglyceride containing 1.7 g of medium-chain fatty acids) led to significant decreases in body weight and fat relative to LCT in 82 adults.[96] Matsuo et al.[97] found similar effects in a study using a similar design. MCTs may suppress appetite relative to LCT, as they are more readily absorbed and oxidized. They are also more ketogenic than LCT, and it has been suggested that ketones act as appetite suppressants.

There is some preliminary evidence that ketone bodies (specifically beta-hydroxybutyrate) are appetite suppressants when given orally,[98] and this may enhance compliance when subjects attempt to lose weight using very low-calorie diets. Currently there is little evidence that degree of fatty acid esterification influences appetite and EI.[99,100] It has been suggested that polyunsaturates (PUFAs) are protective against obesity, since they are more readily mobilized and oxidized and may influence gene expression of appetite-controlling peptides.[101] Recent work in humans suggests that saturated fats are less satiating than mono- or polyunsaturates.[102,103] An intriguing study in humans has reported that supplementation with very high levels of gamma-linolenate (at 5 g/day compared to 5 g/day olive oil) significantly reduced weight gain over 12 months after extensive weight reduction using very low-calorie diets.[104] Currently there are few or no reports on the effects of structured lipids on appetite and energy balance. It has been suggested that diglycerides may reduce weight gain due to high fat intakes relative to triglycerides. The evidence is currently sketchy. We have found no effect of diglycerides on appetite or energy balance either within or between days. However, the position of the fatty acid side chains may be of importance. Maki et al. found that incorporation of 1,3 diglyceride oil into a weight-reducing diet increased weight and fat loss in 131 obese subjects over 24 weeks, compared to normal triglyceride.[105] While significant, the differences were modest, amounting to a 1.1% greater weight loss for the diglyceride treatment. In the future, specific nutrients could be tailored to exert quantitatively significant effects on appetite control, tissue deposition, and energy balance. In this context, it is of note that certain isomers of conjugated linoleic acid (CLA) can be used to influence appetite and tissue deposition in animals[106] and perhaps humans.[107] The effects of CLA are not entirely understood but appear to be near pharmacological in nature. In a series of studies Riserus et al.[114–116] have examined the impact of both mixed isomers and the *trans*-10,*cis*-12 CLA isomer on anthropometry, lipid, and glucose metabolism and markers of lipid peroxidation. They found that CLA may slightly decrease body fat in humans but has no effect on weight or body mass index. It does however have deleterious effects on insulin sensitivity, blood glucose, and serum lipids and increases lipid peroxidation. Belury et al. did find that plasma levels of administered CLA mixtures were inversely associated with body weight in subjects with type 2 diabetes.[108] Petridou et al. found that 45-day supplementation with CLA had no effect on weight or body fat of young healthy women.[109] The initial promise shown by CLA as being capable of limiting weight gain does not appear to have been fulfilled. As in many of the above examples unusual lipids or structured triglycerides have biologically curious effects, but little impact on appetite and energy balance in humans. However, it can be envisaged that in the future structured lipids could be developed to combine some of the individually modest effects of fat type on appetite and feeding behavior.

16.7.1 The Fat Paradoxes

The apparently ambivalent effects of fat have generated a phenomenon referred to as the fat paradox. A fat such as corn oil infused into the ileum or jejunum has been shown to slow gastric emptying, increase feelings of fullness, and reduce food intake in a test meal,[110] whereas similar infusions made intravenously exert no effect on gastric emptying or measures of appetite. Lipid infusions at around 80% of resting energy requirements, over 3 days, produce only partial compensation (43%) of EI.[111] These findings imply that potent fat-induced satiety signals are generated by pre-absorptive rather than postabsorptive physiological responses. In addition, a number of short- and medium-term studies have demonstrated high energy intakes with high-fat foods.[5,88,89] How can these two features be reconciled? It appears that, in normal feeding, the stomach controls the rate at which nutrients are delivered to the duodenum on an approximately caloric basis. Thus the high levels of satiety seen in gastrointestinal infusions studies may well be due to supraphysiological saturation of satiety mechanisms arising from the small intestine.

In recent years a second fat paradox has become apparent. Despite the fact that the fat content of the diet has been reduced over the last decade, there appears to have been no decrease in the prevalence of obesity in Western society. Part of this could be because the more we tell people what to eat the more they tell us they are eating what we want to see. Part of it may be due to the increasingly sedentary environment we live in. It is also likely that the low-fat food revolution has produced a range of lower-fat foods that are not much lower in ED than their full-fat counterparts, and are as, if not more, appealing as the foods they were designed to replace. In addition, both portion size and the proportion of EI from liquids has increased over this time. All of these factors would tend to produce the patterns in obesity prevalence that exist and also illustrate the mulitfactorial nature of the dietary determinants of EI.

16.8 ALCOHOL

Alcohol is exceptional in that its ingestion can stimulate food intake and so induces countercompensatory increases in EI.[112,113] Given that alcohol is also a drug with depressant effects on the CNS, this is not surprising. This is illustrated by the work of de Castro and Mattes,[85,113] who suggest that, in moderate drinkers at least, the energy derived from alcohol is added to the energy derived from other sources. de Castro has shown that EI is higher on days when alcohol is consumed than on days when it is not and that as EI from alcohol rises there is no compensatory reduction in food intake. Mattes has suggested, from a meta-analysis of several studies, that alcohol appears to stimulate EI.[85] Thus there is some evidence that alcohol promotes excess EI by increasing, or at least failing to suppress on a caloric basis, EI from other food sources.

16.9 THE COMBINED EFFECTS OF MACRONUTRIENTS AND ENERGY DENSITY ON ENERGY INTAKE

In considering the nutritional determinants of EI in 102 free-living adults, self-recording their food intake for 7 days, both macronutrients and ED determine EI in subjects consuming their normal diets.[19] The notion that ED alone drives EI is oversimplified. Multifactorial models appear more appropriate to explain nutritional determinants of feeding. This is illustrated in Figure 16.7. It is recommended that modeling work such as this be extended in order to better appreciate and predict the way in which the nutritional characteristics of the diet affect EI in people at large. Since differences between subjects can account for almost half of the variance in the relationships between food composition and EI (Figure 16.7), models should help to identify key factors that predict a significant proportion of intersubject variation in feeding behavior.

On balance, foods that are energy dense, high in fats, sugars, and rapidly assimilated starches, and that are low in protein and fiber are conducive to higher levels of EI. An apparent paradox is that, while water lowers the ED of the diet, higher levels of water intake *per se* seem to have little impact on overall EI. What does appear to be important is the way in which water is bound into the food matrix. Thus foods that have a high intrinsic water content such as meat, fish, fruit, and vegetables are all low in ED, and this decreases the rate at which they are digested and assimilated. It is also known that when water intake is not sufficient (when people are dehydrated), they eat less. Despite these intriguing observations, there is a remarkable paucity of data examining the relationship between fluid and food intake and how this impacts on overall energy balance.

16.9.1 Supporting the Human Knowledge Base with Complementary Studies in Animal Models

There are a number of areas where research in animal models can extend and complement the work that has been conducted in humans. Many laboratory studies in animals and humans carefully control individual dietary factors. However, it would be useful to examine the impact of multiple dietary treatments on body composition and putative molecular mechanisms of weight control over long periods. An example would be to compare high- and low-protein and high- and low-carbohydrate diets in a 2×2 design. In this way it would be possible to use animal models to inform human studies as to which combinations of dietary attributes best promote weight stability in *ad libitum*-feeding animals.

It is perhaps important to attempt to disentangle the influence of environmental (unregulated) and physiological (regulated) influences on long-term energy balance and body weight.

Because a great deal of compensatory responses involve the process of learning, it would be valuable to increase our understanding of the longer-term effects of dietary manipulations on feeding behavior and energy balance when animals and humans have the opportunity to learn the consequences of consuming diets of different compositions. Furthermore, given that in the absence of learning it is very easy to use diet composition and energy density to alter energy balance, it would be extremely valuable to ascertain the rate and extent of compensation over time for such manipulations.

In humans, the present recommended rate of weight loss is 1 to 2 pounds per week. However, we need a better understanding of the relationship between the rate of weight loss, the composition of weight loss, its impact on functional outcomes, and subsequent weight regain. Is rapid weight loss really deleterious and, if so, why and to what extent?

Animal models would be invaluable in gaining a better understanding of the mechanisms of protein-induced satiety. It is also becoming important to understand whether the apparent effect of high-protein diets requires a particularly low carbohydrate intake or whether carbohydrate is merely acting as another energy-providing substrate. Additionally, the relatively high throughput of research in small animals might accelerate our ability to test the effects of novel carbohydrates, starches, and fibers on satiety, nutrient absorption, and energy balance. In this context, it is becoming necessary to work out what correlates of a low glycemic index might be associated with lower energy intakes. These include the starch, fiber, and sugar content of foods, physical properties of the food, and degree of preparation.

Finally, animal models will be of great value in helping us improve our appreciation of the relationship between nutritional and sensory attributes of foods in promoting excess energy intakes and how these dietary attributes might be manipulated to limit excess energy intake.

16.10 CONCLUSIONS

The current lack of consensus regarding how macronutrients influence appetite, feeding behavior, and weight control is not primarily due to a lack of evidence. It is largely due to the interpretation of that evidence. There has been a tendency in the literature for one- or two-factor models to supersede each other, as a means to translate research into user-friendly messages that consumers can digest and assimilate (for example, low-fat messages, low-carbohydrate messages). However, the dietary determinants of energy intake and weight control are multifactorial. Models that embrace this complexity explain more of the variance in energy intake and body weight and give a truer reflection of how diet composition impacts on energy balance. A key challenge to the scientific community is to develop ways to translate the relatively complicated messages arising from the results of their research into policy messages that consumers can use and trust as a means of navigating through their food environment, toward a healthier body weight.

REFERENCES

1. WHO, Diet, Nutrition and the Prevention of Chronic Disease, World Health Organization, Geneva, 1990.
2. Hill, R.J. and Davies, P.S.W., The validity of a 4 day weighed food record for measuring energy intake in female classical ballet dancers, *Eur. J. Clin. Nutr.*, 1999, 53(9), 752.
3. Blundell, J.E. and Stubbs, R.J., High and low carbohydrate and fat intakes: Limits imposed by appetite and palatability and their implications for energy balance, *Eur. J. Clin. Nutr.*, 1999, 53 (Suppl. 1), S148.
4. Stubbs, R.J., Macronutrient effects on appetite, *Int. J. Obes.*, 1995, 19 (Suppl. 5), S11.
5. Stubbs, R.J. et al., Covert manipulation of dietary fat and energy density: Effect on substrate flux and food-intake in men eating *ad libitum*, *Am. J. Clin. Nutr.*, 1995, 62(2), 316.
6. WHO, Obesity: Preventing and Managing the Global Epidemic, World Health Organization, Geneva, 2000, p. 1.
7. Garrow, J., *Obesity and Related Diseases*, Churchill Livingstone, London, 1988.
8. Kant, A.K. et al., Proportion of energy intake from fat and subsequent weight change in the NHANES I Epidemiologic Follow-up Study, *Am. J. Clin. Nutr.*, 1995, 61, 11.
9. Stubbs, R.J. and O'Reilly, L.M., Carbohydrate and fat metabolism, appetite, and feeding behavior in humans, in *Neural Control of Macronutrient Selection*, Berthoud, H.R. and Seeley, R.J., Eds., CRC Press, Boca Raton, FL, 1998, p. 165.
10. Gill, A., *The Journey Back from Hell. Conversations with Concentration Camp Survivors*, Harper Collins, London, 1994.
11. Mercer, J.G. and Speakman, J.R., Hypothalamic neuropeptide mechanisms for regulating energy balance: From rodent models to human obesity, *Neurosci. Biobehav. Rev.*, 2001, 25(2), 101.
12. DEFRA, National Food Survey 2000, Department for Environment, Food and Rural Affairs, London, 2001.
13. Stephen, A.M. and Sieber, G.M., Trends in individual fat consumption in the United Kingdom 1900–1985, *Br. J. Nutr.*, 1994, 71, 775.
14. Johnson, R.K. and Frary, C., Choose beverages and foods to moderate your intake of sugars: The 2000 Dietary Guidelines for Americans — What's all the fuss about? *J. Nutr.*, 2001, 131(10), 2766S.
15. Zizza, C., Siega-Riz, A.M., and Popkin, B.M., Significant increase in young adults' snacking between 1977–1978 and 1994–1996 represents a cause for concern! *Prev. Med.*, 2001, 32(4), 303.
16. Cavadini, C., Siega-Riz, A.M., and Popkin, B.M., US adolescent food intake trends from 1965 to 1996, *West. J. Med.*, 2000, 173(6), 378.
17. Stubbs, R.J., Appetite, feeding behaviour and energy balance in human subjects, *Proc. Nutr. Soc.*, 1998, 57(3), 341.
18. Holland, B. et al., *The Composition of Foods*, 5th ed., The Royal Society of Chemistry and Ministry of Agriculture, Fisheries and Food, Cambridge, 1991.
19. Stubbs, J., Ferres, S., and Horgan, G., Energy density of foods: Effects on energy intake, *Crit. Rev. Food Sci. Nutr.*, 2000, 40(6), 481.
20. Drewnowski, A., What factors influence the energy density of the diet? *Obes. Res.*, 2000, 8, O43.
21. Crowe, T.C. et al., Energy density of foods and beverages in the Australian food supply: Influence of macronutrients and comparison to dietary intake, *Eur. J. Clin. Nutr.*, 2004, 58(11), 1485.
22. La Fontaine, H.A. et al., Two important exceptions to the relationship between energy density and fat content: foods with reduced-fat claims and high-fat vegetable-based dishes, *Public Health Nutr.*, 2004, 7(4), 563.

23. Stookey, J.D., Energy density, energy intake and weight status in a large free-living sample of Chinese adults: exploring the underlying roles of fat, protein, carbohydrate, fiber and water intakes, *Eur. J. Clin. Nutr.*, 2001, 55(5), 349.
24. Cox, D.N., Perry, L., and Moore, P.B., Measurements of energy density from lean and obese consumers' self reported dietary intakes: Variation and associations with other dietary components, *Proc. Nutr. Soc.*, 1999, 58(1), 7A.
25. Stubbs, R.J. and Whybrow, S., Energy density, diet composition and palatability: influences on overall food energy intake in humans, *Physiol. Behav.*, 2004, 81(5), 755.
26. McCrory, M.A. et al., Dietary determinants of energy intake and weight regulation in healthy adults, *J. Nutr.*, 2000, 130 (2S Suppl.), 276S.
27. Rolls, B.J., The role of energy density in the overconsumption of fat, *J. Nutr.*, 2000, 130 (2S Suppl.), 268S.
28. Prentice, A.M., Manipulation of dietary fat and energy density and subsequent effects on substrate flux and food intake, *Am. J. Clin. Nutr.*, 1998, 67, 535S.
29. Mazlan, N. et al., Effects of increasing increments of fat and sugar-rich snacks into the diet on energy and macronutrient intake in lean and overweight men, *Br. J. Nutr.*, 2006, 96, 596.
30. Whybrow, S. et al., Effects of two-weeks' mandatory snack consumption on energy intake and energy balance, *Obes. Res.*, 2007, 15(3), 673.
31. Yeomans, M.R., Weinberg, L., and James, S., Effects of palatability and learned satiety on energy density influences on breakfast intake in humans, *Physiol. Behav.*, 2005, 86(4), 487.
32. Levitsky, D.A., The non-regulation of food intake in humans: hope for reversing the epidemic of obesity, *Physiol. Behav.*, 2005, 86(5), 623.
33. de Castro, J.M., Macronutrient relationships with meal patterns and mood in the spontaneous feeding-behavior of humans, *Physiol. Behav.*, 1987, 39(5), 561.
34. Geliebter, A.A., Effects of equicaloric loads of protein, fat, and carbohydrate on food intake in the rat and man, *Physiol. Behav.*, 1979, 22, 267.
35. de Graaf, C., Schreurs, A., and Blauw, Y.H., Short-term effects of different amounts of sweet and nonsweet carbohydrates on satiety and energy intake, *Physiol. Behav.*, 1993, 54, 833.
36. Miller, M.G. and Teates, J.F., Acquisition of dietary self-selection in rats with normal and impaired oral sensation, *Physiol. Behav.*, 1985, 34(3), 401.
37. de Graaf, C. et al., Short-term effects of different amounts of protein, fats, and carbohydrates on satiety, *Am. J. Clin. Nutr.*, 1992, 55, 33.
38. Hill, A.J. and Blundell, J.E., Comparison of the action of macronutrients on the expression of appetite in lean and obese human subjects, *Ann. N.Y. Acad. Sci.*, 1989, 575, 529.
39. Hill, A.J. and Blundell, J.E., The effects of a high-protein or high-carbohydrate meal on subjective motivation to eat and food preferences, *Nutr. Behav.*, 1986, 3, 133.
40. Barkeling, B., Rossner, S., and Bjorvell, H., Effects of a high-protein meal (meat) and a high-carbohydrate meal (vegetarian) on satiety measured by automated computerized monitoring of subsequent food intake, motivation to eat and food preferences, *Int. J. Obes.*, 1990, 14, 743.
41. Booth, D.A., Chase, A., and Campbell, A.T., Relative effectiveness of protein in late stages of appetite suppression in man, *Physiol. Behav.*, 1970, 5(11), 1299.
42. Lyle, L.D., Control of eating behavior, in *Nutrition and the Brain,* Wurtman, R.J. and Wurtman, J.J., Eds., Raven Press, New York, 1977.
43. Kyriazakis, I., Emmans, G.C., and Whittemore, C.T., Diet selection in pigs choices made by growing pigs given foods of different protein concentrations, *Anim. Prod.*, 1990, 51, 189.

44. Kyriazakis, I. and Emmans, G.C., Selection of a diet by growing pigs given choices between foods differing in contents of protein and rapeseed meal, *Appetite*, 1992, 19(2), 121.
45. Millward, D.J., A protein-stat mechanism for the regulation of growth and maintenance of the lean-body mass, *Nutr. Res. Rev.*, 1995, 8, 93.
46. Stubbs, R.J. and Elia, M., Macronutrients and appetite control with implications for the nutritional management of the malnourished, *Clin. Nutr.*, 2001, 20, 129.
47. Keys, A. et al., *The Biology of Human Starvation*, University of Minnesota Press, Minneapolis, 1950.
48. Dulloo, A.G., Jacquet, J., and Girardier, L., Poststarvation hyperphagia and body fat overshooting in humans: A role for feedback signals from lean and fat tissues, *Am. J. Clin. Nutr.*, 1997, 65(3), 717.
49. Dulloo, A.G., Jacquet, J., and Girardier, L., Autoregulation of body composition during weight recovery in human: The Minnesota Experiment revisited, *Int. J. Obes.*, 1996, 20(5), 393.
50. Westerterp-Plantenga, M.S. et al., High protein intake sustains weight maintenance after body weight loss in humans, *Int. J. Obes.*, 2004, 28(1), 57.
51. Whybrow, S. et al., Protein supplementation subsequent to weight-loss: Effects on body weight, unpublished.
52. Pellett, P.L. and Young, V.R., The effect of different levels of energy intake on protein metabolism and of different levels of protein intake on energy metabolism: a statistical evaluation from the published literature, in *Protein-Energy Interactions*, Proceedings of an IDECG workshop, Scrimshaw, N.S. and Schurch, B., Eds., International Dietary Energy Consultancy Group. Switzerland, 1992.
53. Elia, M., Stubbs, R.J., and Henry, C.J.K., Differences in fat, carbohydrate, and protein metabolism between lean and obese subjects undergoing total starvation, *Obes. Res.*, 1999, 7(6), 597.
54. Skov, A.R. et al., Randomized trial on protein vs carbohydrate in *ad libitum* fat reduced diet for the treatment of obesity, *Int. J. Obes.*, 1999, 23(5), 528.
55. Brehm, B.J. et al., A randomized trial comparing a very low carbohydrate diet and a calorie-restricted low fat diet on body weight and cardiovascular risk factors in healthy women, *J. Clin. Endocrinol. Metab.*, 2003, 88(4), 1617.
56. Stern, L. et al., The effects of low-carbohydrate versus conventional weight loss diets in severely obese adults: one-year follow-up of a randomized trial, *Ann. Intern. Med.*, 2004, 140(10), 778.
57. Samaha, F.F. et al., A low-carbohydrate as compared with a low-fat diet in severe obesity, *N. Engl. J. Med.*, 2003, 348(21), 2074.
58. Foster, G.D. et al., A randomized trial of a low-carbohydrate diet for obesity, *N. Engl. J. Med.*, 2003, 348(21), 2082.
59. Weigle, D.S. et al., A high-protein diet induces sustained reductions in appetite, *ad libitum* caloric intake, and body weight despite compensatory changes in diurnal plasma leptin and ghrelin concentrations, *Am. J. Clin. Nutr.*, 2005, 82(1), 41.
60. Yudkin, J., *Pure, White and Deadly*, Viking, London, 1986.
61. Stubbs, R.J., Mazlan, N., and Whybrow, S., Carbohydrates, appetite and feeding behavior in humans, *J. Nutr.*, 2001, 131(10), 2775S.
62. Flatt, J.P., The difference in storage capacities for carbohydrate and for fat, and its implications in the regulation of body weight, *Ann. N.Y. Acad. Sci.*, 1987, 499, 104.
63. Astrup, A. and Raben, A., Carbohydrate and obesity, *Int. J. Obes.*, 1995, 19 (Suppl. 5), S27.
64. Hill, J.O. and Prentice, A.M., Sugar and body weight regulation, *Am. J. Clin. Nutr.*, 1995, 62 (Suppl.), S264.

65. Bolton-Smith, C. and Woodward, M., Dietary composition and fat to sugar ratios in relation to obesity, *Int. J. Obes.,* 1994, 18, 820.
66. Gibney, M.J. et al., Consumption of sugars, *Am. J. Clin. Nutr.,* 1995, 62 (Suppl. 1), 178S.
67. Foundation, I.F.I.C., *Review: Uses and Nutritional Impact of Fat Reduction Ingredients,* International Food Information Council Foundation, Washington, DC, 1997.
68. Leveille, G.A. and Finley, J.W., Macronutrient substitutes — Description and uses, in *Nutritional Implications of Macronutrient Substitutes,* Anderson, G.H., Rolls, B.J., Steffen, D.G., Eds., New York Academy of Sciences, New York, 1997, p. 11.
69. Stubbs, R.J. et al., Covert manipulation of energy density of high carbohydrate diets in "pseudo free-living" humans, *Int. J. Obes.,* 1998, 22(9), 885.
70. Stubbs, R.J., Harbron, C.G., and Prentice, A.M., Covert manipulation of the dietary fat to carbohydrate ratio of isoenergetically dense diets: effect on food intake in feeding men *ad libitum, Int. J. Obes.,* 1996, 20, 651.
71. Horgan, G.W., Whybrow, S., and Stubbs, R.J., Fat and carbohydrate do not displace each other in the diet, *Proc. Nutr. Soc. Lond.,* 2006, 65(OCA/B), 82A (abstract).
72. Bingham, S.A., Patterns of dietary fibre consumption in humans, in *CRC Handbook of Dietary Fiber in Human Nutrition,* Spiller, G.A., Ed., CRC Press, Boca Raton, FL, 1993, p. 509.
73. Howarth, N.C., Saltzman, E., and Roberts, S.B., Dietary fiber and weight regulation, *Nutr. Rev.,* 2001, 59(5), 129.
74. Drewnowski, A., Taste preferences and food intake, *Annu. Rev. Nutr.,* 1997, 17, 237.
75. Mazlan, N., Horgan, G., and Stubbs, R.J., Mandatory snacks rich in sugar, starch or fat; effect on energy and nutrient intake, *Int. J. Obes.,* 2001, 25 (Suppl. 2), S54.
76. Raben, A., Macdonald, I., and Astrup, A., Replacement of dietary fat by sucrose or starch: Effects on 14d *ad libitum* energy intake, energy expenditure and body weight in formerly obese and never-obese subjects, *Int. J. Obes.,* 1997, 21(10), 846.
77. Hirsch, E. and Walsh, M., Effect of limited access to sucrose on overeating and patterns of feeding, *Physiol. Behav.,* 1982, 29(1), 129.
78. Kanarek, R.B. and Marks-Kaufman, R., Developmental aspects of sucrose-induced obesity in rats, *Physiol. Behav.,* 1979, 23(5), 881.
79. Rogers, P.J. et al., Uncoupling sweet taste and calories: comparison of the effects of glucose and three intense sweeteners on hunger and food intake, *Physiol. Behav.,* 1988, 43, 547.
80. Raben, A. et al., Sucrose compared with artificial sweeteners: different effects on *ad libitum* food intake and body weight after 10 wk of supplementation in overweight subjects, *Am. J. Clin. Nutr.,* 2002, 76(4), 721.
81. Levine, A.S. and Billington, C.J., Dietary fiber: Does it affect food intake and body weight? in *Appetite and Body Weight Regulation: Sugar, Fat and Macronutrient Substitutes,* Fernstrom, J.D. and Miller, G.D., Eds., CRC Press, Boca Raton, FL, 1994, p. 191.
82. Blundell, J. and Burley, V., Satiation, satiety and the action of fibre on food intake, *Int. J. Obes.,* 1987, 11 (Suppl.), 9.
83. Burley, V. and Blundell, J., Action of dietary fibre on the satiety cascade, in *Dietary Fibre: Chemistry, Physiology and Health Effects,* Kritchevsky, D., Bobfield, C., and Anderson, J.W., Eds., Plenum Press, New York, 1990, p. 227.
84. Stevens, J., Does dietary fiber affect food-intake and body-weight? *J. Am. Diet. Assoc.,* 1988, 88(8), 939.
85. Mattes, R.D., Dietary compensation by humans for supplemental energy provided as ethanol or carbohydrate in fluids, *Physiol. Behav.,* 1996, 59(1), 179.
86. Fryer, J.H., The effects of a late-night caloric supplement upon body weight and food intake in man, *Am. J. Clin. Nutr.,* 1958, 6(4), 354.
87. Raben, A. et al., A randomized 10 week trial of sucrose vs artificial sweeteners on body weight and blood pressure after 10 weeks, *Obes. Res.,* 2001, 9, 86S.

88. Duncan, K.H., Bacon, J.A., and Weinsier, R.L., The effects of high and low energy density diets on satiety, energy intake, and eating time of obese and nonobese subjects, *Am. J. Clin. Nutr.*, 1983, 37, 763.
89. Lissner, L. et al., Dietary-fat and the regulation of energy intake in human subjects, *Am. J. Clin. Nutr.*, 1987, 46, 886.
90. Foltin, R.W. et al., Caloric compensation for lunches varying in fat and carbohydrate content by humans in a residential laboratory, *Am. J. Clin. Nutr.*, 1990, 52, 969.
91. Foltin, R.W. et al., Caloric, but not macronutrient, compensation by humans for required-eating occasions with meals and snacks varying in fat and carbohydrate, *Am. J. Clin. Nutr.*, 1992, 55(2), 331.
92. Lawton, C.L. et al., Dietary-fat and appetite control in obese subjects weak effects on satiation and satiety, *Int. J. Obes.*, 1993, 17(7), 409.
93. Lissner, L. and Heitmann, B.L., Dietary-fat and obesity evidence from epidemiology, *Eur. J. Clin. Nutr.*, 1995, 49(2), 79.
94. Green, S.M. and Blundell, J.E., Subjective and objective indices of the satiating effect of foods, Can people predict how filling a food will be? *Eur. J. Clin. Nutr.*, 1996, 50, 798.
95. Stubbs, R.J. and Harbron, C.G., Covert manipulation of the ratio of medium- to long-chain triglycerides in isoenergetically dense diets: Effect on food intake in *ad libitum* feeding men, *Int. J. Obes.*, 1996, 20, 435.
96. Kasai, M. et al., Effect of dietary medium- and long-chain triacylglycerols (MLCT) on accumulation of body fat in healthy humans, *Asia Pac. J. Clin. Nutr.*, 2003, 12(2), 151.
97. Matsuo, T. et al., Effects of a liquid diet supplement containing structured medium- and long-chain triacylglycerols on body fat accumulation in healthy young subjects, *Asia Pac. J. Clin. Nutr.*, 2001, 10(1), 46.
98. Rich, A.J., Chambers, P., and Johnston, I.D.A., Are ketones an appetite suppressant? *J. Parenter. Enter. Nutr.*, 1988, 13, 7S (abstract).
99. Johnstone, A.M. et al., Breakfasts high in monoglyceride or triglyceride: No differential effect on appetite or energy intake, *Eur. J. Clin. Nutr.*, 1998, 52(8), 603.
100. Johnstone, A.M. et al., Overfeeding fat as monoglyceride or triglyceride: effect on appetite, nutrient balance and the subsequent day's energy intake, *Eur. J. Clin. Nutr.*, 1998, 52(8), 610.
101. Storlien, L.H., Dietary fats and insulin action, *Int. J. Obes.*, 1998, 22, S46 (abstract).
102. Lawton, G.L. et al., The degree of saturation of fatty acids influences post-ingestive satiety, *Br. J. Nutr.*, 2000, 83(5), 473.
103. French, S. et al., The effect of fatty acid composition on intestinal satiety in man, *Int. J. Obes.*, 1998, 22, S82.
104. Phinney, S. et al., Gamma linolenate reduces weight regain following weight loss by very low calorie diets in humans, *Int. J. Obes.*, 1998, 22, S64.
105. Maki, K.C. et al., Consumption of diacylglycerol oil as part of a reduced-energy diet enhances loss of body weight and fat in comparison with consumption of a triacylglycerol control oil, *Am. J. Clin. Nutr.*, 2002, 76(6), 1230.
106. Dugan, M.E.R. et al., The effect of conjugated linoleic acid on fat to lean repartitioning and feed conversion in pigs, *Can. J. Anim. Sci.*, 1997, 77(4), 723.
107. Atkinson, R.L. et al., Clinical Implications for CLA in the Treatment of Obesity, in Program of the Annual Meeting, National Nutritional Foods Association, San Antonio, TX, 1998.
108. Belury, M.A., Mahon, A., and Banni, S., The conjugated linoleic acid (CLA) isomer, t10c12-CLA, is inversely associated with changes in body weight and serum leptin in subjects with type 2 diabetes mellitus, *J. Nutr.*, 2003, 133(1), 257S.
109. Petridou, A., Mougios, V., and Sagredos, A., Supplementation with CLA: isomer incorporation into serum lipids and effect on body fat of women, *Lipids*, 2003, 38(8), 805.

110. Welch, I.M., Sepple, C.P., and Read, N.W., Comparisons of the effects on satiety and eating behavior of infusion of lipid into the different regions of the small-intestine, *Gut,* 1988, 29(3), 306.
111. Gil, K.M. et al., Parenteral-nutrition and oral intake effect of glucose and fat infusions, *J. Parenter. Enter. Nutr.,* 1991, 15(4), 426.
112. Westerterp-Plantenga, M.S. and Verwegen, C.R.T., The appetizing effect of an aperitif in overweight and normal-weight humans, *Am. J. Clin. Nutr.,* 1999, 69(2), 205.
113. de Castro, J.M. and Orozco, S., Moderate alcohol intake and spontaneous eating patterns of humans evidence of unregulated supplementation, *Am. J. Clin. Nutr.,* 1990, 52(2), 246.
114. Risérus, U. et al., Supplementation with trans10, *cis*12-conjugated linoleic acid induces hyperproinsulinaemia in obese men: close association with impaired insulin sensitivity, *Diabetologia*, 47(6), 1016, 2004.
115. Risérus, U., Berglund, L., and Vessby, B., Conjugated linoleic acid (CLA)-reduced abdominal adipose tissue in obese middle-aged men with signs of the metabolic syndrome: a randomised controlled trial, *Int. J. Obes.*, 25(8), 1129, 2001.
116. Raben, A., Should obese patients be counselled to follow a low glycaemic index diet? No, *Obes. Res.*, 3, 245, 2002.

17 Mineral Micronutrient Status and Food Intake: Studies with Animal Models

John Beard

CONTENTS

17.1 INTRODUCTION

The main emphasis of this chapter on micronutrients and food intake will be the specificity of the relationship between mineral deficiency and changes in neural function, food intake, and efficiency of energy utilization. A common theme amongst nearly all animal model studies of nutrient deprivation, and in particular in rodents, is the observation of poor growth and an apparent anorexia. This raises the question of whether a common pathway exists in which decreased total food intake is the outcome, regardless of whether the nutrient deficiency is iron, zinc, selenium, or other micronutrients. Individuals with a single nutrient deficiency either continue to grow and consume body stores, leading to an eventual reduction in body function (Type I nutrients), or they can reduce growth velocity, leading to a conservation of the nutrient and thus reduce the daily requirement for that nutrient. This is referred to as a Type II nutrient pattern.[1] The reduction in appetite that accompanies the Type II nutrient response is believed to be due to a hypothalamic–pituitary based reduction in growth hormone and adrenal cortical release and to changes in activity of the hypothalamic-pituitary-thyroid axis. A consistent finding in most controlled animal studies of single nutrient deficiencies is a reduction in feed efficiency. What is unclear, and is apparently not being pursued by investigators, is the source of the biological signal that tells the body to become less efficient at converting dietary macronutrients to stored or utilized calories. Is this a strategy to try to derive more "essential micronutrient" from an increased consumption of total dietary components? Or, is it that all of these micronutrients influence a single or small number of key regulators of food intake? The sections in this chapter will attempt to explore specific mechanisms associating mineral deficiencies with changes in food intake or feed efficiency, primarily through animal experimentation, but the current literature does not allow resolution of this fundamental question.

17.2 IRON

17.2.1 Function

The topic of iron deficiency and neural functioning has been the focus of a number of recent reviews.[2–4] The rate at which individual tissues and cellular organelles within those tissues develop a true "deficit" in iron is dependent on the rate of turnover of iron-containing proteins, the intracellular mechanisms for recycling iron, and the rate of delivery of iron to tissue from the plasma pool.[5] The manifestations of this depletion of essential body iron, apart from the well-known anemia, are significant decreases in mitochondrial iron–sulfur content, in mitochondrial cytochrome content, and in total mitochondrial oxidative capacity.[5] Iron is not only an essential element and important nutrient, but also a potent toxin. Thus, an elegant system has evolved that regulates the delivery of iron to brain cells and has as its major known components the plasma protein transferrin and its receptor. Iron is an essential component of a number of general cellular functions as well as having functions more specific to neurological activity such as myelin formation and the synthesis of dopamine, serotonin, catecholamines, and possibly gamma amino butyric acid

(GABA).[2,4,6] When iron is stored, it is incorporated into ferritin with a heterogeneous distribution in the brain determined by both anatomical region and cell type.

17.2.2 Sequelae

Iron is a cofactor for tyrosine hydroxylase, tryptophan hydroxylase, xanthine oxidase, and ribonucleoside reductase. Thus the expectation would be that nutritional iron deficiency will lead to decreased activities of these enzymes; however, this is not the consistent observation. When brain iron levels are reduced by as much as 40% with dietary restriction in postweanling rats, there is no change in the activity of tyrosine hydroxylase, tryptophan hydroxylase, monoamine oxidase, succinate hydroxylase, or cytochrome c oxidase.[7] Whole-brain concentrations of norepinephrine (NE) and dopamine (DA) are unaltered by iron deficiency, while concentrations of serotonin and 5-hydroxyindole acetic acid are decreased.[8,9] *In vivo* microdialysis demonstrates that caudate putamen interstitial DA and NE are significantly elevated in awake freely moving iron-deficient (ID) rats,[10] and the rise in extracellular DA with the onset of the dark cycle and feeding behavior is much greater in striatum of ID rats than in controls.[11] Dopamine receptors (DR) are also affected by dietary iron deficiency in mice and rats (see Beard and Connor[2] for a recent review). The degree of reduction in D_2R is generally 20 to 25% in the caudate putamen and prefrontal cortex, while changes in nucleus accumbens and ventral tegmentum are much smaller. Functionality and cell surface expression of these receptors is affected by diurnal cues, and changes in receptor expression have been shown to affect food intake behavior.[12] Yehuda and Mostofsky[13] have recently reported an elevation in cholecystokin-8 (CCK-8) in iron-deficient (ID) rats that also exhibit a decrease in food intake and reduced D_2R density. Treatment with a CCK antagonist was successful at ameliorating the effects of iron deficiency on food intake, providing strong evidence for a functional relationship between iron deficiency and the CCK-food intake regulation loop.[13] Raising iron levels above normal in mice increases expression of the enzyme nitric oxide synthase (NOS) in the paraventricular nucleus (PVN) and lateral area (LHA) of the hypothalamus.[14] Expression of NOS in these areas has been related to control of food intake.[15]

The reduced growth in ID rats was initially attributed to anorexia, but with the inclusion of careful measures of food intake and weight-matched control groups it has been possible to show that ID results not in a reduced food intake, but rather a reduced feed efficiency.[10,16–22] There is an approximate 10% decrease in caloric efficiency in the ID and anemic rats that has been attributed to increased NE turnover, increased metabolic rate, and alterations in thyroid hormone function.[17,23,24] The ID animals actually consume more food than weight-matched controls, and it has been shown that the reduced levels of thyroid hormone are not due to the food restriction,[25,26] because changing the type of carbohydrate in the diet alters hepatic thyroxine monodeiodinase activity, but does not alter the feeding behavior of the rats.[16,17]

The human relevance of these studies is that iron deficiency is the most prevalent nutrient deficiency in the world[27] with as many as 50% of children under 5 years and 60 to 70% of pregnant women affected. There are numerous reports that ID and anemic individuals have a "poor appetite"[28] and particular cravings for ice or dirt.[29,30]

Indeed, studies in Zambia and Kenya have shown that iron supplements and anti-helminthic treatment improve appetite and growth in children,[31,32] suggesting that an improvement in iron status is related to an improvement in total dietary intake. While ferritin, a plasma marker of iron status, is associated with appetite in infants, there is no correlation between ferritin and serum leptin levels.[33]

17.2.3 Summary

Feeding an iron-deficient diet to rodents reduces essential iron in specific brain regions, and a majority of evidence suggests that the primary impact is on monoaminergic systems and GABAergic systems.[2] While specific aspects of appetite have not been examined in animal models, there is suggestive evidence that hypothalamic nuclei as well as hypothalamic-pituitary-adrenal and hypothalamic-pituitary-thyroid axis functioning are affected by iron deficiency.[34] Human studies consistently point toward an improvement in appetite with an improvement in iron status, but again, specific studies regarding the effect of iron status on food choice or on volume of food consumed have not been published.

17.3 IODINE

17.3.1 Function

On a worldwide basis, iodine deficiency and the resultant disorders are as prevalent as iron deficiency and lead to a dramatic impairment in brain development and functioning.[35,36] More than 70% of the body's iodine content is concentrated in the thyroid gland and is associated with the various iodoproteins that are the storage, precursor, or secreted forms of thyroid hormone, thyroxine (T4) and tri-iodothyronine (T3). Consumption of an iodine-deficient diet in rats is associated with a reduction in deiodinase activity and circulating thyroid hormones and a decrease in food intake, but maintenance of T3 concentrations in most tissues.[37,38] Prolonged iodine deficiency and limited thyroid hormone availability to the brain during development leads to neurological damage.[39,40]

17.3.2 Sequelae

The neurological defects associated with early-life iodine deficiency are predominantly in the cerebral cortical association areas, basal ganglia, and motor control pathways.[39,40]

Consistent observations are a decreased number of neurons, irregular arrangement of cells, larger ventricles, and a decreased numbers of dendrites from pyramidal cells in the cortical motor area.[40,41] Thyroid hormones are essential for normal neuroblastogenesis; especially affected are the interhemispheric connections of the anterior commissure, corpus collosum, and callosal connections. Many of these deficits are reversed by iodine replacement; there is, however, there is a persistent low density of synapses in the cortex of iodine-replaced fetuses. In other animal studies, fetal hypothyroidism has been associated with alterations in neurotransmitter metabolism as evidenced by a decrease in protein kinase C, ornithine decarboxylase, choline acetyltransferase, and DOPA decarboxylase.[41] Thus, there is a critical period in which iodine is required for normal development, and if a nutritional deficiency extends beyond this time point not all alterations in function can be reversed by iodine administration. There is no other identified role for iodide apart from thyroid hormone metabolism; therefore, it is the secondary deficiency in thyroid hormones that leads to alterations in CNS function in iodine-deficient animals.[40] In iodine-adequate conditions, fasting in rodents is associated with a change in thyroid releasing hormone (TRH) and control of thyroid stimulating hormone (TSH) secretion; the PVN neurons that control TRH secretion are influenced by neuropeptide Y (NPY) levels,[39] which increase during fasting, and an associated change in neural regulation of the Type II 5′-deiodinase enzyme in brain tissue.[39]

17.3.3 Summary

The inhibition of growth and the neurological consequences of iodine deficiency appear to be the global result of a failure to produce appropriate amounts of thyroid hormone to control neurogenesis and neurological function. Specific studies in animal models relating iodine deficiency to appetite feedback signals are lacking. Observations in humans with severe iodine deficiency characterize the individuals with neurological cretinism as having mental deficiency, deafness, mutism, and motor disorders accompanied by basal ganglia calcification.[42,43] The duration and timing of hypothyroidism during development may be critical in determining the severity of the symptoms and whether they can be reversed by iodine replacement.

17.4 SELENIUM

17.4.1 Function

Selenium functions generally revolve around selenium-dependent glutathione peroxidase (GPX) and the selenocysteine-containing enzymes.[44] While many of the effects of selenium deficiency can be attributed to a loss of GPX activity, not all consequences are clearly linked to this important component of the system that protects against oxidative stress. Cellular GPX isozymes are thought to play a role in the regulation of peroxide concentrations, which in turn are tightly connected to consumption of polyunsaturated fatty acids (PUFA) and neuronal functioning.[45] The conversion of thyroxine to the active hormone, T3, is dependent on the selenocysteine-containing enzyme Type I 5′-deiodinase, but the brain possesses another isoform, Type II deiodinase, which is not selenium dependent.[46] Thus, despite a functional state of hypothyroidism elsewhere in the body, the brain may be protected in selenium deficiency. In combination with iodine deficiency, selenium status may play a role in the pathogenesis of myxedematous cretinism. As noted above in the section on iodine metabolism, hypothyroidism in the developing brain leads to disorders of neural process growth.[41,47]

17.4.2 Sequelae

Selenium deficiency alters monoamine neurotransmitter metabolism in the caudate putamen or substantia nigra in adult rats.[48,49] Selenium-dependent GPX activities in these brain regions are significantly decreased, but a specific role for selenium or GPX activity in brain regions associated with feeding behavior has not been investigated. An animal model frequently used in the early studies of selenium was the chick.[50,51] In these studies selenium-deficient chicks showed a rapid rise in feed intake after administration of selenomethionine. Protein content of the diet, however, may have confounded the interpretation of the results.[52] More recently, Swiss investigators have observed that selenium-deficient laying hens show a preference for feed containing high concentrations of selenium, but there is no relation between this behavior and serum biomarkers of oxidative stress.[53,54] Selenium deficiency is known to decrease feed efficiency and growth in broiler chickens, but this has been clearly shown to be secondary to changes in thyroid hormone biology and not to specific regulation by selenium.[55] The oxidative stress caused by selenium deficiency may also impair function of the hypothalamic-pituitary-adrenal axis. Basal corticosterone levels are normal in selenium-deficient rats, but long-term infusion of adrenocorticotropic hormone (ACTH) fails to elicit a normal corticosterone response. Because corticosterone stimulates leptin secretion, leptin levels are also low in the selenium-deficient animals.[56] These results suggest an alteration in the stress-responsiveness and regulation of the hypothalamic-pituitary-adrenal axis secondary to oxidative stress in animals with lower GPX activity, but it is unlikely that low leptin levels influence energy intake of the animals, because a drop in leptin concentration would be expected to increase food intake, whereas selenium deficiency is associated with decreased food intake.

17.4.3 Summary

Changes in food intake, feed efficiency, and growth of animals that are selenium deficient appear to result from secondary changes in thyroid hormone metabolism that are caused by inadequate levels of selenium-dependent enzymes critical to the prevention of oxidative stress. Although selenium deficiency has been shown to change GPX levels and neurotransmitter function in some areas of the brain, the relationship between selenium status and integrity of function in nuclei associated with the control of food intake has not been investigated. Unlike iodine deficiency, changes in neurological function of selenium-deficient individuals cannot be directly attributed to impaired thyroid hormone production because of the presence of a non-selenium-dependent deiodinase in the brain.

17.5 ZINC

17.5.1 Function

In contrast to the relatively few functional roles described for selenium with regard to CNS function and appetite, zinc is one of the most ubiquitous nutrients. It is a constituent of more than 200 enzymes, and its incorporation into zinc finger transcription factors may account for 15 to 20% of all gene expression in the human genome.[57] A zinc deficiency leads to both primary and secondary alterations in brain function due to low rates of DNA synthesis, a reduced number of polyribosomes, and impaired zinc finger-regulated gene transcription.[58] Zinc is present in ionized form in presynaptic vesicles at concentrations as high as 300 μ*M* and is localized in glutaminergic cells.[59] Zinc-containing pathways are limited to the forebrain, and the best characterized are mossy fiber projections running from hippocampal granule cells to the CA3 pyramidal neurons.[59] The neurochemistry of zinc has recently been reviewed by Frederickson et al.[60] It is released when cells are depolarized[61] and inhibits postsynaptic activation of GABA-A and *N*-methyl-d-aspartate (NMDA) receptors,[62] which possess zinc-specific binding sites.[63] There is active presynaptic reuptake of zinc,[64] but in the presence of glutamate, the ion can also enter postsynaptic cells through ion channels and may be released inside cells in response to cellular stress.[60] The role of endogenous zinc in regulating neural function remains unclear, but it appears to be important in the packaging of excitatory amino acids, the synchronization of release of GABA from neurons, and modulation of activity of GABA-A receptors.[65] Zinc concentration in the brain is highest in the hippocampus, but zinc deprivation has the greatest effect on the development and functioning of the cerebellum and Purkinje cells.[66] Zinc provides an opportunity for control of membrane excitability by depressing postsynaptic action when firing rates become very high.[67]

17.5.2 Sequelae

Poor zinc status has been associated with a failure to grow, anorexia, poor immune function, and cognitive deficits due to the myriad of functions that this metal has in the biology of nearly all cells. Similar characteristics of poor appetite are present in zinc-deficient animals, and the ability to control experimental conditions has allowed a number of investigators to explore potential mechanistic associations between zinc and food intake.[68,69] There are several reports of increased levels of NPY mRNA expression in the hypothalamus of zinc-deplete rats,[70,71] but there is no consensus on an increase in hypothalamic NPY protein concentration,[70,72] and there does not appear to be any change in sensitivity to exogenous NPY[73] that could account for the reduced food intake in conditions of increased NPY expression. Microdialysis studies suggest that zinc deficiency prevents release of endogenous NPY[72] and that this might contribute to the hypophagia of zinc-deficient rats. Rat studies also demonstrate a relationship between brain zinc depletion and reduced hypothalamic monoamine release[72,74] and also with reduced sensitivity to[75] and blunted stimulatory effects of opioids on food intake in zinc-deplete rats, possibly due to changes in receptor sensitivity.[76] There is a decreased preference for carbohydrate in zinc-deficient animals that may account for 100% of their drop in food intake, compared with zinc-adequate controls,[72] which cannot be attributed to changes in hypothalamic norepinephrine concentrations,[74] but could be associated with changes in NPY activity.[77]

The appetite regulation system has been explored by Shay and colleagues for a number of years from a different perspective. Young rats fed a zinc-deficient diet reduce their food intake by up to 50% within a week. Interestingly, within several more days there is an increase in food intake followed by a reduction. This cycle continues with a duration of approximately 3 to 4 days but is quickly normalized by replacing dietary zinc.[71,78] Recent microarray analysis of cDNA in the pituitary of zinc-deficient, zinc-adequate, and zinc-overloaded rats shows a strong correlation between pituitary zinc concentrations and gene expression for NPY, melanin concentrating hormone, ghrelin, calcitonin gene-related product, and serotonin,[79] suggesting that gene expression of potent appetite-regulating neuropeptides is altered by zinc deficiency, but these results need to be confirmed for tissues known to be involved in the control of food intake.

Several investigators have looked for an association between zinc status and leptin. Serum leptin is lower in zinc-deficient than zinc-replete humans[80] or animals, but this may be secondary to the reduction in food intake.[81] Measurement of leptin expression and release from adipose tissue taken from zinc-adequate, zinc-deficient, and rats pair-fed to the zinc-deficient rats showed the same level of leptin mRNA expression in adipose tissue from zinc-deficient and pair-fed rats, supporting the notion that the low circulating concentrations of leptin are secondary to the reduced food intake of zinc-deficient animals. There was, however, a lower rate of leptin secretion from adipose tissue from zinc-deficient than pair-fed rats, indicating an additional zinc-dependent aspect of leptin secretion.[82] If peripheral release of leptin is zinc sensitive, then this may represent an aspect of zinc-induced dysregulation of appetite that is not based on a direct effect on CNS function.

17.5.3 Summary

The significant body of literature relating zinc nutriture to control of food intake provides much stronger evidence for an association between micronutrient requirements and maintenance of normal food intake than is available for most other micronutrients.[69] Animal studies and molecular investigations are identifying changes in structure and function in enterocytes, hypothalamic and other neural centers, the pituitary, and adipocytes. Thus signals of energy balance from adipocytes in addition to fundamental aspects of neuropeptide synthesis and release in the hypothalamus may contribute to the reduction in food intake of zinc-deficient animals.

17.6 COPPER

17.6.1 Function

Copper is essential for normal development of the central nervous system, both in terms of regulating neuropeptide synthesis and in protecting tissue from oxidative damage. Copper is a cofactor for the free radical scavenger superoxide-dismutase (SOD) and thus plays a key role in antioxidant processes.[83] The importance of copper as an antioxidant component of SOD is displayed by the phenotype of neurodegeneration with long-term deficiency.[84–86] Copper is also a component of cuproenzymes such as dopamine β-mono-oxygenase, tyrosinase, monoamine oxidase, and peptidylglycine-α-amidating monoxygenase (PAM), and a deficiency in copper is associated with a deficiency in activity.[87] These enzymes are essential for neurotransmitter biosynthesis, posttranslational modification, and neuropeptide metabolism.[84] The potential importance for PAM in food intake regulation becomes clear when we realize that it is involved in the posttranslation modification (amination of a glycine residue) of neuropeptides such as CCK, NYP, and ghrelin. Copper transporters across cell membranes and chaperone proteins have been described and are important for moving copper from the extracellular space to the more protected oxidative environment of subcellular compartments.[88] Selective deletions of copper transporters or chaperone proteins reveal changes in mitochondrial energy metabolism that contribute to abnormal CNS development and functioning.

17.6.2 Sequelae

There is much less evidence for a relationship between food intake or appetite and copper status than is available for zinc, but as with most other metal deficiencies, there is a reduction in food intake and weight gain of animals fed a copper-deficient diet.[89,90] Copper deficiency increases NPY mRNA levels in the olfactory bulb, but this is not associated with a change in NPY protein levels or a change in food intake.[91] Other studies with rats have focused on production and release of CCK from the exocrine pancreas.[92] CCK is a satiety signal, released from the gastrointestinal tract in response to nutrient ingestion, and one of its functions is to stimulate protein secretion from the exocrine pancreas by activating high-affinity vagal CCK-A receptors.[93] Pancreatic acini isolated from rats that had been fed either a copper-deficient or copper-adequate diet for 4 weeks had a low density of CCK-A receptors, a low amylase content, and a reduced CCK-8-stimulated release of amylase.[92] In contrast, an earlier study with copper-deficient rabbits found significant reductions in acinar cell amylase content, but no detriment in CCK-stimulated amylase release, suggesting different species sensitivity or response to copper depletion in the exocrine pancreas.[94]

Numerous studies have tried to find an association between serum copper and serum leptin. Cross-sectional studies show a positive correlation between serum leptin and serum copper concentrations,[95,96] but intervention studies in humans or animal models have failed to provide evidence of an association, other than the likelihood that both are a response to cytokines released during inflammation.[97,98]

17.6.3 Summary

The literature on copper and food intake is sparse, in part because of the low prevalence of copper deficiency in human populations and the relatively recent discovery of an abundant number of copper transporter and chaperone proteins. There are suggestions of a relationship between copper deficiency and function of the exocrine pancreas due to changes in CCK responsiveness. The identification, in the past 3 years, of a number of copper-dependent enzymes and intriguing evidence of possible copper-dependent alterations in neuropeptide production in hypothalamic centers known to influence food intake may provide the basic information needed to stimulate investigators to explore potential roles of copper in food intake regulation.

17.7 CONCLUSIONS

The focus of this brief review of selected metals reveals a general lack of understanding with the fundamental mechanisms that are activated as animals become deficient in a single micronutrient. In some cases, such as zinc, there is a substantial literature that points to alterations in both the origins of the appetite signals in the periphery as well as the hypothalamic centers that control food intake. In most other cases of metal micronutrient deficiency there is insufficient evidence to make a strong case for a particular site of action regarding the cause of the reduced food intake, although there is some evidence that changes in food intake can result from disruption of endocrine function caused by the micronutrient deficiency.

A majority of the evidence for an association between specific changes in mineral metabolism and abnormal food intake or efficiency of energy utilization comes from animal studies. The benefit of these models is that it is possible to manipulate a single micronutrient while keeping all other aspects of the diet constant, whereas micronutrient deficiencies in humans are often associated with multiple dietary insufficiencies, making it difficult to tease out responses that can be attributed to a specific nutrient. Other obvious advantages are the duration of exposure to deficient diets may be reduced, and tissue sampling can be more invasive in animal models. Importantly, because mineral deficiencies during specific stages of development and growth can cause permanent impairment of function, it would not be ethical to investigate anything other than replacement strategies in human subjects. New genomic tools are becoming available to help identify novel proteins in the metabolism of metal micronutrients and metabolomic and proteomic analyses are also providing new information on potential causes of appetite dysregulation in single-nutrient deficiency states. This new technology will hopefully facilitate progress in understanding the complex mechanisms that relate mineral status to systems that determine what, when, and how much to eat.

REFERENCES

1. Golden, M.H., Specific deficiencies versus growth failure: Type I and type II nutrients, *SCN News,* 12, 10, 1995.
2. Beard, J.L. and Connor, J.R., Iron status and neural functioning, *Annu. Rev. Nutr.,* 23, 41, 2003.
3. Lozoff, B. and Georgieff, M.K., Iron deficiency and brain development, *Semin. Pediatr. Neurol.,* 13, 158, 2006.
4. Rouault, T.A. and Cooperman, S., Brain iron metabolism, *Semin. Pediatr. Neurol.,* 13, 142, 2006.
5. Dallman, P.R., Manifestations of iron deficiency, *Semin. Hematol.,* 19, 19, 1982.
6. Hill, J.M., Iron concentration reduced in ventral pallidum, globus pallidus, and substantia nigra by GABA-transaminase inhibitor, gamma-vinyl GABA, *Brain Res.,* 342, 18, 1985.
7. Youdim, M.B., Iron deficiency effects on brain function, *Public Health Rev.,* 28, 83, 2000.
8. Yehuda, S. and Youdim, M.B., Brain iron: A lesson from animal models, *Am. J. Clin. Nutr.,* 50, 618, 1989.
9. Youdim, M.B., Ben-Shachar, D., and Yehuda, S., Putative biological mechanisms of the effect of iron deficiency on brain biochemistry and behavior, *Am. J. Clin. Nutr.,* 50, 607–615, 1989.
10. Beard, J.L. et al., Altered monamine metabolism in caudate-putamen of iron-deficient rats, *Pharmacol. Biochem. Behav.,* 48, 621, 1994.
11. Nelson, C. et al., *In vivo* dopamine metabolism is altered in iron-deficient anemic rats, *J. Nutr.,* 127, 2282, 1997.
12. Roitman, M.F. et al., Dopamine mediation of the feeding response to violations of spatial and temporal expectancies, *Behav. Brain Res.,* 122, 193, 2001.
13. Yehuda, S. and Mostofsky, D.I., The effects of an essential fatty acid compound and a cholecystokinin-8 antagonist on iron deficiency induced anorexia and learning deficits, *Nutr. Neurosci.,* 7, 85, 2004.

14. Kim, M.J. et al., Increased expression of hypothalamic NADPH-diaphorase neurons in mice with iron supplement, *Biosci. Biotechnol. Biochem.*, 69, 1978, 2005.
15. Morley, J.E. et al., Leptin and neuropeptide Y (NPY) modulate nitric oxide synthase: Further evidence for a role of nitric oxide in feeding, *Peptides*, 20, 595, 1999.
16. Smith, S.M., Johnson, P.E., and Lukaski, H.C., *In vitro* hepatic thyroid hormone deiodination in iron-deficient rats: effect of dietary fat, *Life Sci.*, 53, 603, 1993.
17. Smith, S.M. and Lukaski, H.C., Type of dietary carbohydrate affects thyroid hormone deiodination in iron-deficient rats, *J. Nutr.*, 122, 1174, 1992.
18. Chen, Q., Connor, J.R., and Beard, J.L., Brain iron, transferrin and ferritin concentrations are altered in developing iron-deficient rats, *J. Nutr.*, 125, 1529, 1995.
19. Beard, J.L., Zhan, C.S., and Brigham, D.E., Growth in iron-deficient rats, *Proc. Soc. Exp. Biol. Med.*, 209, 65, 1995.
20. Tobin, B.W., Beard, J.L., and Kenney, W.L., Exercise training alters feed efficiency and body composition in iron deficient rats, *Med. Sci. Sports Exerc.*, 25, 52, 1993.
21. Strube, Y.N., Beard, J.L., and Ross, A.C., Iron deficiency and marginal vitamin A deficiency affect growth, hematological indices and the regulation of iron metabolism genes in rats, *J. Nutr.*, 132, 3607, 2002.
22. Dhur, A., Galan, P., and Hercberg, S., Effect of decreased food consumption during iron deficiency upon growth rate and iron status indicators in the rat, *Ann. Nutr. Metab.*, 34, 280, 1990.
23. Brigham, D.E. and Beard, J.L., Effect of thyroid hormone replacement in iron-deficient rats, *Am. J. Physiol.*, 269, R1140, 1995.
24. Beard, J.L., Tobin, B.W., and Smith, S.M., Effects of iron repletion and correction of anemia on norepinephrine turnover and thyroid metabolism in iron deficiency, *Proc. Soc. Exp. Biol. Med.*, 193, 306, 1990.
25. Erikson, K.M. et al., Iron deficiency decreases dopamine D1 and D2 receptors in rat brain, *Pharmacol. Biochem. Behav.*, 69, 409, 2001.
26. Hess, S.Y. et al., Iron deficiency anemia reduces thyroid peroxidase activity in rats, *J. Nutr.*, 132, 1951, 2002.
27. World Health Organization and Centers for Disease Control and Prevention, Assessing the iron status of populations, World Health Organization, Geneva, Switzerland, 6–8 April 2004.
28. Tympa-Psirropoulou, E. et al., Nutritional risk factors for iron-deficiency anaemia in children 12 to 24 months old in the area of Thessalia in Greece, *Int. J. Food Sci. Nutr.*, 56, 1, 2005.
29. Osman, Y.M., Wali, Y.A., and Osman, O.M., Craving for ice and iron-deficiency anemia: A case series from Oman, *Pediatr. Hematol. Oncol.*, 22, 127, 2005.
30. Hurtig, J., Iron-deficient patients craving ice fairly common behavior, *ONS News*, 20, 3, 2005.
31. Stoltzfus, R.J. et al., Low dose daily iron supplementation improves iron status and appetite but not anemia, whereas quarterly anthelminthic treatment improves growth, appetite and anemia in Zanzibari preschool children, *J. Nutr.*, 134, 348, 2004.
32. Lawless, J.W. et al., Iron supplementation improves appetite and growth in anemic Kenyan primary school children, *J. Nutr.*, 124, 645, 1994.
33. Topaloglu, A.K. et al., Lack of association between plasma leptin levels and appetite in children with iron deficiency, *Nutrition*, 17, 657, 2001.
34. Weinberg, J. et al., Long-term effects of early iron deficiency on consummatory behavior in the rat, *Pharmacol. Biochem. Behav.*, 14, 447, 1981.
35. De Benoist, B. and Delange, F., [Iodine deficiency: Current situation and future prospects]. *Sante*, 12, 9, 2002.
36. Vanderpas, J., Nutritional epidemiology and thyroid hormone metabolism, *Annu. Rev. Nutr.*, 26, 293, 2006.

37. Obregon, M.J. et al., The effects of iodine deficiency on thyroid hormone deiodination, *Thyroid,* 15, 917, 2005.
38. Janssen, K.P. et al., Thyroid function and deiodinase activities in rats with marginal iodine deficiency, *Biol. Trace Elem. Res.,* 40, 237, 1994.
39. Peeters, R. et al., Regional physiological adaptation of the central nervous system deiodinases to iodine deficiency, *Am. J. Physiol. Endocrinol Metab.,* 281, E54, 2001.
40. Pemberton, H.N., Franklyn, J.A., and Kilby, M.D., Thyroid hormones and fetal brain development, *Minerva Ginecol.,* 57, 367, 2005.
41. Georgieff, M.K., Nutrition and the developing brain: nutrient priorities and measurement, *Am. J. Clin. Nutr.,* 85, 614S, 2007.
42. Boyages, S.C., Primary pediatric hypothyroidism and endemic cretinism, *Curr. Ther. Endocrinol. Metab.,* 5, 94, 1994.
43. Boyages, S.C. and Medeiros-Neto, G., Pathogenesis of myxedematous endemic cretinism, *J. Clin. Endocrinol. Metab.,* 81, 1671, 1996.
44. Behne, D. and Kyriakopoulos, A., Mammalian selenium-containing proteins, *Annu. Rev. Nutr.,* 21, 453, 2001.
45. Schafer, K. et al., Effects of selenium deficiency on fatty acid metabolism in rats fed fish oil-enriched diets, *J. Trace Elem. Med. Biol.,* 18, 89, 2004.
46. Kyriakopoulos, A. et al., Detection of small selenium-containing proteins in tissues of the rat, *J. Trace Elem. Med. Biol.,* 14, 179, 2000.
47. Arthur, J.R. et al., Selenium and iodine deficiencies and selenoprotein function, *Biomed. Environ. Sci.,* 10, 129, 1997.
48. Castano, A. et al., Increase in dopamine turnover and tyrosine hydroxylase enzyme in hippocampus of rats fed on low selenium diet, *J. Neurosci. Res.,* 42, 684, 1995.
49. Castano, A. et al., Low selenium diet increases the dopamine turnover in prefrontal cortex of the rat, *Neurochem. Int.,* 30, 549, 1997.
50. Bunk, M.J. and Combs, G.F., Jr., Effect of selenium on appetite in the selenium-deficient chick, *J. Nutr.,* 110, 743, 1980.
51. Bunk, M.J. and Combs, G.F., Jr., Evidence for an impairment in the conversion of methionine to cysteine in the selenium-deficient chick, *Proc. Soc. Exp. Biol. Med.,* 167, 87, 1981.
52. Zhou, Y.P. and Combs, G.F., Jr., Effects of dietary protein level and level of feed intake on the apparent bioavailability of selenium for the chick, *Poult. Sci.,* 63, 294, 1984.
53. Zuberbuehler, C.A., Messikommer, R.E., and Wenk, C., Choice feeding of selenium-deficient laying hens affects diet selection, selenium intake and body weight, *J. Nutr.,* 132, 3411, 2002.
54. Zuberbuehler, C.A. et al., Effects of selenium depletion and selenium repletion by choice feeding on selenium status of young and old laying hens, *Physiol. Behav.,* 87, 430, 2006.
55. Jianhua, H., Ohtsuka, A., and Hayashi, K., Selenium influences growth via thyroid hormone status in broiler chickens, *Br. J. Nutr.,* 84, 727, 2000.
56. Chanoine, J.P., Wong, A.C., and Lavoie, J.C., Selenium deficiency impairs corticosterone and leptin responses to adrenocorticotropin in the rat, *Biofactors,* 20, 109, 2004.
57. Liuzzi, J.P. and Cousins, R.J., Mammalian zinc transporters, *Annu. Rev. Nutr.,* 24, 151, 2004.
58. Rutherford, J.C. and Bird, A.J., Metal-responsive transcription factors that regulate iron, zinc, and copper homeostasis in eukaryotic cells, *Eukaryot. Cell,* 3, 1, 2004.
59. Ruiz, A. et al., Endogenous zinc inhibits GABA(A) receptors in a hippocampal pathway, *J. Neurophysiol.,* 91, 1091, 2004.
60. Frederickson, C.J., Koh, J.Y., and Bush, A.I., The neurobiology of zinc in health and disease, *Nat. Rev. Neurosci.,* 6, 449, 2005.

61. Assaf, S.Y. and Chung, S.H., Release of endogenous Zn2+ from brain tissue during activity, *Nature,* 308, 734, 1984.
62. Vogt, K. et al., The actions of synaptically released zinc at hippocampal mossy fiber synapses, *Neuron,* 26, 187, 2000.
63. Smart, T.G., Xie, X., and Krishek, B.J., Modulation of inhibitory and excitatory amino acid receptor ion channels by zinc, *Prog. Neurobiol.,* 42, 393, 1994.
64. Minami, A. et al., Inhibition of presynaptic activity by zinc released from mossy fiber terminals during tetanic stimulation, *J. Neurosci. Res.,* 83, 167, 2006.
65. Takeda, A. et al., Response of hippocampal mossy fiber zinc to excessive glutamate release, *Neurochem. Int.,* 50, 322, 2007.
66. Wall, M.J., A role for zinc in cerebellar synaptic transmission? *Cerebellum,* 4, 224, 2005.
67. Takeda, A. et al., Enhanced excitability of hippocampal mossy fibers and CA3 neurons under dietary zinc deficiency, *Epilepsy Res.,* 63, 77, 2005.
68. Shay, N.F. and Mangian, H.F., Neurobiology of zinc-influenced eating behavior, *J. Nutr.,* 130, 1493S, 2000.
69. Levenson, C.W., Zinc regulation of food intake: new insights on the role of neuropeptide Y, *Nutr. Rev.,* 61, 247, 2003.
70. Lee, R.G. et al., Zinc deficiency increases hypothalamic neuropeptide Y and neuropeptide Y mRNA levels and does not block neuropeptide Y-induced feeding in rats, *J. Nutr.,* 128, 1218, 1998.
71. Selvais, P.L. et al., Cyclic feeding behaviour and changes in hypothalamic galanin and neuropeptide Y gene expression induced by zinc deficiency in the rat, *J. Neuroendocrinol.,* 9, 55, 1997.
72. Huntington, C.E. et al., Zinc status affects neurotransmitter activity in the paraventricular nucleus of rats, *J. Nutr.,* 132, 270, 2002.
73. Williamson, P.S. et al., Neuropeptide Y fails to normalize food intake in zinc-deficient rats, *Nutr. Neurosci.,* 5, 19, 2002.
74. Buff, C.E., Shay, N.F., and Beverly, J.L., Noradrenergic activity in the paraventricular nucleus and macronutrient choice during early dark onset by zinc deficient rats, *Nutr. Neurosci.,* 9, 189, 2006.
75. Essatara, M.B. et al., Zinc deficiency and anorexia in rats: the effect of central administration of norepinephrine, muscimol and bromerogocryptine, *Physiol. Behav.,* 32, 479, 1984.
76. Essatara, M.B. et al., The role of the endogenous opiates in zinc deficiency anorexia, *Physiol. Behav.,* 32, 475, 1984.
77. Welch, C.C. et al., Preference and diet type affect macronutrient selection after morphine, NPY, norepinephrine, and deprivation, *Am. J. Physiol.,* 266, R426, 1994.
78. Rains, T.M. et al., Growth hormone-releasing factor affects macronutrient intake during the anabolic phase of zinc repletion: total hypothalamic growth hormone-releasing factor content and growth hormone-releasing factor immunoneutralization during zinc repletion, *Nutr. Neurosci.,* 4, 283, 2001.
79. Sun, J.Y. et al., Effect of zinc on biochemical parameters and changes in related gene expression assessed by cDNA microarrays in pituitary of growing rats, *Nutrition,* 22, 187, 2006.
80. Mantzoros, C.S. et al., Zinc may regulate serum leptin concentrations in humans, *J. Am. Coll. Nutr.,* 17, 270, 1998.
81. Gaetke, L.M. et al., Decreased food intake rather than zinc deficiency is associated with changes in plasma leptin, metabolic rate, and activity levels in zinc deficient rats, *J. Nutr. Biochem.,* 13, 237, 2002.
82. Ott, E.S. and Shay, N.F., Zinc deficiency reduces leptin gene expression and leptin secretion in rat adipocytes, *Exp. Biol. Med. (Maywood),* 226, 841, 2001.
83. Rossi, L. et al., Copper imbalance and oxidative stress in neurodegeneration, *Ital. J. Biochem.,* 55, 212, 2006.

84. Madsen, E. and Gitlin, J.D., Copper deficiency, *Curr. Opin. Gastroenterol.,* 23, 187, 2007.
85. Zucconi, G.G. et al., Copper deficiency elicits glial and neuronal response typical of neurodegenerative disorders, *Neuropathol. Appl. Neurobiol.,* 33, 212, 2007.
86. Levenson, C.W., Trace metal regulation of neuronal apoptosis: from genes to behavior, *Physiol. Behav.,* 86, 399, 2005.
87. Prohaska, J.R. and Broderius, M., Plasma peptidylglycine alpha-amidating monooxygenase (PAM) and ceruloplasmin are affected by age and copper status in rats and mice, *Comp. Biochem. Physiol. B Biochem. Mol. Biol.,* 143, 360, 2006.
88. Bourre, J.M., Effects of nutrients (in food) on the structure and function of the nervous system: update on dietary requirements for brain. Part 1: micronutrients, *J. Nutr. Health Aging,* 10, 377, 2006.
89. Frank, A., Danielsson, R., and Jones, B., Experimental copper and chromium deficiency and additional molybdenum supplementation in goats. II. Concentrations of trace and minor elements in liver, kidneys and ribs: haematology and clinical chemistry, *Sci. Total Environ.,* 249, 143, 2000.
90. Frank, A., Anke, M., and Danielsson, R., Experimental copper and chromium deficiency and additional molybdenum supplementation in goats. I. Feed consumption and weight development, *Sci. Total Environ.,* 249, 133, 2000.
91. Rutkoski, N.J. et al., Regulation of neuropeptide Y mRNA and peptide concentrations by copper in rat olfactory bulb, *Brain Res. Mol. Brain Res.,* 65, 80, 1999.
92. Miller, S.T. et al., Chronic dietary Cu(2+)-deficiency alters cholecystokinin signal transduction in isolated rat pancreatic acini, *J. Assoc. Acad. Minor Phys.,* 11, 21, 2000.
93. Li, Y., Hao, Y., and Owyang, C., High-affinity CCK-A receptors on the vagus nerve mediate CCK-stimulated pancreatic secretion in rats, *Am. J. Physiol.,* 273, G679, 1997.
94. Alvarez, C., Garcia, J.F., and Lopez, M.A., Exocrine pancreas in rabbits fed a copper-deficient diet: structural and functional studies, *Pancreas,* 4, 543, 1989.
95. Koury, J.C. et al., Plasma zinc, copper, leptin, and body composition are associated in elite female judo athletes, *Biol. Trace Elem. Res.,* 115, 23, 2007.
96. Olusi, S. et al., Serum copper levels and not zinc are positively associated with serum leptin concentrations in the healthy adult population, *Biol. Trace Elem. Res.,* 91, 137, 2003.
97. Chen, M.D. et al., Plasma concentrations of leptin and selected minerals do not differ in Type 2 diabetic patients with or without sulfonylurea inefficacy, *Diabetes Nutr. Metab.,* 13, 284, 2000.
98. Lee, S.H., Engle, T.E., and Hossner, K.L., Effects of dietary copper on the expression of lipogenic genes and metabolic hormones in steers, *J. Anim. Sci.,* 80, 1999, 2002.

18 Minerals and Food Intake: A Human Perspective

Dorothy Teegarden and Carolyn Gunther

CONTENTS

18.1 INTRODUCTION

The regulation of food intake has an important impact on the development of diseases throughout the world. The incidence of obesity continues to grow worldwide despite efforts to identify the macronutrient composition of diets effective in reducing overall energy intake and subsequent fat mass or in preventing fat accumulation. It has been proposed that certain minerals may impact body fat accumulation and that appetite may play a role in modulating this effect. On the other hand, deficiencies of specific minerals may also reduce food intake, leading to anorexia or malnutrition. Therefore, it is important to understand the role of minerals in regulating food intake in humans and how this regulation may impact human disease.

It is curious to consider that nonenergy-supplying nutrients such as minerals may regulate food intake or appetite. One suggestion is that mammals may have evolved to respond to specific dietary components that act as an indicator of dietary availability. Thus, when food is plentiful, a mineral present in the diet, such as calcium, acts as the signal to reduce body fat mass accumulation. On the other hand, when food is scarce, the lower calcium in the diet may serve as an indicator to promote fat mass accumulation, protecting the body against the scarcity of food. Therefore, teleologically, dietary mineral content may function as an indicator of energy nutrient availability and regulate physiological processes and food intake to appropriately respond to the energy availability in the environment.

The mechanisms by which dietary intake of minerals regulate physiological processes such as food intake must also be considered. In some cases, the specific essential roles of minerals is to function as cofactors influencing how a mineral impacts physiological processes. Alternatively, certain minerals, such as calcium, can participate in eliciting hormonal responses. The hormones may in turn function to regulate the physiological processes secondary to the intake of the mineral.

The impact of minerals on food intake can be directly assessed measuring food intake or compensatory food intake, or associations between intake and nutritional status. On the other hand, measures of the response of mediators of food intake behavior (e.g., leptin, cholycystokinin [CCK], neuropeptide Y [NPY], and ghrelin) to mineral intake may provide insights into potential regulation of food intake and also mechanistic information. However, the regulation of food intake is a complex interaction of hormonal and neuronal controls in addition to learned behaviors that may override the natural cues to control food intake.

This review addresses the current knowledge of the impact of minerals on food intake in humans by several minerals: zinc, calcium, iron, and iodine. Overall, there is little available information on specific effects of minerals on food intake in humans. The minerals included for discussion in this review are based on those for which there is a body of literature in humans. These specific minerals also provide examples of several important factors that should be considered, such as types of studies used, mechanisms explored, and direct versus indirect effects of the minerals on appetite.

18.2 ZINC

18.2.1 Introduction

Zinc is the most actively studied mineral in regards to regulation of food intake.[1,2] Zinc is an essential mineral for humans and required for several physiological processes, including growth, immunity, reproduction, and optimal immunity. Zinc functions as a cofactor for a wide range of enzymes involved in cell division, protein synthesis, and carbohydrate metabolism as well as the activity of hormones such as glucagon, insulin, growth hormone, and thyroid hormone. Zinc is also critical for gastrointestinal structure and function. Zinc deficiency results in dwarfism and hypogonadism. Zinc deficiency also promotes poor appetite and reduced food intake in animals and humans,[1,2] but the mechanisms in humans are not defined.

18.2.2 Mechanisms of Reduced Food Intake: Animal Models

The effect of dietary zinc deficiency in reducing food intake has been extensively investigated in animal models, particularly rats, and less well in humans.[1,2] Although this review is focused on humans, the research in animals contributes to understanding the mechanisms in humans. Zinc deficiency appears to induce characteristic eating behaviors that lead to reduced food intake in rats. Zinc-deficient rats transiently increase their food consumption on a cyclical basis every 3 to 4 days, delay the timing of their first meal of their dark cycle compared to zinc-adequate animals, and eat fewer meals.[3] In addition, intake of carbohydrates is reduced, whereas protein and fat intakes remain stable. Within 1 day of refeeding a zinc-adequate diet, carbohydrate intake is restored with a transient increase in protein intake.[4] Thus, nutrient selection of food and specific feeding behaviors are altered by zinc deficiency, leading to overall decreased food intake.

A variety of physiological mechanisms including neurotransmitter and endocrine secretions have been explored as potential mediators of zinc-induced anorexia, including norepinephrine, gama-aminobutyric acid, dopamine, dinorphin, and galanin, without consistent results.[2,5] Rats fed a zinc-deficient diet for 6 weeks reduced food intake compared to a zinc-adequate diet.[6] In this study, mRNA expression of peptide hormones that inhibit food intake (calcitonin gene-related product, serotonin, and cholecystokinin) were increased in the pituitary of rats fed a zinc-deficient diet compared to those fed a zinc-adequate diet. Ghrelin was unchanged, and the melanin-concentrating hormone, which normally stimulates food intake, was increased in the zinc-deficient compared to the zinc-adequate diets.[6] Thus, zinc deficiency reduces food intake in rats, potentially by regulating several hormones that control feeding behavior, but the specific events mediated by zinc to alter levels of the peptide hormones, or the role of these hormones in regulating food intake needs to be clarified.

The regulation of neuropeptide Y (NPY) may also play a role in zinc-mediated reduction in food intake. NPY is elevated in zinc deficiency and food restriction.[7] Zinc deficiency induces hypothalamic NPY mRNA in the hypothalamus of zinc-deficient rats and NPY peptides are increased in the arcuate nucleus and paraventricular nucleus in zinc-deficient rats.[8] These results seem inconsistent with the reduction in food intake mediated by zinc deficiency. However, NPY levels are equivalent in pair-fed rats, suggesting that NPY regulation is secondary to reduced food intake, not directly due to zinc deficiency.[2] The release of NPY during food restriction is significantly impaired in zinc-deficient animals, which may be a mechanism for causing anorexia (described in detail below). On the other hand, there may be a resistance to NPY in zinc deficiency, leading to high NPY levels, but reduced feed intake. However, zinc-deficient and zinc-adequate rats responded similarly to exogenous NPY applied to the paraventricular nucleus by increasing food intake, suggesting that elevated NPY during zinc deficiency is a response to restore food intake levels toward normal rather than a resistance to NPY.[8] Thus, zinc deficiency promotes reduced food intake in rats,[1,2] but the mechanism(s) underlying this effect has not been clearly defined.

18.2.3 Reduced Food Intake and Hypogeusia: Humans

Reduced food intake, described by Prasad as poor appetite, is an accepted consequence of insufficient zinc intake.[9–12] In addition, hypogeusia or decreased sensitivity to taste is associated with low zinc status.[12–14] For example, poor appetite and impaired taste acuity in young subjects (4 to 6 years) were associated with decreased concentration of zinc in hair.[15] In addition, zinc supplementation in these children reversed the abnormalities.[15] Hemodialysis is associated with zinc deficiency and hypogeusia[16,17] and has been used as a model for zinc deficiency in humans. A 12-week double-blind crossover placebo-controlled trial in 12 dialysis patients with hypogeusia demonstrated that zinc supplementation reduced the recognition and determination threshold level for all four taste qualities.[18] The results of a double-blinded placebo-controlled trial in 22 patients undergoing hemodialysis for 6 months demonstrated that the threshold of taste detection for salt, sweet, and bitter, but not sour, improved with zinc supplementation. The impact of zinc supplementation on symptoms of hypogeusia was also examined in a double-blind, randomized, cross-over-design trial in patients (N = 106, men and women).[19] The results of this study demonstrated that zinc supplementation was not effective in improving symptoms of hypogeusia of unknown origin. Overall, the results showed that, although zinc is not effective at improving hypogeusia induced by other causes, zinc status plays a role in taste acuity. Therefore, hypogeusia induced by zinc deficiency may be a contributing factor to reduced food intake in humans.

The role of the enzyme parotid saliva gustin/carbonic anhydrase VI, a zinc-dependent enzyme, has also been explored to determine how zinc affects taste functions.[20] Saliva gustin/carbonic anhydrase VI enzyme is considered responsible for maintenance of taste bud function. In this study, 14 patients with decreased saliva gustin/carbonic anhydrase VI secretion were treated with zinc supplementation for 4 to 6 months. Secretion of saliva gustin/carbonic anhydrase VI increased in 10 of 14 supplemented patients (categorized as responders). These 10 responders also experienced an improvement in taste acuity and a reduction in dysgeusia. There was no increase in secretion of the enzyme in the remaining four patients (nonresponders), and no improvement in taste acuity was reported. These results may provide support for a direct link, through the zinc-dependent saliva gustin/carbonic anhydrase VI enzyme, between zinc status and taste acuity. Further studies are warranted to explore the role of this enzyme in a zinc-dependent reduction in food intake.

18.2.4 Zinc and Anorexia Nervosa

Because it is evident that zinc deficiency reduces food intake in humans, it has been proposed that zinc deficiency may be a causative factor contributing to, or useful in, treatment of eating disorders such as anorexia nervosa.[21–24] The prevalence of eating disorders in postpubescent females is estimated to be 5 to 10%. The mortality rate for anorexia nervosa is estimated to be 10% occurring within 10 years of diagnosis, the highest of any psychiatric diagnosis, and the leading cause of death in young females 15 to 24 years of age.[25] Therefore, it is critical to identify factors that may prevent or alleviate anorexia nervosa, including a potential role for zinc intake.

The relationship between zinc and anorexia nervosa in humans has been investigated using several approaches including similarity in symptoms, dietary intakes and status measures for zinc, and clinical zinc supplementation intervention trials in anorexics. Hallmark symptoms of zinc deficiency are noted in anorexia nervosa, including weight loss, appetite loss, specific forms of dermatitis, amenorrhea, and depression.[26] Women have a high risk for deficiencies of zinc as assessed by dietary intake assessment.[27,28] However, the results of studies that assess zinc status in anorexic or bulimic patients are controversial, with several showing a relationship,[29–34] while other studies have shown no relationship.[35–37] These inconsistent results may be due to the lack of sensitive measures to assess zinc deficiencies in humans.[38] In addition, zinc supplementation during recovery of patients with anorexia has shown better weight gain compared to unsupplemented controls[33,34,39–41] Thus, there is evidence that zinc deficiency may play a role in anorexia nervosa, and zinc supplementation may aid in recovery of weight gain of anorexics.

18.2.5 Zinc Regulation of Leptin

A potential mechanism underlying zinc-induced reduction in food intake that has been explored in humans is the impact of leptin, which decreases appetite. However, levels of serum leptin are reduced during zinc deficiency, and zinc supplementation raises serum leptin levels, as well as IL-2 and TNF-α, of zinc-depleted men (n = 9).[42] Obese subjects have higher leptin and lower zinc plasma values than their lean controls. A complication in these studies is that leptin, produced in adipose tissue, may reflect changes in adipose stores induced by zinc deficiency as opposed to a regulation directly by zinc. However, in human adipose tissue, zinc treatment significantly increased leptin production, suggesting that zinc stimulates leptin synthesis.[43] Thus, there appears to be an interaction between zinc status and leptin levels, but the interaction is complex and requires further investigation.

18.3 CALCIUM

18.3.1 Introduction

In addition to the well-established role of calcium in bone metabolism, recent studies suggest that calcium intake may also influence other physiological factors. Evidence suggests that higher calcium intakes may lead to reduced fat accumulation or enhance fat mass loss during energy restriction.[44] Some evidence,[45–49] but not all,[50] supports a relationship between dietary calcium intake and body fat accumulation. On the other hand, a one-year dairy product intervention trial[51] did not lead to changes in fat accumulation in healthy young women. A 6-month follow up of this trial demonstrated a significant impact of 18-month intake of calcium with lower body fat accumulation.[49] These results suggest that if calcium has an impact on body fat accumulation, the effect is small but may be significant in the long term. The evidence for calcium enhancing fat mass loss during energy restriction is also contradictory.[52–57] The discrepancies and the small effect observed in epidemiological and intervention studies demonstrates a need to identify potential mechanisms that contribute to the effect in order to determine if, and when, dietary calcium will impact body composition.

Several mechanisms have been proposed to contribute to the impact of calcium on body composition. These include increased energy loss through increased expression of uncoupling proteins, increased lipid oxidation[58–60] or decreased availability of energy by the formation of fecal calcium:fatty acid soaps, reducing the absorption of fats.[61] In addition, it has been proposed that calcium may reduce food intake through reduced appetite, contributing to lower body fat mass or body weight.

18.3.2 Calcium and Dietary Intake

The evidence indicating that calcium influences intake in humans is controversial. A critical issue with many of the studies on calcium consumption and body composition is that the primary source of calcium is dairy products. Dairy protein and other dairy components[62] have also been implicated in regulating body composition and food intake or mediators of food intake, and this complicates the interpretation of many studies. Barr et al.[50] found that elderly people compensated well for the energy contained in three daily servings of milk by reducing food intake from other sources. The satiety value of yogurt and cheese has been determined empirically to be higher than that of many similar foods.[63] However, Almiron-Roig et al. demonstrated that intake of milk was not associated with compensation for the energy contained in the milk consumed.[64]

Another study investigated the impact of a 7-day dairy product intervention on food intake.[65] Participants (18 to 50 years, BMI 25 to 32 kg/m^2, n = 60, equal numbers of men and women) with either habitual low or high intake of calcium were enrolled. Subjects were instructed to consume either a low dairy (one serving dairy product/day) or three portions of dairy products/day for 7 days with a 7-day washout between test periods in a randomized crossover design. No other requirements for intake were given; thus, this study tested the ability of the participants to compensate for the addition of dairy products to their usual intakes. Estimated dietary intakes were assessed daily and appetitive measurements assessed by a computerized system throughout the day. Male participants consumed significantly more calories with the high-dairy intervention diet (approximately 200 kcal/day) compared to the low-dairy diet. Men with high habitual dairy intake reduced their intake of energy from other sources by 31%, but men with low habitual dairy intake did not compensate for the extra dairy intake, but increased 12% more than would be predicted by the addition of two dairy products in the diet. Female participants also compensated for the additional intake from the high-dairy product intervention, but the compensation was not complete. Women with high habitual calcium intake reduced energy intake by 72% of the dairy load from other sources when consuming the high-dairy product intake, and women with low habitual intake reduced energy intake from other sources by 50% of the dairy load. There were no significant differences in ratings of hunger, fullness, desire to eat, or preoccupation with foods between intervention groups. The results of this study suggest that, in contrast to the hypothesis that dairy products may lead to a reduction in food intake, there is incomplete compensation for the energy intake of the dairy products, or potentially an increased energy intake with a low habitual intake of calcium in men. This study does not specifically test the effect of calcium on dietary compensation, but rather dairy products, and dairy products contain many components that are hypothesized to regulate food intake. However, the negative effects support the hypothesis that calcium intake does not significantly reduce food consumption.

18.3.3 Calcium and Food Intake: Mechanisms

The response of specific satiety regulators to dietary calcium provide insights that can be applied to the overall response in humans. Intake of meals containing dairy products increased cholecystokinin (CCK) levels within a 6-hour period more than nondairy product meals in women (39 ± 6 years, n = 10), but not men (31 ± 10 years, n = 14) in a randomized crossover-design study.[66] CCK mediates meal termination and possibly early phase satiety at least in part through its effects on gastric emptying. Subjective satiety response to the test meals was assessed using visual analog scales (VAS) over the 6-hour period following meal consumption. In contrast to the CCK response, the VAS analysis suggested that the nondairy-product meals suppressed hunger more strongly than the dairy-products meals. Within the VAS analysis, the "desire to eat" was lower following consumption of the nondairy-product meals compared to the dairy-product-containing meals. Thus, the nondairy meals were more satiating than the dairy product. Again, it is important to note that this study investigates the impact of dairy product, not calcium specifically, on CCK response and appetitive responses.

Few studies have directly assessed the impact of calcium consumption on food intake. Lorenzen et al.[61] investigated the acute impact of calcium from various levels of dairy product supplementation in a randomized, controlled crossover-design study. In this study, male subjects (n = 18) were between 18 and 50 years old (25.7 ± 1.2 years) and overweight (27.1 ± 0.4 BMI, range 24 to 31 kg/m^2). The four isocaloric test meals consisted of three with dairy products as the calcium source: low calcium (68 mg), medium calcium (350 mg), and high calcium (793 mg). The fourth meal consisted of a calcium supplement with a meal containing whey, casein, and lactose; thus, all four meals contained equivalent levels of dairy protein. Blood was drawn at intervals for 7 hours following meal consumption, followed by an *ad libitum* meal with instructions to eat until "comfortable satisfaction," and energy intake from this meal was estimated. A 3-week washout period occurred between test meals. The results demonstrated that, consistent with an increase in fecal fat loss noted previously by these authors,[67] the area under the curve (AUC) for serum chylomicron-associated triglycerides was reduced after intake of the medium- and high-calcium meals compared to the low-calcium meal. There were no significant differences in AUC by meal in CCK, ghrelin, glucose, GLP-1, PYY, or insulin following test meals. The lack of response to dietary calcium is in contrast to that of Schneeman et al.,[66] where the product tested was nondairy compared to dairy products. The current study[61] is modified by the calcium content with equivalent levels of dairy components. Thus, the CCK response in the Schneeman et al. study[66] may be due to the dairy product component. In the study by Lorenzen et al.,[61] the high-calcium meal was more palatable than the low-calcium or supplement meal, and the subsequent *ad libitum* meal smelled better and was more visually appealing after intake of the high-calcium meal compared to the low-calcium meal. There was no significant difference in energy intake from the *ad libitum* meal following consumption of the test meals. In theory, the increase in palatability may promote an increase in food intake or lack of compensation, similar to that noted in the study by Hollis and Mattes.[65] Cumulatively, these results are consistent with studies in rodents which demonstrate no changes in food intake with low or high calcium intakes,[68,69] and suggest that calcium intake does not influence food intake.

The mechanism by which any dietary mineral may regulate food intake is potentially through hormones regulated by the dietary component. Thus, understanding calcium metabolism will aid in investigating potential mechanisms and lead to insights in the relationship between calcium intake and regulation of food intake. The most studied role played by calcium is in bone metabolism and intracellular regulation of signaling pathways. Serum calcium levels are controlled in a very tight range. Low calcium intake leads to a reduction in serum calcium, which in turn is sensed at the parathyroid gland by a specific calcium receptor. The activated receptor induces the synthesis and release of parathyroid hormone (PTH). PTH acts on the renal 1α-25 hydroxyvitamin D hydroxylase to increase serum levels of 1,25-dihydroxyvitamin D (1,25D), the active form of vitamin D. PTH and 1,25D function to increase serum calcium at the level of the bone, intestine, and kidney. In contrast, with high calcium intakes, the serum levels of PTH and 1,25D are suppressed, and calcitonin levels are increased. Therefore, the potential regulation of food intake by calcium may include the regulation of hormones.

Consistent with a hormonal regulation, evidence from animal studies demonstrates that calcitonin reduces food intake.[70–73] Subcutaneous and intracerebral injections of calcitonin inhibited feeding in rats, suggesting that calcitonin acts directly on the central nervous system.[74] Calcitonin also dramatically reduced feed intake in monkeys (90%) for 3 to 5 days and in rats in a dose-related manner over 24 hours.[75] However, to date little information on the impact of calcitonin on food intake in humans is available, and the physiological relevance is not clear. The impact of calcium on food intake with calcitonin as a mediator has also not been investigated.

18.3.4 Summary

In summary, the results of studies investigating an impact of calcium intake on food intake are controversial. There are no studies that directly show that calcium alone alters food intake. Some studies suggest that hormones which reduce food intake (CCK) are increased by calcium intake, but others do not. Cumulatively, these results suggest that calcium intake is not likely to have a significant impact on food intake. The size effects noted for the impact of calcium on weight or fat mass accumulation are small (less than 100 kcal/day), and it may be difficult, or impossible, to measure such small effects on food intake, appetite, or even hormonal changes.

18.4 IRON

18.4.1 Introduction

The physiological functions of iron have been well described, and the primary symptom of iron deficiency is anemia.[76] Another symptom of iron deficiency is loss of appetite.[77–79] Iron supplementation in African preschoolers improved appetite compared to a placebo as reported by the mother; however the improvement was similar to a deworming medicine.[80] The authors acknowledged that the questionnaire was not validated, and the mothers may not have fully understood the instructions. Although the level of supplementation did not affect mild to moderate anemia, it improved measures of anemia in those who were severely anemic at baseline and positively impacted motor and language development.[81] In another trial, girls 1 to 18 years of age (n = 203) participated in a random placebo-controlled trial of iron and folic acid combined supplementation.[82] The supplementation improved iron status, and the subjects' hunger rating increased according to both the subjects and the mothers.[83] The results of these studies are ambiguous, as the level of supplementation may not have been adequate to achieve meaningful differences in the first study, and the perceived improvements in intake may be due to an overall improvement in health. Separation of physiological and neurological consequences of anemia induced by iron or other cosupplemented factors has not been clearly addressed.

18.4.2 Mechanism

The mechanism by which iron status may influence food intake has been explored in one study by investigating the relationship between iron status and the hormones, ghrelin[84] and leptin[85] in children (n = 108, approximately 4-years-old) categorized into quartiles of iron deficiency. A significant positive correlation was identified between iron status and levels of ghrelin.[84] Decrease in ghrelin levels in iron deficiency anemia can lead to loss of appetite and a decreased desire to eat diverse foods, with a resultant delay in growth and development. This study supports the idea that iron may influence ghrelin levels, which in turn may impact food intake. However, these results are associative and lack cause-and-effect characterization. In addition, ghrelin is only one of numerous hormonal influences on appetite and food intake. In summary, there is no direct evidence that iron specifically influences food intake in humans.[86,87]

18.5 IODINE

There is little data on the impact of iodine in regulating food intake. Iodine is an essential component of thyroid hormones, which are essential for skeletal growth and neurological development.[88,89] Iodine deficiency leads to hypothyroidism, an increase in thyroid stimulating hormones (TSH), and goiter.[90] Clearly, iodine deficiency, particularly *in utero,* infants, and children, leads to irreversible neurological and cognitive deficits manifested in mental retardation, visual problems, and stunted growth. However, direct association of iodine insufficiency or deficiency with food intake has not been described in humans.

Since iodine is critical for maintenance of optimal levels of thyroid hormones, it is worth considering the possible impact of these hormones on food consumption behaviors. Thyroid hormones, which increase the basal metabolic rate and thermogenesis, have been reported to be one factor regulating leptin, with alterations in thyroid status potentially leading to compensatory changes in leptin. To this end, the relationship between thyroid status and leptin levels was explored in patients (n = 65) with thyroid cancer before and after ablation and thyroid suppressive treatments.[91] Serum leptin levels increased significantly from the hypothyroid to the subclinical hyperthyroid state, and serum leptin levels significantly correlated with free thyroxine index or FT4, and TSH (all $P < 0.05$), even when controlled for BMI and body fat. Thus, circulating thyroid hormone may play a role in regulating leptin metabolism independent of BMI and body fat. Therefore, iodine may influence food intake through thyroid metabolism.

18.6 SUMMARY

There is little evidence supporting a role for most minerals in modulating food intake. Zinc deficiency may play a role in reducing food intake and in the development of anorexia nervosa. In contrast, calcium intake does not appear to control food intake, though this hypothesis has been explored in a number of studies. There is little evidence for, or against, either iron or iodine having a direct role in regulating food intake in humans.

Overall, the direct role of minerals in food intake in humans has not been explored. Although a symptom of deficiency of several minerals (zinc, iodine, iron) is reduced food intake, it is not clear if this is a direct effect of the mineral or a secondary effect of the physiological consequences and poor health elicited by the deficiency. This issue of assessing direct effect is very difficult to delineate in humans.

The development of deficiency versus insufficiency is a factor that is not considered in many studies relating nutritional factors with physiological. Overt deficiency for several minerals, such as iron and zinc, is prevalent worldwide. However, insufficiency is also prevalent worldwide, and this condition should also be addressed in studies. Further, adaptation to specific intakes occurs with most minerals, and this information has often been neglected in considering responses to supplementation.

In conclusion, zinc deficiency is associated with poor appetite and reduced food intake, and the evidence supports that calcium intake does not regulate food intake in humans. There is little evidence available investigating the role of other minerals on food intake. The results of the impact of the minerals selected for this review on food intake are consistent between studies employing humans and the animal models. The physiological consequences of the mineral deficiencies (or insufficiencies) are difficult to dissect from a direct effect of the mineral on food intake. Finally, few mechanistic studies investigating the role of minerals in regulating food intake in humans are currently available.

REFERENCES

1. Jing, M.Y., Sun, J.Y., and Weng, X.Y., Insights on zinc regulation of food intake and macronutrient selection, *Biol. Trace Elem. Res.,* 115 (2), 187, 2007.
2. Shay, N.F. and Mangian, H.F., Neurobiology of zinc-influenced eating behavior, *J. Nutr.,* 130 (5S Suppl.), 1493S, 2000.
3. Rains, T.M. et al., Food intake patterns are altered during long-term zinc deficiency in rats, *Physiol. Behav.,* 65 (3), 473, 1998.
4. Rains, T.M. and Shay, N.F., Zinc status specifically changes preferences for carbohydrate and protein in rats selecting from separate carbohydrate-, protein-, and fat-containing diets, *J. Nutr.,* 125 (11), 2874, 1995.
5. Essatara, M.B. et al., Zinc deficiency and anorexia in rats: The effect of central administration of norepinephrine, muscimol and bromerogocryptine, *Physiol. Behav.,* 32 (3), 479, 1984.
6. Sun, J.Y. et al., Effect of zinc on biochemical parameters and changes in related gene expression assessed by cDNA microarrays in pituitary of growing rats, *Nutrition,* 22 (2), 187, 2006.
7. Levenson, C.W., Zinc regulation of food intake: New insights on the role of neuropeptide Y, *Nutr. Rev.,* 61 (7), 247, 2003.
8. Lee, R.G. et al., Zinc deficiency increases hypothalamic neuropeptide Y and neuropeptide Y mRNA levels and does not block neuropeptide Y-induced feeding in rats, *J. Nutr.,* 128 (7), 1218, 1998.
9. Prasad, A.S., Zinc: the biology and therapeutics of an ion, *Ann. Intern. Med.,* 125 (2), 142, 1996.
10. Prasad, A.S., Discovery of human zinc deficiency and studies in an experimental human model, *Am. J. Clin. Nutr.,* 53 (2), 403, 1991.
11. Prasad, A.S., Clinical, biochemical and nutritional spectrum of zinc deficiency in human subjects: an update, *Nutr. Rev.,* 41 (7), 197, 1983.
12. Van Wouwe, J.P., Clinical and laboratory assessment of zinc deficiency in Dutch children. A review, *Biol. Trace Elem. Res.,* 49 (2–3), 211, 1995.
13. Buzina, R. et al., Zinc nutrition and taste acuity in school children with impaired growth, *Am. J. Clin. Nutr.,* 33 (11), 2262, 1980.
14. Heyneman, C.A., Zinc deficiency and taste disorders, *Ann. Pharmacother.,* 30 (2), 186, 1996.
15. Hambidge, K.M. et al., Low levels of zinc in hair, anorexia, poor growth, and hypogeusia in children, *Pediatr. Res.,* 6 (12), 868, 1972.
16. Reyes, A.J. et al., Diuretics and zinc, *S. Afr. Med. J.,* 62 (11), 373, 1982.
17. Russell, R.M., Cox, M.E., and Solomons, N., Zinc and the special senses, *Ann. Intern. Med.,* 99 (2), 227, 1983.
18. Sprenger, K.B. et al., Improvement of uremic neuropathy and hypogeusia by dialysate zinc supplementation: a double-blind study, *Kidney Int. Suppl.,* 16, S315, 1983.
19. Henkin, R.I. et al., A double blind study of the effects of zinc sulfate on taste and smell dysfunction, *Am. J. Med. Sci.,* 272 (3), 285, 1976.
20. Henkin, R.I., Martin, B.M., and Agarwal, R.P., Efficacy of exogenous oral zinc in treatment of patients with carbonic anhydrase VI deficiency, *Am. J. Med. Sci.,* 318 (6), 392, 1999.
21. Tannhauser, P.P., Anorexia nervosa: a multifactorial disease of nutritional origin? *Int. J. Adolesc. Med. Health,* 14 (3), 185, 2002.
22. Patrick, L., Eating disorders: a review of the literature with emphasis on medical complications and clinical nutrition, *Altern. Med. Rev.,* 7 (3), 184, 2002.
23. Birmingham, C.L. and Gritzner, S., How does zinc supplementation benefit anorexia nervosa? *Eat. Weight. Disord.,* 11 (4), e109, 2006.

24. Su, J.C. and Birmingham, C.L., Zinc supplementation in the treatment of anorexia nervosa, *Eat. Weight. Disord.,* 7 (1), 20, 2002.
25. Sullivan, P.F., Mortality in anorexia nervosa, *Am. J. Psychiatry,* 152 (7), 1073, 1995.
26. Bakan, R., The role of zinc in anorexia nervosa: Etiology and treatment, *Med. Hypotheses,* 5 (7), 731, 1979.
27. Hadigan, C.M. et al., Assessment of macronutrient and micronutrient intake in women with anorexia nervosa, *Int. J. Eat. Disord.,* 28 (3), 284, 2000.
28. Bakan, R. et al., Dietary zinc intake of vegetarian and nonvegetarian patients with anorexia nervosa, *Int. J. Eat. Disord.,* 13 (2), 229, 1993.
29. Katz, R.L. et al., Zinc deficiency in anorexia nervosa, *J. Adolesc. Health Care,* 8 (5), 400, 1987.
30. Casper, R.C. et al., An evaluation of trace metals, vitamins, and taste function in anorexia nervosa, *Am. J. Clin. Nutr.,* 33 (8), 1801, 1980.
31. Lask, B. et al., Zinc deficiency and childhood-onset anorexia nervosa, *J. Clin. Psychiatry,* 54 (2), 63, 1993.
32. McClain, C.J. et al., Zinc status before and after zinc supplementation of eating disorder patients, *J. Am. Coll. Nutr.,* 11 (6), 694, 1992.
33. Humphries, L. et al., Zinc deficiency and eating disorders, *J. Clin. Psychiatry,* 50 (12), 456, 1989.
34. Birmingham, C.L., Goldner, E.M., and Bakan, R., Controlled trial of zinc supplementation in anorexia nervosa, *Int. J. Eat. Disord.,* 15 (3), 251, 1994.
35. Kopala, L.C. et al., Olfactory identification ability in anorexia nervosa, *J. Psychiatry Neurosci.,* 20 (4), 283, 1995.
36. Van Binsbergen, C.J. et al., Nutritional status in anorexia nervosa: Clinical chemistry, vitamins, iron and zinc, *Eur. J. Clin. Nutr.,* 42 (11), 929, 1988.
37. Misra, M. et al., Nutrient intake in community-dwelling adolescent girls with anorexia nervosa and in healthy adolescents, *Am. J. Clin. Nutr.,* 84 (4), 698, 2006.
38. Wood, R.J., Assessment of marginal zinc status in humans, *J. Nutr.,* 130 (5S Suppl.), 1350S, 2000.
39. Safai-Kutti, S., Oral zinc supplementation in anorexia nervosa, *Acta Psychiatr. Scand. Suppl.,* 361, 14, 1990.
40. Yamaguchi, H. et al., Anorexia nervosa responding to zinc supplementation: A case report, *Gastroenterol. Jpn.,* 27 (4), 554, 1992.
41. Bryce-Smith, D. and Simpson, R.I., Case of anorexia nervosa responding to zinc sulphate, *Lancet,* 2 (8398), 350, 1984.
42. Mantzoros, C.S. et al., Zinc may regulate serum leptin concentrations in humans, *Am. Coll. Nutr.,* 17 (3), 270, 1998.
43. Chen, M.D., Song, Y.M., and Lin, P.Y., Zinc may be a mediator of leptin production in humans, *Life Sci.,* 66 (22), 2143, 2000.
44. Teegarden, D., The influence of dairy product consumption on body composition, *J. Nutr.,* 135 (12), 2749, 2005.
45. Lin, Y.C. et al., Dairy calcium is related to changes in body composition during a two-year exercise intervention in young women, *J. Am. Coll. Nutr.,* 19 (6), 754, 2000.
46. Loos, R.J. et al., Calcium intake is associated with adiposity in Black and White men and White women of the HERITAGE Family Study, *J. Nutr.,* 134 (7), 1772, 2004.
47. Davies, K.M. et al., Calcium intake and body weight, *J. Clin. Endocrinol. Metab.,* 85 (12), 4635, 2000.
48. Jacqmain, M. et al., Calcium intake, body composition, and lipoprotein-lipid concentrations in adults, *Am. J. Clin. Nutr.,* 77 (6), 1448, 2003.
49. Eagan, M.S. et al., Effect of 1-year dairy product intervention on fat mass in young women: 6-month follow-up, *Obesity (Silver Spring),* 14 (12), 2242, 2006.

50. Barr, S.I. et al., Effects of increased consumption of fluid milk on energy and nutrient intake, body weight, and cardiovascular risk factors in healthy older adults, *J. Am. Diet. Assoc.,* 100 (7), 810, 2000.
51. Gunther, C.W. et al., Dairy products do not lead to alterations in body weight or fat mass in young women in a 1-y intervention, *Am. J. Clin. Nutr.,* 81 (4), 751, 2005.
52. Zemel, M.B. et al., Regulation of adiposity by dietary calcium, *FASEB J.,* 14 (9), 1132, 2000.
53. Zemel, M.B. et al., Calcium and dairy acceleration of weight and fat loss during energy restriction in obese adults, *Obes. Res.,* 12 (4), 582, 2004.
54. Zemel, M.B. et al., Dairy augmentation of total and central fat loss in obese subjects, *Int. J. Obes. (Lond.),* 29 (4), 391, 2005.
55. Zemel, M.B. et al., Effects of calcium and dairy on body composition and weight loss in African-American adults, *Obes. Res.,* 13 (7), 1218, 2005.
56. Thompson, W.G. et al., Effect of energy-reduced diets high in dairy products and fiber on weight loss in obese adults, *Obes. Res.,* 13 (8), 1344, 2005.
57. Shapses, S.A., Heshka, S., and Heymsfield, S.B., Effect of calcium supplementation on weight and fat loss in women, *J. Clin. Endocrinol. Metab.,* 89 (2), 632, 2004.
58. Melanson, E.L. et al., Effect of low- and high-calcium dairy-based diets on macronutrient oxidation in humans, *Obes. Res.,* 13 (12), 2102, 2005.
59. Gunther, C.W. et al., Fat oxidation and its relation to serum parathyroid hormone in young women enrolled in a 1-y dairy calcium intervention, *Am. J. Clin. Nutr.,* 82 (6), 1228, 2005.
60. Melanson, E.L. et al., Relation between calcium intake and fat oxidation in adult humans, *Int. J. Obes. Relat. Metab. Disord.,* 27 (2), 196, 2003.
61. Lorenzen, J.K. et al., Effect of dairy calcium or supplementary calcium intake on postprandial fat metabolism, appetite, and subsequent energy intake, *Am. J. Clin. Nutr.,* 85 (3), 678, 2007.
62. Pedersen, N.L. et al., Caseinomacropeptide specifically stimulates exocrine pancreatic secretion in the anesthetized rat, *Peptides,* 21 (10), 1527, 2000.
63. Holt, S.H. et al., A satiety index of common foods, *Eur. J. Clin. Nutr.,* 49 (9), 675, 1995.
64. Almiron-Roig, E. and Drewnowski, A., Hunger, thirst, and energy intakes following consumption of caloric beverages, *Physiol. Behav.,* 79 (4–5), 767, 2003.
65. Hollis, J.H. and Mattes, R.D., Effect of increased dairy consumption on appetitive ratings and food intake, *Obesity (Silver Spring),* 15 (6), 1520, 2007.
66. Schneeman, B.O., Burton-Freeman, B., and Davis, P., Incorporating dairy foods into low and high fat diets increases the postprandial cholecystokinin response in men and women, *J. Nutr.,* 133 (12), 4124, 2003.
67. Jacobsen, R. et al., Effect of short-term high dietary calcium intake on 24-hour energy expenditure, fat oxidation, and fecal fat excretion, *Int. J. Obes. (Lond.),* 29 (3), 292, 2005.
68. Zhang, Q. and Tordoff, M.G., No effect of dietary calcium on body weight of lean and obese mice and rats, *Am. J. Physiol. Regul. Integr. Comp. Physiol.,* 286 (4), R669, 2004.
69. Siddiqui, S. et al., Dietary vitamin D and calcium reduce body fat accretion in Wistar rats regardless of dietary energy source, *FASEB J.,* 21, A56, 2007.
70. Uda, K. et al., Stable human calcitonin analogues with high potency on bone together with reduced anorectic and renal actions, *Biol. Pharm. Bull.,* 22 (3), 244, 1999.
71. Levine, A.S. and Morley, J.E., Reduction of feeding in rats by calcitonin, *Brain Res.,* 222 (1), 187, 1981.
72. Morley, J.E. et al., Interrelationships between calcitonin and other modulators of feeding behavior, *Psychopharmacol. Bull.,* 20 (3), 463, 1984.
73. Morley, J.E. et al., The effect of peripheral administration of peptides on food intake, glucose and insulin in wolf pups, *Peptides,* 7 (6), 969, 1986.

74. Freed, W.J., Perlow, M.J., and Wyatt, R.J., Calcitonin: inhibitory effect on eating in rats, *Science,* 206 (4420), 850, 1979.
75. Perlow, M.J. et al., Calcitonin reduces feeding in man, monkey and rat, *Pharmacol. Biochem. Behav.,* 12 (4), 609, 1980.
76. Beard, J.L. and Connor, J.R., Iron status and neural functioning, *Annu. Rev. Nutr.,* 23, 41, 2003.
77. Pollitt, E. and Leibel, R.L., Iron deficiency and behavior, *J. Pediatr.,* 88 (3), 372, 1976.
78. Theuer, R.C., Iron undernutrition in infancy, *Clin. Pediatr. (Phila),* 13 (6), 522, 1974.
79. Judisch, J.M., Naiman, J.L., and Oski, F.A., The fallacy of the fat iron-deficient child, *Pediatrics,* 37 (6), 987, 1966.
80. Stoltzfus, R.J. et al., Low dose daily iron supplementation improves iron status and appetite but not anemia, whereas quarterly anthelminthic treatment improves growth, appetite and anemia in Zanzibari preschool children, *J. Nutr.,* 134 (2), 348, 2004.
81. Stoltzfus, R.J. et al., Effects of iron supplementation and anthelmintic treatment on motor and language development of preschool children in Zanzibar: double blind, placebo controlled study, *Br. Med. J.,* 323 (7326), 1389, 2001.
82. Kanani, S.J. and Poojara, R.H., Supplementation with iron and folic acid enhances growth in adolescent Indian girls, *J. Nutr.,* 130 (2S Suppl.), 452S, 2000.
83. Lawless, J.W. et al., Iron supplementation improves appetite and growth in anemic Kenyan primary school children, *J. Nutr.,* 124 (5), 645, 1994.
84. Akarsu, S. et al., Plasma ghrelin levels in various stages of development of iron deficiency anemia, *J. Pediatr. Hematol. Oncol.,* 29 (6), 384, 2007.
85. Topaloglu, A.K. et al., Lack of association between plasma leptin levels and appetite in children with iron deficiency, *Nutrition,* 17 (7–8), 657, 2001.
86. Chwang, L.C., Soemantri, A.G., and Pollitt, E. Iron supplementation and physical growth of rural Indonesian children, *Am. J. Clin. Nutr.,* 47 (3), 496, 1988.
87. Latham, M.C. et al., Improvements in growth following iron supplementation in young Kenyan school children, *Nutrition,* 6 (2), 159, 1990.
88. Bernal, J. and Nunez, J., Thyroid hormone action and brain development, *Trends Endocrinol. Metab.,* 133, 390, 2000.
89. Delange, F., Iodine deficiency as a cause of brain damage, *Postgrad. Med. J.,* 77 (906), 217, 2001.
90. Markou, K. et al., Iodine induced hypothyroidism, *Thyroid,* 11, 501, 2001.
91. Hsieh, C.J. et al., Serum leptin concentrations of patients with sequential thyroid function changes, *Clin. Endocrinol. (Oxf.),* 57 (1), 29, 2002.

Index

C

H

I

L

M

N

R

S

T

V

W

Y

Z

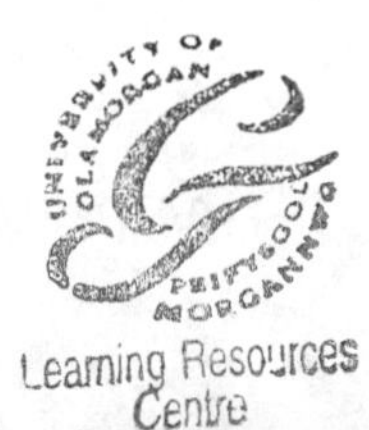